W0090614

LOW-INTENSITY
CBT SKILLS
& INTERVENTIONS

SAGE was founded in 1965 by Sara Miller McCune to support the dissemination of usable knowledge by publishing innovative and high-quality research and teaching content. Today, we publish over 900 journals, including those of more than 400 learned societies, more than 800 new books per year, and a growing range of library products including archives, data, case studies, reports, and video. SAGE remains majority-owned by our founder, and after Sara's lifetime will become owned by a charitable trust that secures our continued independence.

Los Angeles | London | New Delhi | Singapore | Washington DC | Melbourne

LOW-INTENSITY
CBT SKILLS
& INTERVENTIONS

a practitioner's manual

Edited by
PAUL FARRAND

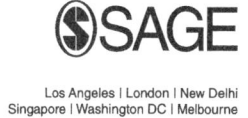

Los Angeles | London | New Delhi
Singapore | Washington DC | Melbourne

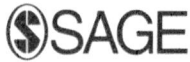

Los Angeles | London | New Delhi
Singapore | Washington DC | Melbourne

SAGE Publications Ltd
1 Oliver's Yard
55 City Road
London EC1Y 1SP

SAGE Publications Inc.
2455 Teller Road
Thousand Oaks, California 91320

SAGE Publications India Pvt Ltd
B 1/I 1 Mohan Cooperative Industrial Area
Mathura Road
New Delhi 110 044

SAGE Publications Asia-Pacific Pte Ltd
3 Church Street
#10-04 Samsung Hub
Singapore 049483

Editor: Susannah Trefgarne
Assistant editor: Ruth Lilly
Production editor: Martin Fox
Copyeditor: William Baginsky
Proofreader: Genevieve Friar
Indexer: Judith Lavender
Marketing manager: Dilhara Attygalle
Cover design: Naomi Robinson
Typeset by: Cenveo Publisher Services

Foreword © David M. Clark, 2020
Editorial arrangement, Introduction, Chapter 1 and 11 © Paul Farrand, 2020
Chapter 2 © Pamela Myles-Hooton, 2020
Chapter 3 © Joshua E.J. Buckman, Rob Saunders, and Steve Pilling, 2020
Chapter 4 © Jeffrey McDonnell, Nichola Kirkland-Davis, and Rachel Newman, 2020
Chapter 5 © Zoe Symons, 2020
Chapter 6 © Katie Lockwood, 2020
Chapter 7 © Chris Williams and Paul Farrand, 2020
Chapter 8 © Paul Chadwick, 2020
Chapter 9 © Faye Small, 2020
Chapter 10 © Aljie van Hoorn, Paul Farrand, and Chris Dickens, 2020
Chapter 12 © Simon Grist, 2020
Chapter 13 © Mark Papworth, 2020
Chapter 14 © Judith Gellatly, Rebecca Pedley, Penny Bee, and Karina Lovell, 2020
Chapter 15 © Faye Small and Katie Lockwood, 2020
Chapter 16 © Georgina Miles, 2020
Chapter 17 © Sophie Brooks, 2020
Chapter 18 © Earlise C. Ward, 2020
Chapter 19 © Alessa Werson, Paul Farrand, and Ken Laidlaw, 2020
Chapter 20 © Paul Farrand and Ursula James, 2020

First published 2020

Apart from any fair dealing for the purposes of research or private study, or criticism or review, as permitted under the Copyright, Designs and Patents Act, 1988, this publication may be reproduced, stored or transmitted in any form, or by any means, only with the prior permission in writing of the publishers, or in the case of reprographic reproduction, in accordance with the terms of licences issued by the Copyright Licensing Agency. Enquiries concerning reproduction outside those terms should be sent to the publishers.

Library of Congress Control Number: 2020937012

British Library Cataloguing in Publication data

A catalogue record for this book is available from the British Library

ISBN 978-1-5264-8682-0
ISBN 978-1-5264-8681-3 (pbk)

At SAGE we take sustainability seriously. Most of our products are printed in the UK using responsibly sourced papers and boards. When we print overseas we ensure sustainable papers are used as measured by the PREPS grading system. We undertake an annual audit to monitor our sustainability.

Contents

About the Editor

Professor Paul Farrand is Director of the Low-Intensity Cognitive Behavioural Therapy (LICBT) clinical portfolio for the training of Psychological Wellbeing Practitioners (PWP) within Clinical Education, Development and Research (CEDAR), Psychology, University of Exeter. He has developed many of the most commonly used LICBT interventions adopted by Improving Access to Psychological Therapies (IAPT) services and is a member of the IAPT Expert Advisory Group, LICBT practitioner workforce development groups and national training and professional body accreditation committees. He is engaged in research and training associated with LICBT in several countries, currently the USA, Saudi Arabia and Sweden. In his clinical practice he has worked as Consultant Psychological Lead within the Oral and Maxillofacial Surgical hospital-based specialty for over 20 years. In recognition of his contribution to psychological therapies training, he was awarded National Teaching Fellowship in 2012.

Penny Bee is a Chair in Applied Mental Health Research at the University of Manchester. She contributes to undergraduate and postgraduate learning. She is co-lead of the Mental Health Research Group, where her main research interests lie in the development and evaluation of innovative models of mental health service delivery.

Sophie Brooks is a Lecturer on the PGCert Evidence Based Psychological Therapies and the PWP Supervision training at Exeter University, having previously worked as a Psychological Wellbeing Practitioner within a local NHS service.

Dr Joshua E.J. Buckman is a Clinical Research Fellow at UCL, his research focuses on personalising treatments for people with common mental disorders, particularly depression. He has worked in IAPT services in a research capacity since 2011 and as a clinician since 2014, providing training and clinical supervision to a range of IAPT clinicians and lecturing on the UCL Low Intensity Cognitive Behavioural Interventions Post Graduate course.

Paul Chadwick is Associate Professor and Deputy Director of the UCL Centre for Behaviour Change. He is also a Consultant Clinical and Health Psychologist specialising in interventions with adults and children with diabetes, obesity, cardiovascular disease and issues affecting sexual health and development.

Chris Dickens is Professor of Psychological Medicine, and the Lead for the Mental Health Research Group at Exeter University. He is a member of the University of Exeter Collaboration for Academic Primary Care, and an honorary Consultant in Psychological Medicine with the Devon Partnership NHS Trust.

Dr Judith Gellatly is a mental health Research Fellow at The University of Manchester. She has managed a number of research trials focusing on the delivery of psychological therapies for common mental health problems, including a multi-centre trial exploring the effectiveness of computerised cognitive behaviour therapy and guided self-help for OCD.

Simon Grist is a Low Intensity CBT Programmes Course Director at the University of Southampton leading a suite of educational programmes delivering CBT training. He originally trained as a Mental Health Nurse and then as a High Intensity CBT therapist.

Ursula James joined the IAPT programme in NHS England in 2016. She worked as an RMN in acute and community mental health care for many years before training in CBT and moving into IAPT services in 2009. She works on policy developments, and clinical delivery of the IAPT programme nationally.

Nicole Kirkland-Davis has worked for the NHS for the past 11 years; she is currently a Clinical Coordinator and Senior CBT Therapist. She is also a Clinical Tutor at UCL on their Low Intensity Cognitive Behavioural Interventions Postgraduate Certificate course.

Ken Laidlaw is a Professor of Clinical Psychology, Director of Postgraduate Research Programmes, and Director of DClinPsy and CAPs Programme, CEDAR, at the University of Exeter.

Katie Lockwood is a practising Psychological Wellbeing Practitioner (PWP) and Lecturer within CEDAR, at the University of Exeter.

Karina Lovell is a Professor of Mental Health (University of Manchester). She is an accredited CBT therapist. She is an NIHR Senior Investigator and a former president of the BABCP. Her programme of research has focused on alternative, accessible and innovative low intensity interventions for common mental health problems.

Dr Jeffrey McDonnell is a Clinical Psychologist with experience of working in Primary and Secondary Care services using cognitive behavioural approaches to assess and treat a variety of presenting problems. He currently works as a Teaching Fellow and Clinical Tutor on University College London's Postgraduate Course in Low Intensity Cognitive Behavioural Interventions.

Georgina Miles is a Psychological Wellbeing Practitioner (PWP) and tutor with the Clinical Psychology Unit at the University of Sheffield. She teaches on both the PWP and Education Mental Health Practitioner (EMHP) courses.

Pamela Myles-Hooton worked in the NHS for 20 years and at the University of Reading for 11 years. From 2019 she has worked on a number of projects including authoring a blended learning training programme in evidence-based low intensity interventions for NHS Education for Scotland.

Rachel Newman is the Joint Director of the London IAPT programme at UCL.

Dr Mark Papworth is a consultant clinical psychologist and Course Director of Newcastle University's PGCert in Low Intensity Psychological Therapies (seconded by

Tees, Esk and Wear Valleys NHS Trust). He also works in private practice in Newcastle at Psychology Northeast. He is the lead author of 'Low Intensity Cognitive Behaviour Therapy: A Practitioner's Guide'.

Dr Rebecca Pedley is a research associate within the Division of Nursing, Midwifery and Social Work at the University of Manchester. Her PhD used mixed methods to develop and test a measure of illness perceptions in OCD. She currently leads an RfPB funded study which explores how to better support parents of children with OCD.

Professor Steve Pilling is a Professor of Clinical Psychology & Clinical Effectiveness at UCL.

Dr Rob Saunders is a Senior Research Associate at UCL, focusing on the use of data to improve healthcare delivery and the measurement of clinical needs in mental health settings.

Faye Small has been working within the field of IAPT since 2009, with a previous background in mental health and counselling. Faye has also qualified as both a PWP and High Intensity CBT practitioner and is now the Programme Lead on the PGCert Psychological Therapies Practice (LICBT) within CEDAR at the University of Exeter.

Dr Zoe Symons is a Lecturer at Exeter University. She teaches on courses covering evidence-based low intensity treatments for common mental health problems.

Dr Alje van Hoorn is an Academic Clinical Fellow at the University of Exeter and a Psychiatrist and Mental Health practitioner for the NHS.

Dr Earlise C. Ward is a licensed psychologist and Associate Professor at the University of Wisconsin-Madison, School of Nursing. Her main clinical and research interest is in effectiveness of culturally adapted depression treatments. Dr Ward uses her clinical expertise, and research findings to develop culturally adapted depression treatments for African American adults with depression.

Alessa Werson was formerly a Psychological Wellbeing Practitioner at NHS IAPT Wellbeing Service Welwyn and Hatfield. She is now a Graduate Research Assistant at the University of Exeter.

Professor Chris Williams is an award-winning author, and Emeritus Professor of Psychosocial Psychiatry at the University of Glasgow, Scotland, UK and a Fellow of the Royal College of Psychiatrists and Honorary Fellow of BABCP. He is Director of Five Areas Ltd and author of the popular www.llttf.com website.

Foreword

David M. Clark

Low-intensity CBT interventions have had a profound impact on the provision of psychological therapy for common mental health problems in the UK and in many other countries. It has long been recognised that cognitive-behaviour therapy is effective in the treatment of depression and anxiety related problems. However, public provision was held back by the high cost of traditional face-to-face CBT. Starting in 2004, the National Institute of Health and Social Care Excellence (NICE) issued a series of clinical guidelines that suggested a way forward. Emerging research suggested that many people with mild to moderate depression and/or anxiety might benefit from interventions that involved less therapist input (hence 'low intensity') but still faithfully imparted the CBT skills that patients would find helpful for managing their emotional difficulties. This opened up the concept of a cost effective 'stepped care' system in which a substantial proportion of people would start treatment with a low-intensity intervention. Many should find that the low-intensity intervention alone met their needs. Some would find that, although helpful, low-intensity intervention alone was insufficient and subsequent 'stepping up' to a more traditionally delivered high-intensity CBT or other therapy would be required.

In 2006 the UK Department of Health funded two pilots to examine whether: low-intensity interventions could be offered at scale in routine services; could achieve the outcomes achieved in previously published randomised controlled trials; and could be incorporated within an integrated stepped care system. The pilots (which were in Doncaster and Newham) were a resounding success (Clark, Layard, Smithies, Richards, Suckling, and Wright, 2009). Overall outcomes were in line with what one might expect for CBT and large numbers of people were treated, with the provision of low-intensity interventions being critical to helping large numbers of people.

Building on the success of the Doncaster and Newham pilots, the UK government announced the creation of a national stepped care therapy programme called Improving Access to Psychological Therapy (IAPT). From small beginnings in 2008, IAPT has now grown to a point where it provides a course of treatment to around

605,000 people a year, with the government committed to expanding to almost 1 million people each year by 2024. A unique session by session outcome monitoring system tracks patients' progress throughout low- and high-intensity therapy. Outcomes are in line with expectation. Approximately five in every ten treated patients recover and seven in every ten show substantial and worthwhile improvement. Low-intensity CBT continues to be at the heart of the programme and has shown its worth year in and year out.

Of course, low-intensity CBT can only achieve excellent clinical outcomes if its practitioners are well-trained, have acquired the necessary clinical skills, are well-supported by regular supervision, and work in services that pay attention to the well-being of their staff as well as that of their clients. This is where the excellent *Low-intensity CBT Skills and Interventions: A Practitioner's Manual* so wonderfully hits the spot. Paul Farrand, one of the leading originators of low-intensity work, has assembled an outstanding group of authors, all of whom are LICBT experts. Together they have produced a comprehensive series of chapters that take students, experienced practitioners and teachers through all aspects of the LICBT practitioner role. The key concepts underpinning low-intensity work and how it differs from more traditional delivery of CBT are clearly articulated. It is a different and important way of working and this is made very clear. The manual then provides invaluable guidance on how to conduct low-intensity assessments and to support patients through the full range of NICE recommended low-intensity therapies. The social context in which interventions are delivered is crucial and suitable adaptions for particular populations are clearly described. An invaluable practitioner manual.

David M. Clark

National Clinical and Informatics Advisor for IAPT; Professor of Experimental Psychology, University of Oxford

Acknowledgements

Several people are always in the background when taking on the huge endeavour of editing such a substantial text. Paula, my wife, for keeping things running when I locked myself away to focus on editing, my kids Ollie, Ellis and Amélie for keeping me grounded, my mum Muriel and my sisters Julie and Wendy for fostering my Australian directness. While sometimes getting me in hot water, it has generally served me well. Finally, Professor Eugene Mullan for being my mentor but mostly a friend, enjoy your retirement.

Online Resources

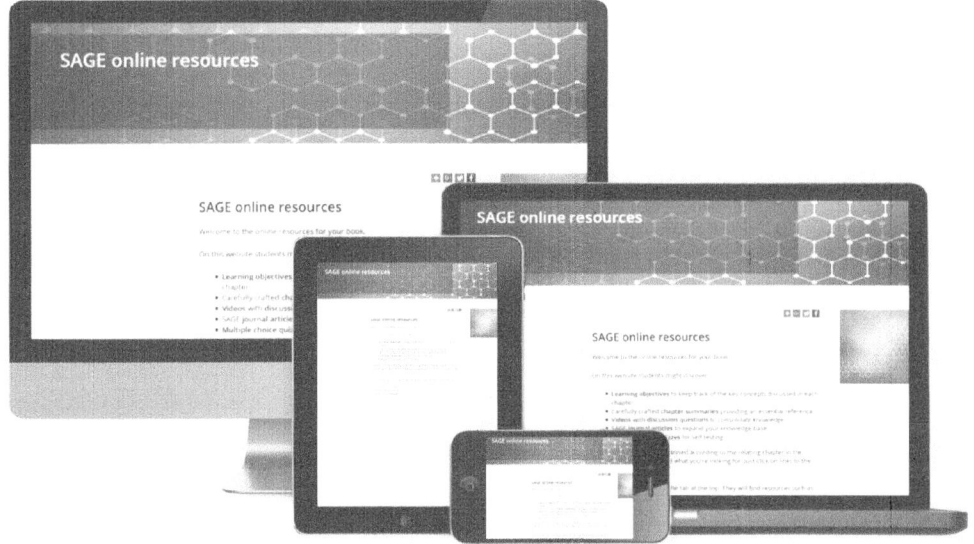

Low-Intensity CBT Skills and Interventions: A Practitioner's Manual is supported by online resources to aid study and assist in teaching, which are available at https://study.sagepub.com/farrand.

Worksheet templates and short exercises for a patient to work through independently or a practitioner and patient to work through together.

Weblinks to Psychological Wellbeing Practitioners (PWP) workbooks that can be used in low-intensity training and practice with patients. They cover topics such as 'Managing Your Worry', 'Unhelpful Thoughts', 'Facing Your Fears' and support the specific interventions described in the chapters.

Worksheet Templates

6.1   Example of a relapse prevention worksheet
9.1   Reflection record for use in clinical skills supervision
11.1   Behavioural activation schedule
11.2   Example of a classifying activity worksheet
11.3   Example of an activity grading worksheet

Workbooks and Resources

The worksheets and workbooks are Clinical Education, Development and Research (CEDAR), Psychology, University of Exeter interventions: http://cedar.exeter.ac.uk/.

Obsessive Compulsive Disorder: A Self-Help Book (Lovell and Gega, 2011) is from the University of Manchester: http://man.ac.uk/Fyl12C.

Introduction

Pedagogic Approach

Paul Farrand

The pedagogic approach adopted within *Low-Intensity CBT Skills and Interventions* has been organised and informed by the seminal work of Professor James Bennett-Levy. Professor Bennett-Levy's research has made a significant contribution to evidence-informed training for the psychological therapies workforce and has no doubt contributed to improving the effectiveness of cognitive behavioural therapy (CBT) in practice.

Cognitive Model of Skills Development

The *Cognitive Model of Skills Development* (Bennett-Levy, 2006) highlights the role of three systems – Declarative, Procedural, Reflective (DPR) – associated with competency development.

Declarative Knowledge

- 'Knowing that' represents factual knowledge the low-intensity CBT (LICBT) practitioner has regarding:
  o *common factors* that form the basis of the clinical method
  o *specific factors* representing the theoretical foundation and specific competences upon which the LICBT clinical method and interventions are based.
- It is predominantly delivered using didactic pedagogic approaches such as lectures, clinical skills supervision and directed-learning activities such as reading.

- There are increasing opportunities to deliver declarative knowledge through online technology-enhanced learning methods within a blended learning approach (Graham, 2006).
- It presents opportunities to inform a component of university-directed or self-directed learning incorporated into standardised delivery.

Procedural Knowledge

- 'Knowing how to, and when to' apply *specific factor skills* associated with the clinical method (see Parts 2 and 3).
- Although there may be a declarative element to procedural knowledge, pedagogic approaches that facilitate the transfer of declarative to procedural knowledge are required. *Active* pedagogic approaches include simulated structured role-plays, directly observed or recorded specific factor practice and clinical skills supervision of *live* patient clinical sessions.
- Development of procedural knowledge is ongoing.
- It is stimulated when the practitioner is required to apply already acquired procedural skills to newly experienced clinical challenges or adapt practice to accommodate patients with diversity.
- Developing procedural knowledge is often implicit, with practitioners not fully aware of the application of common or specific factors.
- Training providers and supervisors need to ensure that pedagogic approaches supporting the development of specific factors have an element of observation. This may require training providers to ensure an appropriate staff–student ratio to enable trainees get an appropriate level of feedback.
- Reflection is the key system for facilitating ongoing competence development required for *professional expertise*.

Reflection

- Making the implicit explicit enables the implicit nature of the development of procedural knowledge to be made explicit (Bennett-Levy, 2003).
- Ongoing reflective practice has a seminal role in distinguishing expert from novice practitioners (Skovholt and Rønnestad, 2001).
- There is additional potential to enhance practitioner resiliency (Skovholt and Rønnestad, 2001) and further opportunities for reflection in LICBT with the provision of case management alongside clinical skills supervision (Farrand et al., 2016).
- Reflective questions are used throughout each chapter to stimulate personal reflection on salient, and at times, challenging points.

Closing the Gap between the DPR systems

Self-practice/self-reflection (SP/SR; Bennett-Levy et al., 2001) offers effective ways to close the gap between the three systems associated with the DPR model. The focus of SP/SR, including reflection on the personal self, enables trainees to learn from the application of procedural skills whilst reflecting on any personal impact that skills application may have on them. This enables trainees to more effectively put themselves in the patients' shoes, facilitating competency development by enabling them to anticipate challenges when directly experiencing specific factors associated with the LICBT clinical method. Tools such as blogs to support written reflections following self-practice have been used to enable trainers to address commonly occurring themes or share reflections as the basis of classroom discussion (Farrand et al., 2010). This approach can be particularly helpful when the delivery of training includes university-directed or self-directed learning components.

Assessing Your Understanding

An 'Assessing Your Understanding' section is included at the end of each chapter to help you appreciate your understanding of declarative knowledge and continue to develop procedural competency. Multiple-choice, extended-matching or essay questions and case studies are included at the end of each chapter to enable you to assess your declarative knowledge. These are supplemented by SP/SR activities to help you continue to develop clinical competency during, or following, training, to stimulate continuing professional development and facilitate the transition from novice to expert (Bennett-Levy et al., 2009). Reflection points included within each chapter are included to stimulate reflection on key areas.

1

Low-Intensity Cognitive Behavioural Therapy

Revolution Not Evolution

Paul Farrand

Learning Objectives

By the end of this chapter you should be able to:

- Appreciate the context justifying the emergence of low-intensity CBT
- Critically evaluate the fundamental characteristics of low-intensity CBT
- Demonstrate a critical awareness of the evidence base supporting low-intensity CBT and methodological limitations
- Critically appraise differences between low- and high-intensity CBT
- Demonstrate an awareness of key challenges associated with low-intensity CBT

Background

On a worldwide scale, mental health service delivery is associated with under-investment, excessive waiting times, lack of choice, significant demands on patients, large workforce variation and poorly informed by the evidence base (Ngui et al., 2010). This has resulted in increased demands for parity of esteem between mental and physical healthcare to improve access to evidence-based treatment, meet patient aspirations, provide high-quality care and give equal status to training and practice (Royal College of Psychiatrists, 2013). Across England, efforts to achieve parity of esteem resulted in the publication of the *No Health without Mental Health* (Department of Health, 2011) mental health strategy. This strategy identifies long-term ambitions to transform mental healthcare with *Closing the Gap: Priorities for Essential Change in Mental Health* (Department of Health, 2014) translating these ambitions into short-term action. To achieve these ambitions, however, it was recognised that a new mental health programme would be required for implementation across England.

The IAPT Programme

The IAPT programme represents the first national implementation of a mental health programme to make evidence-based psychological therapies available to every adult needing them for the treatment of common mental health problems 'at the right time and in the right place' (Seward and Clark, 2010: 480).

Key Point

The main drivers justifying development and implementation of the IAPT programme for the treatment of common mental health problems (Seward and Clark, 2010) have been:

- Justice-based care arising from the personal impact of mental health problems on patients (Layard and Clark, 2015)
- A strong clinical evidence-base determined by the National Institute for Health and Clinical Excellence (NICE) informing mental health treatment
- A powerful economic case to address societal and lost productivity costs associated with mental health problems calculated to be in the region of £7-10 billion (Centre for Economic Performance, 2006)
- Recognition that solely focusing on increasing the availability of the high-intensity mental health workforce was no longer a viable option (Bennett-Levy et al., 2010).

These drivers created a strong *'constellation of rationale and evidence'* providing the initial momentum to justify and establish the IAPT programme (Seward and Clark, 2010: 480). The IAPT programme is now informing similar service developments on a worldwide scale in countries such as the USA (Chapter 20), Hong Kong and Sweden.

Stepped Care

Prior to development of the IAPT programme it became apparent that achieving long-term ambitions to transform mental healthcare and meet epidemic level demands for treatment would require a fundamental change in the organisation of mental health treatment (Richards, 2010a). The change was to develop a mental health stepped care delivery model enabling service delivery to be least restrictive (Bower and Gilbody, 2005; van Straten et al., 2015). Lower demands would be placed on patients in terms of costs and personal inconvenience and on service providers through the utilisation of a different workforce at Steps 2 and 3 of the stepped care model (Richards, 2010a). Rather than relying solely on high-intensity Step 3 face-to-face psychological therapists, the revolution in service delivery spearheaded the evolution of a new Step 2 LICBT psychological therapies practitioner workforce.

Key Point

The core characteristics associated with stepped care implemented within the IAPT programme (Richards, 2010a) are:

- The mental health psychological practitioner workforce supporting evidence-based low-intensity CBT at Step 2 and therapies workforce delivering evidence-based high-intensity psychological therapies at Step 3
- Assessment is undertaken at Step 2 unless knowledge of the mental health difficulty at referral suggests it is unlikely to be consistent with NICE Guidelines for Step 2 treatment
- The pivotal role of NICE guidelines to inform evidence-based clinical decision-making regarding selection of the appropriate step for the treatment of common mental health problems
- As determined by NICE, patients receive the least restrictive evidence-based psychological therapy to promote recovery
- Outcome measures are systematically taken at every session to inform ongoing treatment decisions and support self-correction whereby patients not responding adequately will be supported to step up to a NICE evidence-based high-intensity treatment
- Stepped care models should accommodate stepping down where a less intensive treatment becomes appropriate.

What is Low-Intensity CBT?

CBT is an evidence-based psychological therapy with a strong evidence-base for the treatment of common mental health problems, alongside several severe and enduring mental health problems such as psychosis and schizophrenia (NICE, 2014a). How-ever, without unsustainable increases in the levels of funding (Layard et al., 2007) it is unlikely to radically improve access to evidence-based psychological therapy when only available within a traditional high-intensity CBT (HICBT) format. Revo-lution not evolution in the delivery of CBT was therefore required, leading to the implementation of CBT in the form of supported low-intensity CBT (LICBT) self-help interventions. Whilst LICBT has been implemented within Stepped Care (Richards, 2010a) and alongside wider organisational systems such as case-management super-vision (Chapter 9) within the IAPT programme, it represents a fundamental shift in the delivery of CBT in its own right and shares common characteristics.

Key Point

The core characteristics of LICBT are:

- Use of CBT-informed self-help resources to deliver CBT techniques (Richards, 2004)
- Delivery through a variety of CBT self-help mediums, primarily within written, computer-ised (cCBT) or internet-based (iCBT) formats (Chapter 7) with increasing research now focusing on other delivery formats such as video-mediated, e-mail and based around apps
- CBT self-help interventions supported by an LICBT psychological practitioner workforce
- A Step 2 LICBT psychological practitioner workforce competent in supporting patients to use CBT self-help interventions
- Briefer session times required to support the patient to use LICBT techniques deliv-ered through CBT self-help interventions
- Adoption of CBT self-help interventions for the treatment of common mental health problems directly informed by the evidence base.

Continued developments in the evidence-base still make a single definition captur-ing the key characteristics of LICBT elusive (Bennett-Levy et al., 2010). However, with respect to the IAPT programme, consensus concerning core characteristics of LICBT is beginning to emerge.

Evidence Base

Consistent with HICBT, a large evidence base supports the implementation of LICBT in the form of guided written CBT, cCBT and iCBT self-help interventions. This has informed the clinical evidence base for LICBT treatment of common mental health problems determined by NICE (National Collaborating Centre for Mental Health, 2018). For a comprehensive review of the evidence base, see Bennett-Levy et al. (2010).

Interventions

There are over 30 systematic reviews and 50 controlled trials demonstrating the effectiveness of CBT self-help interventions for the treatment of common mental health problems (Delgadillo, 2018). Systematic reviews comparing guided CBT self-help with face-to-face psychological therapies have identified no significant differences in treatment effectiveness or drop-out up to one year post assessment (Cuijpers et al., 2010). However, variability in effect size across studies highlights the need for further research to recognise moderators that may be associated with effectiveness (Delgadillo, 2018). Research to date has identified clinical moderators to include mental health condition, support type and patients with existing depression rather than those at risk (Farrand and Woodford, 2013). Research moderators include unclear allocation concealment, observer-rated outcome measures and comparisons with waiting-list control groups (Gellatly et al., 2007). With respect to guided self-help, moderators associated with session length, delivery mode or therapist background were not related to effectiveness. Very few studies have examined the effectiveness of cCBT across conditions (Carlbring et al., 2018).

Delivery and Support

The evidence base regarding ways to improve access through the provision of choice regarding cCBT, iCBT (Ritterband et al., 2010), telephone-based (T-CBT; Mohr et al., 2012), video teleconferencing (Varger et al., 2019) or email to support LICBT (Hadjistavropoulos, 2018) is encouraging. A systematic review comparing face-to-face with iCBT demonstrated no difference in effectiveness (Carlbring et al., 2018). Additionally, no differences emerged regarding drop-out that has previously been identified to be a challenge for internet-based interventions (Christensen et al., 2009). Evidence has also demonstrated the utility of T-CBT (Bee et al., 2008). In a randomised controlled trial comparing high-intensity face-to-face with T-CBT there was little difference in effectiveness post treatment with lower attrition with T-CBT (Mohr et al., 2012). However, caution should be exercised given that treatment gains were better maintained with face-to-face CBT following the end of treatment.

Acceptability

Excluding a study examining a CBT self-help intervention based on behavioural activation for armed forces veterans (Chapter 20; Farrand et al., 2019a), little research has examined the acceptability of written CBT self-help interventions (Lewis et al., 2012). However, good levels of acceptability have been demonstrated regarding the delivery of therapy over the telephone (Lovell et al., 2006; Ludman et al., 2007) and patients' experience of cCBT for depression (Rost et al., 2017). However, methodological challenges arising from qualitative research in this area have been associated with difficulties defining user acceptance and variations in measurement (Rost et al., 2017). Furthermore, whilst some patients have expressed a preference for cCBT, the majority are generally ambivalent (Knowles et al., 2015). A complex relationship is therefore likely to exist between patients' preferences expressed towards delivery format and support type (Bee et al., 2010). This has reinforced requirements to promote choice of support type within a stepped care model (Bower and Gilbody, 2005).

Key Point

Evidence-based conclusions associated with LICBT:

- Guided CBT self-help is as effective as face-to-face psychological therapies for the treatment of common mental health difficulties, excluding post-traumatic stress disorder (PTSD) and social anxiety.
- More research is needed to recognise other moderators that may be associated with greater effectiveness.
- Use of cCBT, ICBT and T-CBT offers the opportunity to improve access without reducing effectiveness.
- Good levels of acceptability are associated with T-CBT and cCBT, although methodological limitations should currently limit conclusions from being generalised.

Differences between HICBT and LICBT

Whilst both are grounded within a CBT model and directly informed by the evidence base, significant differences exist between HICBT and LICBT beyond time taken to deliver the intervention. Awareness of wider differences related to the clinical method and workforce is especially important if confusion between LICBT and Brief CBT is to be avoided. Brief CBT is a variation of HICBT with delivery of techniques condensed as a result of greater specificity and flexibility afforded to the therapist following treatment protocols (Hazlett-Stevens and Craske, 2004).

Clinical Method

With both low- and high-intensity CBT based on a CBT model, the most obvious (often only!) difference identified by many is related to the dose of therapy (National Collaborating Centre for Mental Health, 2018) received by the patient. However, whilst a CBT model informs the clinical model within both high- and low-intensity CBT, several additional clinical features differentiate them (Table 1.1).

Table 1.1 Main differences between High- and Low-Intensity CBT

Category	Difference	Definition
Clinical method	Therapeutic dose	Amount of therapeutic resource (session length, number of sessions) recommended to bring about change
	'Here and now' v. 'Longitudinal' cognitive behavioural formulation	Focus of the low-intensity CBT clinical method and treatment on the patient's presenting problem being experienced rather than on an appreciation of developmental factors
	Specific factor skills employed when questioning	Type of skills employed to reach an understanding of the patient's mental health difficulties
	Single-strand v. Multi-strand intervention	The number of CBT 'techniques/interventions' adopted in the treatment of a patient's mental health difficulty
Workforce	Responsibilities	Roles and responsibilities undertaken by a low-intensity psychological practitioner workforce compared to a high-intensity therapist
	Supervision	Differences in the type and characteristics of supervision received

Therapeutic Dose

Within HICBT the optimal dose of therapy is typically in excess of ten weekly 60-minute treatment sessions recommended by NICE for the appropriate common mental health problem. However, following an assessment in the region of 40 minutes, an average of five to eight briefer support sessions is typically received with LICBT (Bennett-Levy et al., 2010), thereby making better use of scarce resources (van Straten et al., 2015). Using NICE guidelines (National Collaborating Centre for Mental Health, 2018) to inform delivery of different doses of CBT, LICBT represents a way to achieve high-volume working that helps to improve access and democratise CBT (Bennett-Levy et al., 2010). Although treatment dose directly provided by the practitioner is lower in LICBT, it is likely that patients themselves spend similar amounts of time engaging with the interventions as with HICBT (van Straten et al., 2015). This possibility arises as a result of the increased emphasis on patients to engage with self-help interventions between sessions; engagement with HICBT is often limited to completing homework set.

Here and Now v. Longitudinal Cognitive Behavioural Formulation

During an LICBT assessment, the practitioner employs a range of common factor and questioning skills (Chapter 5; Richards and Whyte, 2011) to gain an understanding of features associated with the patient presentation in the here and now (Chapter 2). This informs the cognitive-behavioural model shared with the patient and informs

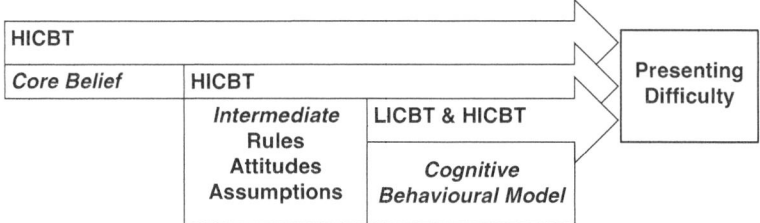

Figure 1.1 High- and low-intensity CBT formulation

selection of the appropriate CBT self-help intervention (Chapter 4). Within HICBT, however, a greater range of questioning skills, such as the downward arrow technique (Beck, 1995) is employed to inform a longitudinal cognitive-behavioural formulation that extends beyond the here and now (Figure 1.1).

A longitudinal formulation seeks to appreciate the influence of enduring cognitive distortions, such as intermediate – rules, attitudes, assumptions – and core beliefs, on the cognitive model that accounts for the way the presenting problem is impacting on the patient in the here and now (Beck, 1995).

Specific Factor Skills Employed When Questioning

As determined by the longitudinal formulation, HICBT assessment requires several specific factor skills (Chapter 5) to be employed to gain an understanding of the influence that intermediate and core beliefs have on the presenting problem. These include techniques such as continuum methods to evaluate negative schemas (Padesky, 1994). However, beyond skills such as funnelling (Chapters 2 and 6) adopted at both high- and low-intensity CBT, the focus of an LICBT assessment on the *here and now* requires a narrower range of questioning and specific factor skills.

Single-Strand v. Multi-Strand Interventions

LICBT represents a single-strand approach (Turpin et al., 2010) whereby following assessment a clinical decision is reached (Chapters 3 and 4) to adopt a specific CBT self-help intervention from the LICBT toolkit (Part II). The practitioner then supports the patient to engage with the single-strand intervention. This contrasts with HICBT where evidence-based protocols specify the delivery of several different interventions as part of a multi-strand approach. For example, in the treatment of generalised anxiety disorder (GAD), a treatment protocol (Dugas and Robichaud, 2007) informing NICE (2011a) guidelines specifies adopting cognitive restructuring to identify and challenge worry beliefs, problem-solving and exposure to uncertainty. The movement towards an even more elaborated multi-strand approach is now gaining momentum given further developments in third wave HICBT (Hayes and Hoffmann, 2017).

Workforce

Representing movement away from sole reliance on a Step 3 high-intensity CBT therapist workforce, the development and implementation of a Step 2 psychological practitioner role – psychological wellbeing practitioner (PWP) – denotes a core feature of the IAPT programme. Whilst both workforces share generic and basic CBT competences, the CBT and problem-specific competencies associated with assessment and treatment differ (Roth and Pilling, 2007a,b). Within the high-intensity therapist workforce, specific multi-strand CBT interventions are delivered to the patient. This contrasts to competencies held by the Step 2 LICBT psychological therapy practitioner workforce that empowers patients to manage their own recovery by providing them with ongoing support to engage with CBT self-help interventions (Chapter 6). Consequently, different competencies have implications for responsibilities placed on each workforce, making training and supervision of the Step 2 and 3 workforces fundamental to the IAPT programme (Roth and Pilling, 2008).

Responsibilities

Similar to debates within healthcare surrounding responsibilities of assistant practitioners (Wakefield et al., 2010), there has been little clarity regarding how the LICBT psychological therapy practitioner role fits within the wider mental health workforce. However, this is beginning to be addressed through the recent establishment of the Psychological Professions Network (Psychological Professions Network, 2018). Whilst currently non-registered practitioners, professional bodies are now in discussion to establish accreditation criteria to recognise LICBT psychological practitioners as a competency-based and autonomous mental health workforce that make their own treatment decisions. With assistant practitioners or paraprofessionals (Farrand et al., 2009) there is vertical substitution of roles delegated by a professional role higher up the occupational ladder (Nancarrow and Borthwick, 2005). Within the IAPT programme, however, PWPs neither undertake delegated roles nor assist HICBT therapists. The PWP psychological therapy practitioner level role therefore has equal status with that of the HICBT therapist within the stepped care model, with outcomes mutually dependent on both workforces.

Training and Supervision

Within the IAPT stepped care model, significant focus is placed upon ensuring that the Step 2 LICBT and Step 3 psychological therapy workforce have received high-quality competency-based training. Training is informed by a nationally specified HICBT (Liness and Muston, 2011) and LICBT training curriculum (University College London, 2015), itself informed by a CBT competence model (Roth and Pilling, 2007a). LICBT Psychological Therapy Practitioner training is supplemented by educator and student materials (Richards and Whyte, 2011) that have informed several features of this training manual. Ensuring accreditation of trainers and training programmes also helps to enhance fidelity to treatment delivery of LICBT interventions (Hides et al., 2010). Furthermore, separate curricula to inform training for the high- and low-intensity CBT workforce potentially reduces the likelihood of therapeutic drift, helping to maintain evidence-based practice (Waller, 2009). Differences between HICBT and LICBT also exist with respect to the types of supervision received (Chapter 9).

Challenges Encountered

Following the implementation of the IAPT programme, a number of challenges associated with LICBT have been identified. In addition to accounting for an emerging evidence base, overcoming such challenges may serve to enhance an understanding of LICBT and assist in determining a suitable definition (Bennett-Levy et al., 2010).

Clinical Heterogeneity

Whilst based on a CBT model, significant variation exists with respect to the content and delivery of CBT self-help interventions (Lewis et al., 2012). In addition to differences in the content of interventions included within CBT self-help for the treatment of specific common mental health difficulties, variations are also evident regarding the CBT self-help format. Such variation extends beyond differences between the modality to deliver self-help interventions, but also arises with respect to types of written CBT self-help approach. These can vary: intervention specific stand-alone worksheets, intervention specific CBT self-help booklets (e.g. Farrand et al., 2019a), CBT self-help booklets (e.g. Farrand et al., 2019b) and books (e.g. Gilbert, 2009) that target a specific common mental health difficulty and include psychoeducation in addition to worksheets.

Lack of Consensus Regarding Single-Strand Interventions

Although LICBT represents a single-strand approach (Turpin et al., 2010), there is little consensus between researchers, LICBT psychological therapy practitioners and HICBT therapists regarding the composition of single-strand interventions. For example, within *A Recovery Programme for Depression* (Lovell and Richards, 2012), the cognitive restructuring intervention comprises a 'thought diary' to identify unhelpful thoughts and 'evidence table' to challenge them. However, 'as long as the intention is cognitive or schematic change' (Clark, 2013: 2), interventions such as behavioural experiments have also been associated with cognitive restructuring. This approach has been adopted within a cognitive restructuring intervention (Farrand et al., 2019a). However, when using this intervention, consideration needs to be given to ways of supporting the behavioural experiment when undertaken outside the session (Chapter 6). Unlike HICBT, where in-vivo experiments are encouraged (Rouf et al., 2015), supporting interventions outside of a support session are not commonly undertaken in LICBT.

Therapeutic Drift during Support Sessions

Although clear distinctions should be drawn between low- and high-intensity CBT, challenges can be encountered when an LICBT psychological therapy practitioner drifts between supporting single-strand CBT self-help interventions and delivering multi-strand interventions (Waller, 2009). When the practitioner drifts into HICBT, adopting techniques such as downward arrow (Beck, 1995) or continuum methods (Padesky, 1994), challenges to working outside of competencies developed during training (Roth and Pilling, 2007a) or working within constraints imposed by the therapeutic dose is encountered. They may be more likely to arise when the LICBT psychological therapy practitioner drifts into employing HICBT techniques to deliver specific stand-alone worksheets within sessions rather than supporting the patient to work through CBT self-help workbooks between sessions. However, LICBT psychological therapy practitioners losing confidence in the LICBT interventions when patients show little sign of recovery has also been recognised as a factor that can lead to therapeutic drift (Telford and Wilson, 2010).

Therapeutic Drift within CBT Self-Help Interventions

The genesis of self-help as a concept informing self-help books (Smiles, 1859) precedes the development of CBT self-help. Consequently, CBT has been adapted in many different ways to inform the content of the self-help interventions leading to significant heterogeneity. This has resulted in some CBT self-help interventions being more representative of HICBT by adopting multi-strand interventions, longitudinal formulations and techniques to address more enduring cognitive distortions (Beck, 1995). For example, a commonly adopted written CBT self-help book for depression, *Overcoming Depression*, (Gilbert, 2009) includes techniques such as cognitive restructuring but as part of a multi-strand approach including a compassion focus and addressing other difficulties that can be co-morbid with depression, such as anger. Additionally, multi-strand interventions have been adopted within iCBT programmes proposed to be LICBT with support provided by LICBT practitioners (Richards et al., 2018). For example, 'Space from Depression' includes techniques for depression such as behavioural activation, self-control desensitisation and cognitive restructuring alongside techniques used to challenge core beliefs. NICE guidelines for depression are cited as the justification for the approach taken. However, these guidelines highlight these techniques when used as part of a multi-strand approach within HICBT.

LICBT self-help interventions adopting a multi-strand approach is therefore inconsistent with a single-strand approach associated with LICBT. They can drift away from the focus of the difficulties presented in the here and now and address a longitudinal formulation and require a psychological practitioner workforce to drift from the LICBT clinical method.

Reflection Point

What implications for practice when selecting LICBT interventions arise as a consequence of heterogeneity in the CBT clinical method included within self-help interventions?

Whilst there is guidance informing the selection of CBT self-help interventions (Richards and Farrand, 2010; University College London, nd), the focus is largely upon criteria related to presentation, style and the evidence base but it largely fails to address characteristics differentiating low- from high-intensity CBT.

Retention of the LICBT Psychological Therapy Practitioner Workforce

A major challenge experienced by the IAPT programme has been attrition from the PWP, LICBT psychological therapy practitioner workforce (National Collaborating Centre for Mental Health, 2018). Soon after the end of training a significant number of the PWP workforce leave the role, with many seeking to undertake HICBT training to work at Step 3 of the Stepped Care model. High attrition has potential to destabilise services and challenge recovery rates with the workforce largely comprising novice practitioners that have failed to enhance and develop their competencies (Roth and Pilling, 2017). Experiencing a situation such as this with a workforce has the effect of threatening and fragmenting the quality of care (Imison, Castle-Clarke and Watson, 2016). Furthermore, failing to maintain the PWP challenges the economic case used as a justification behind the IAPT programme, threatening long term sustainability. However, development of the Psychological Professions Network, new vocational routes into training such as apprenticeships and developments in Assistant Practitioner roles represents the potential to reduce attrition by improving access to the workforce.

Increased Demands Placed on LICBT Psychological Therapy Practitioners

Working within a high volume LICBT mental health environment having higher patient caseloads alongside shorter contact durations compared with HICBT has the potential to place increased demands on the LICBT psychological therapy practitioner workforce (Richards, 2010b). To ensure safe and effective working with a high volume of patients 'clinical case management' supervision was developed for the LICBT practitioner working within the IAPT programme with clinical skills supervision focused on skills development (Chapter 9; Richards, 2010b). However, whilst both forms of supervision meet four of the purposes of supervision (Turpin and Wheeler, 2011), the fifth function associated with 'Staff Support and the Prevention of Burn-Out' may not be fully realised. Consequently, there may be a failure to support the practitioner to better maintain their own health and well-being or to address any emotional difficulties of their own unrelated to work.

Key Point

Challenges encountered with LICBT:

- Clinical heterogeneity regarding the content and delivery of CBT self-help interventions, self-help format and types of written CBT self-help interventions.
- Lack of consensus exists as to what constitutes single strand with respect to LICBT interventions.
- Therapeutic drift between low- and high-intensity CBT arising with respect to both clinical support sessions and within the CBT self-help interventions.
- High levels of attrition can be experienced with the LICBT psychological therapy practitioner workforce.
- High levels of demands are placed on the LICBT psychological therapy practitioner workforce potentially requiring higher levels of supervision capacity to support staff.

Summary

For many years, service delivery has evolved to meet large increases in demand for mental health treatment. However, simply evolving mental health services has resulted in excessive waiting times, lack of choice and poor connection to the evidence base. Revolution in mental health service delivery based on the implementation of LICBT within Step 2 of a stepped care model has provided a solution to these challenges. This chapter has highlighted that whilst based on a CBT model, key characteristics associated with the LICBT clinical method and workforce serve to distinguish low- from high-intensity CBT with these characteristics addressed more extensively in other chapters. As can be common with revolution however, several new challenges to be addressed have emerged.

Assessing Your Understanding

Declarative

Essay Questions

- Critically evaluate differences between low- and high-intensity CBT for the assessment and treatment of depression.
- Critically evaluate several challenges with low-intensity CBT and propose potential solutions with reference to the literature.

Extended Matching Questions

1. Each answer is worth one mark.
2. There are 15 answers.
3. The question is worth 15 marks.
4. There *is* negative marking.
5. Answer by clearly writing the capital letter associated with each option in the response boxes provided after each question.
6. More response boxes are provided than answers, so you are not required to put an answer in each response box.
7. For each question, only those answers supplied within the appropriate spaces will be marked as correct. If you make an error, put a cross through the space with the answer in it and add a new space with the answer on the appropriate line.

Table 1.2 Theme: Characteristics of Low-Intensity CBT

	Options		
A	Deferred entry	**N**	Stratified delivery
B	Global therapy	**O**	Stepping up
C	NICE-informed treatment decisions	**P**	Case management supervision
D	Therapeutic drift	**Q**	Transference
E	Outcomes taken at every session	**R**	Delivered at Step 4
F	Health technology	**S**	Based on 'specific' factors only
G	Therapist level workforce	**T**	Free word association
H	Downward arrow technique	**U**	Multi-strand interventions
I	Habituation	**V**	Self-correcting
J	Transtheoretical	**W**	Relapse prevention
K	Based on brief CBT interventions	**X**	Lower levels of patient engagement
L	Alexithymia	**Y**	Delivered on average in 8–10 sessions
M	Least restrictive	**Z**	'Longitudinal' assessment

Lead in: Select the 15 most *commonly* identified characteristics associated with Low-Intensity CBT. Each option can be used once, more than once, or not at all.

1. Core characteristics of LICBT

2. Difference between LICBT and HICBT

3. Features of Stepped Care

Worth 15 marks

Procedural

Case Vignette-Based Question

Identify eight examples in the case vignette where the low-intensity CBT psychological therapy practitioner is not working in a manner consistent with low-intensity CBT. (Question worth 16 marks; 2 marks per answer.)

Ellis, a low-intensity CBT psychological therapy practitioner, has recently assessed Ms Lashmay. At the start of the assessment session Ellis introduced herself and her role as a therapist in the Horizon Mental Health Service. Ellis began the assessment by asking Ms Lashmay what brought her to the service for an assessment and soon recognised that Ms Lashmay was possibly struggling with 'social anxiety'. To confirm this

(Continued)

possibility, Ellis said, 'People with social anxiety may worry about saying something stupid. Can I ask what would be so bad about that?' The answer confirmed to Ellis that Ms Lashmay was indeed struggling with social anxiety and introduced the required outcome measures. Ellis fed the outcome measures back and said that because Ms Lashmay only had mild social anxiety, she would work with her delivering evidence-based CBT self-help interventions face to face, usually taking about eight to ten sessions of 60 minutes. Ellis indicated that given that this was based around CBT self-help materials, the time Ms Lashmay would engage with treatment would be less than if Ms Lashmay was to use high-intensity CBT. Ellis recommended a CBT self-help workbook called *Be at Ease with Yourself and Others*. She highlighted the fact that she had used this with other patients who reported finding it really helpful, especially liking the behavioural activation and cognitive restructuring intervention alongside the compassion-focused approach.

1.	2.
3.	4.
5.	6.
7.	8.

Answers to **Assessing Your Understanding** questions can be found in the appendix on p. 333

Further Reading and Resources

Bennett-Levy, J., Richards, D.A., Farrand, P., Christensen, H., Griffiths, K.M., Kavanagh, D.J. et al. (eds) (2010) *Oxford Guide to Low Intensity CBT Interventions*. Oxford: Oxford University Press.

Bower, P. and Gilbody, S. (2005) Stepped care in psychological therapies: access, effectiveness and efficiency: narrative literature review. *British Journal of Psychiatry*, 186, 11–17.

Cuijpers, P., Donker, T., van Straten, A. and Andersson, G. (2010) Is guided self-help as effective as face-to-face psychotherapy for depression and anxiety disorders? A systematic review and meta-analysis of comparative outcome studies. *Psychological Medicine*, 40, 1943–57.

National Collaborating Centre for Mental Health (NCCMH) (2018) *The Improving Access to Psychological Therapies Manual*. Available at www.england.nhs.uk/publication/the-improving-access-to-psychological-therapies-manual (accessed 6 October 2019).

To access the online resources accompanying this chapter, please visit: https://study.sagepub.com/farrand

Part I
Low-Intensity Clinical Method

2

Low-Intensity CBT Assessment

Unlocking the Key to Successful Intervention

Pamela Myles-Hooton

Learning Objectives

By the end of this chapter you should be able to:

- Structure a low-intensity CBT assessment session
- Gather information in a patient-centred way to collaboratively reach a brief and accurate understanding of the patient's main mental health difficulties and impacts
- Undertake an accurate risk assessment
- Apply standardised assessment tools including symptom and other psychometric instruments to inform a problem formulation
- Summarise patient difficulties within a problem statement
- Negotiate SMART end of treatment goals

Background

Before effective delivery of any low-intensity CBT (LICBT) intervention, a comprehensive assessment is required to gain a full understanding of the presenting patient problem and impact. A competent assessment will not only lead to a thorough and accurate understanding of a patient's presenting difficulties and provide a clear indication as to what treatment interventions are appropriate, but also help establish a strong therapeutic relationship. Consistent with the LICBT clinical method, assessments can be undertaken face-to-face, over a media platform, or over the telephone (Chapter 1). There are two main types of overall assessments a practitioner may undertake (NCCMH, 2018).

Key Point

Main types of LICBT assessment:

- Problem formulation: Derive an initial shared understanding of the presenting problems captured in a problem statement and used to inform decision-making and treatment planning.
- Screening/Triage: Undertaken to determine if a person is suitable for a service and if so the appropriate step in the stepped care service delivery model (Chapter 4) and determine if urgency is required during allocation due to elevated levels of risk.

Whilst practitioners may be expected to conduct either of these forms of assessment within service, there is debate surrounding the consistency of screening/triage assessment within LICBT working. Working within the stepped care model of service delivery (Bower and Gilbody, 2005) the assumption is that in the absence of any information suggesting otherwise, patients should undertake an LICBT problem formulation assessment. Following assessment, the patient should continue with treatment at Step 2 where appropriate or be referred to another step consistent with NICE Guidance (NCCMH, 2018). Given service efficiency and cost-benefits associated with this way of working (Chapter 1) resulting in reduced waiting times within the Improving Access to Psychological Therapies programme (IAPT; NCCMH, 2018), it is unclear what additional benefits arise from the LICBT practitioner workforce undertaking screening/triage assessments. Benefits are further questioned given that screening/triage assessments adopted within Stratified Care service delivery models result in patients receiving a greater number of treatment sessions but similar outcomes to stepped care (van Straten et al., 2006).

Questioning Skills

During assessment a competent questioning style is crucial to establish the nature of patient difficulties whilst providing session structure. Asking the right questions in a sensitive manner sets the tone for all future interactions and helps build a strong therapeutic alliance.

Funnelling

When assessing a patient's difficulties, it is generally helpful to use a funnelling approach (Figure 2.1).

Top of the Funnel

Adopting this approach, the LICBT practitioner will start with general, open questions to help the patient start talking about their difficulties (e.g. 'What problems are you experiencing that have led you to seek help?'). The 'Four W' questions can be used as open questions to represent the top of the questioning funnel.

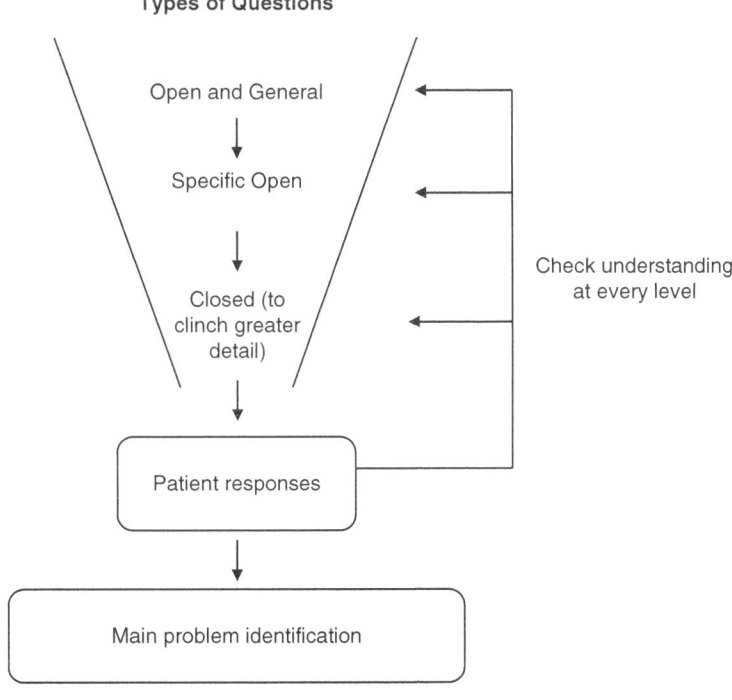

Types of Questions

Open and General

↓

Specific Open

↓

Closed (to clinch greater detail)

↓

Check understanding at every level

Patient responses

↓

Main problem identification

Figure 2.1   Funnelling technique (adapted from Richards and Whyte, 2011)

Key Point

The 'four Ws' questions:

- What is the problem?
- Where does the problem occur?
- With whom is the problem better or worse?
- When does the problem happen?

Moving down the Funnel

When funnelling, ask open questions to request more specific information and begin to move down the funnel (e.g. 'Can you tell me a bit more about how your anxiety is affecting you on a day-to-day basis?'; 'Can you say a bit more about how your low mood has been affecting you?'). Following this approach, the patient chooses the focus of the answers and the practitioner encourages the patient to provide more detail.

Bottom of the Funnel

Closed questions obtain more specific detail (e.g. 'How often do you have problems getting off to sleep at night?'; 'Have you noticed particular situations where you are more likely to experience a panic attack?'). By doing this, the patient is helped to focus on providing a clearer picture of how their problems are affecting them with the LICBT practitioner getting a sense of the frequency, intensity and duration associated with the problem (e.g. 'How often do you experience panic attacks in an average week?'; 'Using a scale of 0–10, where 10 is the most intense and 0 is no symptoms, how severe is your anxiety when you get panicky?'; 'How long do your panic attacks tend to last?').

Problem Formulation Assessment Structure

Within LICBT, completing assessment sessions and deriving a problem formulation typically take 35–40 minutes (Richards and Whyte, 2011) and are delivered using a specific structure comprising a clear beginning, middle and end across six separate but interdependent sections (Table 2.1).

Adopting common factor skills (Chapter 5) and working collaboratively through-out the assessment session will help develop a strong therapeutic alliance to build

Table 2.1 Typical LICBT Assessment Structure (adapted from Richards and Whyte, 2011)

Introduction: Assessment session	• Introductions: Full and preferred names • Brief clear explanation of LICBT practitioner role • Overview and agree session agenda • Confidentiality and informed consent

Information gathering: General presentation	• Elicit information on:
	  ○ Triggers
	  ○ Onset and progress
	  ○ Medication
	  ○ Impact
	  ○ Modifying and maintaining factors
	  ○ Employment status
	  ○ Previous treatments
	  ○ Other current treatments
	  ○ Alcohol consumption and drug use
	• Administration of routine outcome measures

Risk assessment	• Ideation • Intent • Plans • Actions • Prevention • Self-harm • Risk to others • Risk from others • Neglect to self • Neglect of others
Information gathering: Problem formulation	• Emotional symptoms • Behavioural symptoms • Cognitive symptoms • Physical symptoms
Information giving and shared decision-making	• Problem summary • Problem statement • Goal setting • Barriers to goals • Psychoeducation • Treatment options • Support modality
Ending the session	• Session summary • Agree next steps • Arrange next appointment

upon during treatment sessions. It is therefore essential that the assessment is appropriately paced to gain an accurate understanding of the patient's difficulties. When new to this way of working there can be a tendency to become overly focused on a list of questions. However, this can hinder active listening and responsiveness to what the patient is saying. A degree of flexibility to enable a better flow to the session whilst facilitating a specific focus on areas of importance that may arise, in particular risk, is therefore important. When working more flexibly however, consideration should always be given to fundamental characteristics of the LICBT clinical method (Chapter 1).

Introduction to Assessment Session

The importance of making a good introduction to an assessment session can sometimes be overlooked. However, getting off to the right start means it is important to establish realistic patient expectations about the competency of the LICBT practitioner and potential benefits of LICBT. This helps the LICBT practitioner gauge the potential practitioner–patient interaction and determine appropriate common factors (Chapter 5). The benefits of establishing a good introduction is further enhanced given the importance of establishing a relationship with patients that represent some form of diversity (Chapters 18 and 19). For example, when assessing a patient who needs an interpreter, it is important to establish the ground rule that everything that everyone says in the room will be translated. This statement makes it clear that everyone will be included in all communication at all times. This is important so that patients do not ever feel excluded.

Introductions

Whether in person, by telephone or other support modalities, it is essential to establish that the assessment session is being undertaken with the right person. Practitioners should therefore introduce themselves and ascertain the patient's full name and how they would like to be addressed.

Clinical Example

Introduction

'Hello, I'm Delaney Hasbrook but please call me Del. Can I please check your full name?' Followed up with: 'What would you like me to call you?'

Brief Clear Explanation of LICBT Practitioner Role

Once preferred names have been established it is important to orientate the patient to the session, providing a brief description of the role and job title.

Clinical Example

Introducing Role

I'm a low-intensity practitioner here at Busbrook House. What this means is that I help people who are experiencing difficulties such as anxiety and low mood by working together using tried and tested evidence-based interventions that are likely to help the problem. I'll explain later in our session what kinds of interventions I can offer that may be helpful for you. How does that sound?

Overview and Agree Session Agenda

Consistent with high-intensity CBT (HICBT; Beck et al., 1987) it is important to provide an overview of the aims of the session, collaboratively developing an agenda and specifying session length.

Clinical Example

Overviewing Session

Our session will last up to 45 minutes during which time I hope to get an understanding of what brings you here today, which means I will ask you questions about your problem and how it is affecting different areas of your life. There will be lots of opportunities for you to ask questions and by the end of the session, together we will work out next steps. How does that sound?

It is a good idea to find out if this is what the patient is expecting and whether this meets their needs.

Confidentiality and Informed Consent

It is imperative from the outset that confidentiality is accurately explained, with the end of the introductions an ideal time to explain the remits of confidentiality. It is not true to say that the session is completely confidential. The following use of patient information should therefore be highlighted.

Clinical Practice

Confidentiality

- Explain that any information discussed will be handled sensitively and shared only with the team responsible for their care.
- There will be an electronic patient record of each session.
- Outcome measures may become part of an anonymised national database.
- You will regularly discuss patient progress with your supervisor.
- With patient consent, explain that clinical recordings of sessions will be used to inform supervision, giving details about how they will be used.
- Indicate the conditions under which confidentiality will be broken in respect of risk to self or others.

When risk is addressed, it is important that the practitioner is open and transparent with the patient, specifying the conditions under which risk concerns would be disclosed to others.

Clinical Example

Breaking Confidentiality

I will only break confidentiality if there are concerns about immediate or serious risk to, or from others, or to yourself. I would talk to you before taking action so we can come up with a plan of how best to do it. But it is important that you know that there are times when I would be legally bound to break confidentiality.

Having completed introductions, orientating the patient to the session and explaining confidentiality, provide the patient with the opportunity to ask questions and say if they would like to add anything to the agenda for the session.

Information-Gathering: General Presentation

To establish relevant information about the presenting problem, a patient-centred interviewing style is recommended (Richards and Whyte, 2011).

Key Point

Features of a patient-centred approach:

- Treating the patient with dignity and respect
- Acknowledging them as experts by experience
- Being informed by the evidence base and using collaborative decision-making to decide the most acceptable intervention for the presenting problem (Chapter 4).

Triggers

It is important to identify triggers to specific events associated with the presenting problem in the here and now (Chapter 1). For example, 'What sorts of things trigger the panic attacks you are experiencing on a daily basis?'; 'Have you noticed anything that is more likely to lead to a bad night's sleep?'; 'Have you noticed any triggers to your low mood?'.

Onset and Progress

A general understanding regarding events or impacts that may have contributed to the problem in the here and now should be obtained. The presenting problem may have started suddenly (e.g. the end of a significant relationship, redundancy, a panic attack when stuck on a ride) or had a gradual onset (e.g. becoming progressively anxious and worried about things). The progress of the problem may indicate that it has remained the same since it started. The patient may have had periods when the problem was significantly better or worse, or it may have been getting gradually worse over time. It is important to ensure that questioning around onset and progress is used to understand the context associated with the presenting problem only. This is different to finding out what factors may have initially contributed to the onset of the problem that forms part of the assessment to derive a longitudinal cognitive-behavioural formulation undertaken within HICBT (Chapter 1).

Medication

Given the impact medications may have on successful engagement with LICBT interventions, or potential difficulties that may require monitoring, such as those related to risk or withdrawal effects, it is important that the assessment explores medication use for mental and physical health difficulties (Chapter 10).

Clinical Example

Questions Exploring Medication Use

- What medications are being taken?
- What are medications taken for?
- Are medications being taken as prescribed?
  - If not, explore attitudes towards medication taking.
- How long have medications been taken for?
- Have any side-effects been experienced?
  - If evident, explore impact.
  - Has the GP been informed?
- What are the potential benefits of the medication?

If medication is not being taken as prescribed, or side-effects are being experienced and/or difficulties taking them are expressed, the LICBT practitioner should funnel to enquire about the patient's attitude towards medication taking. On these occasions the patient should be encouraged to raise any issues with their GP or other person involved in their care and followed up (Chapter 10).

Impact

The practitioner should try to establish the wider impact of the problem on the patient's life using open questions towards the top of the funnel such as 'How does the problem impact your life?' and then move down the funnel to gain more specific information – 'You say it impacts your sleep. Tell me a bit more about how it does that'. The practitioner should be aware of any impact that has potentially significant consequences if not addressed. If any are identified the patient should be supported to address these. At times this may involve signposting or liaising with other health and social care, charitable or community organisations (Chapter 1). Failure to resolve any impact with potential consequences may serve to maintain the presenting problem and impair treatment (NCCMH, 2018).

Modifying and Maintaining Factors

Factors that make the presenting problem better or worse should be explored. At times these may be desirable and inform subsequent treatment, for example a patient with low mood experiencing relief when they have been walking through the park.

Not all factors giving temporary relief to a problem are helpful, however, and many play a role in maintaining the problem – for instance, a patient reporting their anxiety as significantly lower if they only walk the dogs during the evening (avoidance) or carrying a bottle of water in case they feel faint (safety behaviour).

Employment Status

People with mental or physical health difficulties experience higher risks of unemployment, absenteeism and lower levels of productivity at work (NICE, 2009a). Being in a 'good' job can help maintain or facilitate recovery from mental or physical illness (Modini et al., 2016) – for example, providing opportunities to establish life-routines (Chapter 11), achieve a sense of self-worth or value and income. Questions to address current employment status and attitudes to work may therefore help identify if supporting employment opportunities may be helpful alongside LICBT interventions to further facilitate recovery from mental health difficulties and enhance mental wellbeing. Within the IAPT programme this approach is enhanced through the Psychological Wellbeing Practitioner working collaboratively with an employment advisor (NCCMH, 2018).

Previous Treatments

It is useful to know whether the patient has received previous treatments for the same or similar problems and whether they found particular treatments helpful in any way or they had a negative experience. This can be particularly helpful in recognising any previous challenges the patient may have experienced with LICBT interventions. This may help to inform potential adaptations that could be made (Chapters 18 and 19) or choice of other evidence-based psychological therapies.

Other Current Treatments

The patient may be seeing another mental health professional or a complementary therapy practitioner who is providing homeopathic remedies or interventions. It is useful to find out how helpful the patient is finding any such intervention and how they view its role within the context of their potential work with you.

Alcohol Consumption and Drug Use

Misuse of alcohol or substances can have a significant negative impact on a patient's functioning and adversely impact their ability to engage with treatment. It is therefore worthwhile to ask about any substances the patient is currently taking and the way they believe these may impact on their ability to engage with LICBT. It is important to remember that caffeine is a strong, long-lasting and highly consumed stimulant so should also be specifically asked about, funnelling down to enquire about a potential impact on the patient's ability to sleep (Chapter 17). Arguably, it is unlikely that on first meeting, a person will divulge illicit drug use or overuse of alcohol but it is still worth enquiring about and checking in subsequent sessions.

Administration of Routine Outcome Measures

To ensure the effectiveness and efficiency of the stepped care model of mental health service delivery (Chapter 1) standardised Routine Outcome Measures (ROMs) are systematically taken at every session, informing the IAPT programme Minimum Data Set (MDS; Table 2.2).

Table 2.2 Routine Outcome Measures adopted within the IAPT programme

Problem	Recommended measure	Number of items	Cut-off score	Reference
Depression	PHQ-9	9	10 and above	Kroenke et al. (2001)
General anxiety	GAD-7	7	8 and above	Spitzer et al. (2006)
Phobias	Phobia scales	3	4 and above on any item	Marks and Matthews (1979)
Functioning	Work and Social Adjustment Scale (WASAS)	5	N/A	Mundt et al. (2002)

Whilst initially developed to assess the severity of symptoms associated with Generalised Anxiety Disorder (GAD), the GAD-7 (Spitzer et al., 2006) is adopted as the default measure to address severity across the range of anxiety disorders within the IAPT programme. However, when being used for all anxiety disorders, the measure fails to address the key symptoms to target for specific anxiety disorders. This information can inform clinical decision-making (Chapter 4) to target the most distressing symptoms for the patient. Anxiety-related disorder specific ROMs have therefore been recommended to accompany the MDS within the IAPT programme (Table 2.3; NCCMH, 2018).

Collecting ROMs enables the LICBT practitioner to monitor treatment progress and inform ongoing treatment decisions, supporting 'self-correction' within the stepped care model when necessary (Bower and Gilbody, 2005). Furthermore, their use can be effective in enhancing patient outcomes (Shimokawa, et al., 2010) that can be helpful to highlight to patients when introducing ROMs. Within the IAPT programme, analysis of the ROMs also enables services to be monitored centrally to inform programme and organisational efficiency (Richards, 2010a).

Table 2.3   Anxiety disorder specific Routine Outcome Measures

Problem	Recommended measure	Number of items	Cut-off score	Reference
Agoraphobia	The Agoraphobia-Mobility Inventory (MI)	52	Above an item average of 2.3	Chambless et al. (1985)
Generalised anxiety disorder	Penn State Worry Questionnaire – Short (PSWQ)	16	45 and above	Behar et al. (2003)
Health anxiety	Health Anxiety Inventory – Short Week Version (SHAI)	18	15 and above	Salkovskis et al. (2002)
Obsessive compulsive disorder	Obsessive Compulsive Inventory (OCI)	42	40 and above	Foa et al. (1998)
Panic disorder	Panic Disorder Severity Scale (PDSS)	7	8 and above	Shear et al. (2001)
Post-traumatic stress disorder	Impact of Events Scale (IES) – Revised	22	30 and above	Creamer et al. (2003)
Social anxiety disorder	Social Phobia Inventory	19	19 and above	Connor et al. (2000)

Clinical Example

Introducing Routine Outcome Measures

Monitoring symptoms using a number of tried and tested questionnaires is useful for checking progress and seeing whether what we are doing is helping you with your difficulties. It is useful to start with a baseline so I shall explain each of the measures and then give you feedback on what the scores indicate. Each session I shall ask you to complete the measures and discuss how things are going with your treatment. Many people find it helpful to track their progress and there is research that shows that people receiving feedback on session-by-session measures tend to do better in treatment.

Risk Assessment

It is essential that the patient's level of risk is determined at assessment and given that risk is not static, monitored at every support session (Chapter 6). Novice LICBT practitioners may worry about asking risk-related questions.

Reflection Point

Think about who you would ask for support from if you found yourself worrying a lot about undertaking a risk assessment or enquiring about risk.

However, it has been highlighted that enquiring about suicide could reduce, rather than increase, suicidal ideation (Dazzi et al., 2014). The LICBT practitioner should not be apologetic or embarrassed asking about risk and instead, should introduce it in a positive way.

Clinical Example

Introducing Risk Assessment

I would like to ask you some very specific questions now about your safety. It might be that some areas do not affect you and that's fine, but it's important I ask you anyway. Going forward, I shall ask similar questions to these each session to check whether there have been any changes.

Where appropriate, each area addressed in a full risk assessment should be asked in relation to the present and the past (Table 2.4). Knowing if a patient has made a serious attempt on their life previously is useful to know to inform clinical decision-making around risk in the present.

In the event of serious concerns about risk it is imperative that follow-up questions are asked to work down the funnel and ascertain the current level of risk. Immediate risk issues should be addressed directly, the service risk protocol should be enacted, and the situation raised during the next case management supervision session (Chapter 9).

Information-Gathering: Problem Formulation

A useful way to get a fuller understanding of a patient's presenting difficulty is to ask questions about a recent time the problem happened (e.g. 'Can you tell me about the last time you felt really low?'; 'Can we go through the panic attack you had yesterday so we can see what happened?'). These questions should enable the presenting difficulty to be translated into a LICBT *here and now* problem formulation (Chapter 1). Depending on the LICBT problem formulation model adopted, this will involve targeting questions to address the presenting problem in terms of the main arising symptoms.

Table 2.4   Example questions asked during risk assessment

Area of risk	Example questions
Ideation: Suicidal thoughts	'Do you ever have thoughts of taking your own life?' 'Have you ever felt this way in the past?'
Intent: Active motivation to act	'Have you given any thought to how you might take your own life?' 'How often do you have thoughts of killing yourself?' 'How do you feel when you have these thoughts?' 'How easily can you put these thoughts out of your mind?' 'How strongly do you believe that you would act on these thoughts on a scale of 0–10?'
Plans: Specific action plans	'Have you made any plans to act on these thoughts?' 'Have you acted on these thoughts in the past?'
Actions: Current and past	'Have you taken any steps towards taking your own life?' 'What access do you have to things that you might use to take your own life?' 'What did you use when you attempted to take your own life in the past?'
Prevention: Protective factors, social network, services	'What's keeping you going at the moment?' 'Who do you turn to when you need someone to talk to about things?' 'What stopped you from taking your own life when things got so tough for you last time?'
Self-harm	'Sometimes when people are feeling low, they deliberately hurt themselves as a way of trying to cope. Is this something you have ever tried?' 'Tell me about the last time that happened.'
Risk to others	'I can hear how much you've been hurt by bullies at work and I'm wondering if you've ever felt like hurting these people?' 'Do you ever feel like you may be a risk to other people?' 'When you are feeling suicidal, do you have thoughts of harming or killing others?'
Risk from others	'How safe do you feel from other people?' 'Have you ever felt at risk of harm from someone else?'
Neglect to self	'Do you have everything you need to get on with day-to-day activities?' 'How are you getting on with looking after yourself?'
Neglect of others	'Are you responsible for the care of others (e.g. elderly relative, children, etc.)?' 'Do you have any concerns about your ability to do that at the moment?'

Clinical Example

Questions to Elicit Symptoms of the Presenting Problem

- Physical
  - Do you notice any sensations in your body when you have a panic attack?
  - When you're feeling low, do you notice anything is going on in your body?
- Behavioural
  - Is there anything you do when you notice yourself getting worried?
  - What do you do when you are feeling particularly low?
- Cognitive
  - Have you noticed any words or images go through your mind when you are feeling worried?
  - When you're particularly low, have you noticed any thoughts or pictures that come to mind?

- Emotional
  - When you notice being tired, your legs are heavy and you are off your food, how do you feel emotionally?
  - When you're lying awake, unable to get to sleep, how does that make you feel?

Symptoms explored will vary according to the problem formulation model adopted, between a specific focus on physical (**A**utonomic), **B**ehavioural, **C**ognitive and **E**motional symptoms and description of the wider context within the *Five Parts* (Padesky and Mooney, 1990) or *Five Areas* (Williams and Garland, 2002) approaches. Capturing symptoms in this manner can be a useful way to orientate patients to a CBT-informed approach (Figure 2.2).

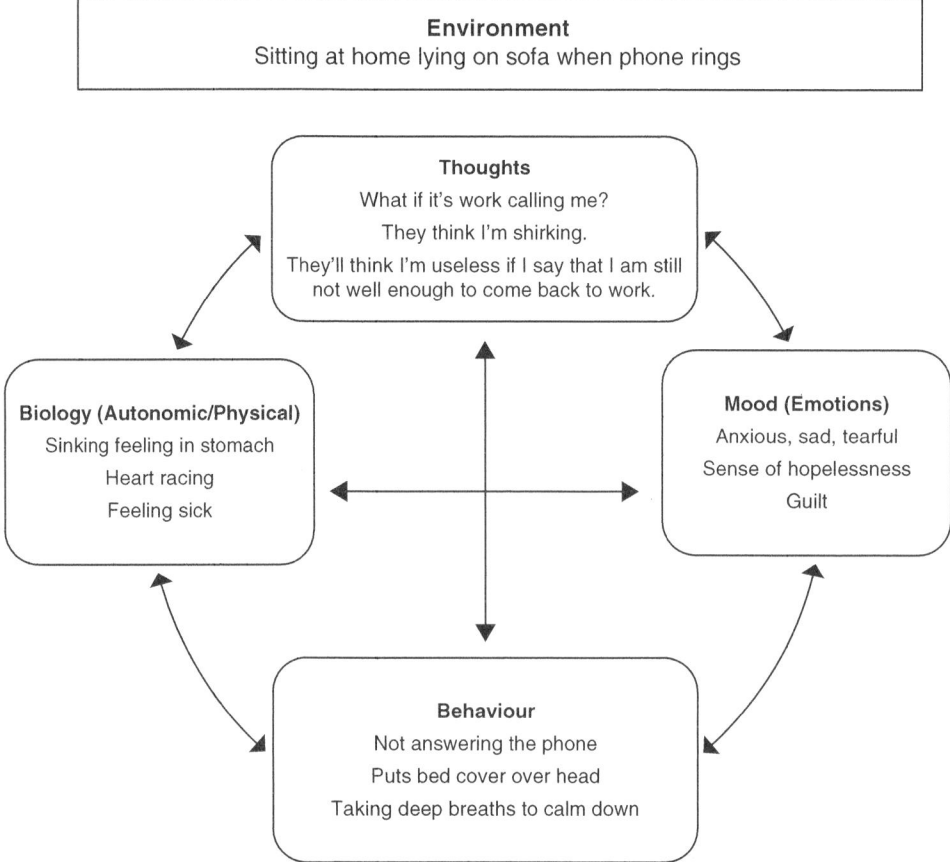

Figure 2.2 Symptoms of presenting problem represented within the Five Parts Model (5-part model adapted with permission of the author, copyright 1986 by the Center for Cognitive Therapy; www.padesky.com)

Information Giving and Shared Decision-Making

Having collaboratively captured the main symptoms that are affecting the patient the assessment moves onto information giving and shared decision-making which is informed by the five parts or five areas model.

Problem Statement

To monitor progress with the patient throughout treatment, facilitate LICBT telephone working (Chapter 1) and form the basis of case management supervision (Chapter 9), a brief and succinct written problem statement associated with the presenting problem in the here and now is developed.

Three key features of the presenting problem are broken down to form the problem statement that is returned to regularly with the patient throughout the treatment period to monitor change:

- Trigger
- Symptoms
- Impact.

Table 2.5 Example problem statements taken from *The CBT Handbook* (reproduced from *The CBT Handbook* (Myles and Shafran, 2015) by kind permission of Little, Brown Book Group)

Problem statements	Dimensions
Example 1 'My main problem is feeling tired all the time and low in mood particularly on waking, leading me to stay in bed; as a result I am finding it difficult to work and see friends and worrying that I can't stop mulling over the break-up and that things will never get any better.'	Trigger – waking Symptoms – feeling tired all the time (physical); low in mood (emotions); staying in bed (behaviour); worrying things will never get better (cognitive) Consequences – difficult to work and see friends
Example 2 'Pressure at work and threat of redundancies are leading me to work very long hours as I feel like I need to prove my worth to my boss, feeling stressed, difficulty sleeping and proneness to headaches; consequently I am left with no energy or time to spend with Jay or to see friends.'	Trigger – pressure at work and threat of redundancies Symptoms – I need to prove my worth to my boss (cognitive); feeling stressed (emotions); difficulty sleeping, headaches, no energy (physical); work very long hours (behavioural) Consequences – lack of time to spend with Jay or see friends
Example 3 'Avoidance of travelling anywhere by bike due to physical symptoms such as racing heart and shaking, and a fear that I'll be knocked off again, leading me to become increasingly restricted about how I get to and from work.'	Trigger – travelling anywhere by bike Symptoms – Avoidance (behaviour); racing heart and shaking (physical); fear (emotions); 'I'll be knocked off again' (cognitive) Consequences – increasingly restricted about getting to and from work

It is not uncommon for patients to present with several problems and when this arises the LICBT practitioner and patient work collaboratively using a 0–100 scale to identify how severe, distressing or impactful each of the problems is. A collaborative decision is then reached to prioritise the problems and identify the first problem to tackle.

Goal-Setting

Agreeing end of treatment SMART goals is an opportunity to reach a collaborative decision regarding what the LICBT single-strand treatment is aiming to achieve.

Key Point

SMART goals are:

- **S**pecific
- **M**easurable
- **A**chievable
- **R**ealistic
- **T**imely.

Using SMART helps to ensure abstract goals (e.g. I want to feel better around people) are operationalised (e.g. Be able to go out with friends twice a week for a minimum of three hours by the end of treatment), and unrealistic goals (e.g. I want to never feel anxious again) are addressed so that they can become achievable.

Barriers to Goals

During assessment the practitioner will explore any barriers that may surround engagement with the LICBT intervention adopted. The COM-B model (Chapter 8; Michie et al., 2011) is commonly used by LICBT practitioners to address practical barriers to engagement throughout subsequent sessions (Chapter 6).

Psychoeducation

The LICBT practitioner will already have begun psychoeducation with the introduction of the problem formulation model adopted to demonstrate links between symptoms that the patient may not have previously been aware of. Depending on the

LICBT intervention adopted, psychoeducation may either be included within the workbook (e.g. Farrand et al., 2019b), or be available as handouts or online resources (www.nhs.uk/conditions).

The practitioner uses psychoeducation to provide information to help the patient better understand their presenting problems. In addition to conveying factual information about the patient's presenting problem it is generally useful to provide resources such as booklets and handouts that may be readily available in your workplace or signposting to an online resource.

Treatment Options

Decision-making informing the treatment options offered will be dependent on the presenting problem, evidence base and the provision of choice (Chapter 4). Typical options are drawn from the single-strand LICBT interventions, intervention format (booklets, computerised CBT, worksheets), support modality (face-to-face, telephone; Chapter 7) and signposting to other services (statutory, community, charitable) which may include employment support advisors. Availability across options may, however, be dictated by the mental health service.

Ending the Session

At the end of the assessment session, the LICBT practitioner should employ short capsule summaries to address three main areas to ensure the patient is able to engage with treatment between sessions.

Clinical Practice

Areas Addressed

- Session summary: Summarise the session, asking the patient what they will take away from the session and if they have any questions.
- Next steps: Identify what the patient has understood to be undertaken between sessions to form the basis of the following support sessions (Chapter 6).
- Arrange next session: Agree when, where, and the support modality for the following support session where appropriate.

Prepare information collected around these areas to form the basis of the next case management supervision session (Chapter 9).

Summary

This chapter has provided an overview of a typical structure for an LICBT assessment session, highlighting the importance it represents as the first step to successful collaborative working. The assessment session provides an opportunity to build a strong therapeutic relationship while establishing a clear understanding of the patient's presenting difficulties in the here and now. The use of ROMs is key to measuring progress and should be administered during the assessment session to provide a baseline against which to measure progress within subsequent support sessions (Chapter 6). Working collaboratively to develop a problem formulation to capture the patient's presenting difficulties and inform a problem statement and determining SMART goals inform clinical decision-making (Chapter 4) for subsequent LICBT treatment.

Assessing Your Understanding

Declarative

Multiple Choice Questions

1. Questioning in an assessment should: [Select all that apply]
   (a) Move from open to closed questions
   (b) Use open questions throughout to gain a broad understanding
   (c) Use closed questions throughout to clinch lots of detail
   (d) Move from closed to open questions
   (e) Should maintain a structure at all times
2. When is it appropriate to disclose confidential information without the consent of the patient? [Select all that apply]
   (a) If the patient is at risk of harming themselves
   (b) Never
   (c) If the patient is at risk of harming others
   (d) If there are child protection issues
   (e) When the member of the family enquires about a patient
3. The only people outside the care team who should be routinely advised of information disclosed by a patient are: [Select all that apply]
   (a) The patient's immediate family
   (b) The patient's partner

(c) A trusted friend of the patient

(d) All of the above

(e) No-one

Procedural

Self-Practice/Self-Reflection

You are going into an assessment session with Zena. All you know is that she has self-referred for a problem she is experiencing with panic attacks.

- Using the assessment structure, write down at least one question in each section that you might like to ask Zena.
- Reflect how you might feel being asked those questions.
- Revisit your questions and revise them accordingly.
- Reflect on what you learned from this exercise.

Answers to **Assessing Your Understanding** questions can be found in the appendix on p. 333.

Further Reading and Resources

Bennett-Levy, J., Richards, D.A., Farrand, P., Christensen, H., Griffiths, K.M., Kavanagh, D.J., Klein, B., Lau, M.A., Roudfoot, J., Ritterband, L., White, J. and Williams, C. (2010) *Oxford Guide to Low Intensity CBT Interventions.* Oxford: Oxford University Press.

Papworth, M., Marrinan, T. and Martin, B. (2013) *Low Intensity Cognitive Behaviour Therapy: A Practitioner's Guide.* London: SAGE.

Richards, D.A. and Whyte, M. (2011) *Reach Out: National Programme Student Materials to Support the Delivery of Training for Practitioners Delivering Low Intensity Interventions* (3rd edition). London: Rethink.

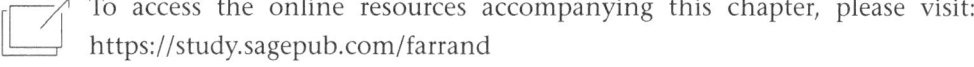 To access the online resources accompanying this chapter, please visit: https://study.sagepub.com/farrand

3

Diagnoses and Problem Descriptors

Labelling Problems, Not People

Joshua E.J. Buckman, Rob Saunders and Stephen Pilling

Learning Objectives

By the end of this chapter you should be able to:

- Demonstrate an awareness of the main diagnoses seen in services that have implemented low-intensity cognitive behavioural therapy
- Critically evaluate diagnostic classifications systems predominantly based on a symptom severity threshold being crossed
- Apply the Probable Diagnosis Decision Support Tool to determine likely diagnoses
- Critically evaluate the clinical value of thorough assessment and the identification of diagnoses for low-intensity cognitive behavioural therapy service users and services

---

Background

Understanding the nature and context of the problems that have brought someone to seek help from psychological therapies services is crucial to the effective delivery of treatment. Central to this is an understanding of how those problems have evolved, the experience of the problems, including current symptoms and the impact of them on functioning. All of these factors help determine a diagnosis. Some people arrive for an assessment with a clear sense of the problems they are struggling with. They may have had a number of previous assessments, received diagnoses and received a number of treatments or therapies. For others, the assessment might be the first time they have been able to talk about their problems in any depth with a health professional. In either case, the language people use to describe their problems may not fit with medical models of disorder and corresponding diagnostic categories, or it may not be thought to be congruent with such diagnoses. It is common for people to talk about 'feeling low', 'stressed' or 'having a panic attack' over and above any other problems being experienced. This may help point towards probable diagnoses but equally may not encompass the range of problems they are having. A good assessment is essential to teasing this apart and better understanding the nature of the presenting problems. In all scenarios, there are three key elements to any assessment in low-intensity CBT (LICBT) services.

Key Point

Key elements to assessment in LICBT services:

*   Developing a shared understanding of the problems that have brought someone to the assessment, rooted in their own personal experiences.
*   Developing an understanding of how those problems might be resolved
*   Agreeing an initial plan to begin resolving those problems.

Some people may arrive at assessment with a clear sense of their problems whereas others may not be able to describe them, be unsure how they have developed or are maintained and become worried that things cannot change. To support people who come to psychological therapy services develop an understanding of their problems that they find useful, LICBT practitioners need to draw on the knowledge and experience they gained through training. This may pertain to the nature of problem presentations, the course of such problems and evidence on the effectiveness of interventions. With this knowledge and experience, LICBT practitioners may reach a probable diagnosis with their patient that can be reviewed after further assessment or treatment.

Reflection Point

Reflect on what it is like when you are unwell and visit a health professional. What role does diagnosis play for you, in terms of your expectations of what is going to happen and for the care you might receive.

When done well, assessments and thoughtful consideration of problems and probable diagnoses, developed collaboratively with patients, can be important interventions in their own right. After the assessment session in psychological therapy services that include LICBT interventions, such as Improving Access to Psychological Therapies (IAPT) services in England (Chapters 1 and 20), approximately 40 per cent of service users do not require or want treatment, are referred on, or are signposted elsewhere. Ensuring that assessments are done well, information is gathered and advice developed on the basis of them is communicated effectively (Chapter 2) is therefore of great importance (Clark, 2018). It provides the framework on which appropriate identification of the LICBT intervention to address the probable diagnosis is made (Part II).

Problem Descriptors

Reaching a probable diagnosis is fundamental to practice in LICBT; the way they are recorded in IAPT is in the form of problem descriptors. The main features upon which the probable diagnosis is reached may then be expressed by patients in the form of a problem statement (Chapter 2).

Key Point

Problem descriptors:

- remain provisional at the start, during and end of treatment
- can be reviewed and amended with further assessment or if the agreed focus of therapy changes
- represent the presenting problem or probable diagnosis as the agreed focus of treatment
- align with *International Classification of Diseases*, 10*th* edition codes – for example, ICD-10 F32 for a depressive episode or F40.1 for social phobia (WHO, 1992)
- inform treatment planning using NICE recommended interventions for the probable diagnosis
- determine the appropriateness of offering an LICBT intervention
- inform the most appropriate LICBT intervention for each probable diagnosis.

Presenting Characteristics of Common Mental Health Disorders (CMDs)

The key characteristics of problems and symptoms identified during assessment (Chapter 2) and summarised in the problem statement inform the recognition and subsequent probable diagnosis using the ICD-10 (WHO, 1992). Those addressed below are focused on common mental health problems receiving a probable diagnosis within a stepped care service delivery model such as provides the organisation structure for the IAPT programme (Chapter 1). However, it should be recognised that people can present with symptoms associated with severe and enduring mental health difficulties. On these occasions the LICBT practitioner would refer the patient to the appropriate step in the stepped care model or follow the service risk protocol when necessary.

Depression

To meet criteria for a diagnosis of depression, symptoms must occur nearly every day and impact functioning in everyday life.

Key Point

Core symptoms:

- Pervasive and persistent low mood (feeling down, depressed or hopeless)
- Anhedonia (a loss of pleasure or interest in usually enjoyable activities)
- Lacking in energy, increased tiredness or fatigue
- Withdrawal from everyday activities.

Common symptoms:

- Reduction in self-esteem or self-confidence
- Poor concentration
- Sleep disturbance (either sleeping more or less than usual)
- Worthlessness
- Guilt
- Significant changes in appetite or weight
- Psychomotor agitation or retardation (moving more restlessly or more slowly than usual)
- Irritability
- Tearfulness
- Decreased libido
- Thoughts that life is not worth living or of suicide.

When reaching a probable diagnosis of depression, symptoms of anxiety can also be common. Therefore, whether depression has impacted functioning and this in turn has led to anxiety or worry, or whether anxiety has led to avoidance of activities leading to depressive symptoms, it is important to determine the primary presenting problem.

Anxiety Disorders

An evidence base exists across a range of anxiety disorders treated with LICBT interventions (Part II) at Step 2 of a stepped care model (Chapter 1). However, the evidence base does not include social anxiety, post-traumatic stress disorder or health anxiety, which should be treated at Step 3. However, it is important that LICBT practitioners are aware of these disorders as they will present at assessment. Before considering specific anxiety disorders it is also important to first appreciate what constitutes a panic attack as this can inform subsequent diagnosis and can occur in the context of many anxiety disorders.

Key Point

Characteristics of a panic attack:

- A sudden period of intense fear or anxiety
- Physical symptoms, such as a pounding heart or shortness of breath
- Is often, but not always, associated with cognitive symptoms such as a belief that something awful is about to happen
- Anxiety peaks around 10 minutes before slowly abating.

Panic attacks occur in the context of many anxiety disorders and therefore should not necessarily lead to a probable diagnosis related to panic disorder. Appropriate use of questioning during assessment should enable triggers to panic attacks to be identified, informing subsequent diagnosis (Chapter 3).

Generalised Anxiety Disorder

Generalised anxiety disorder (GAD) is the most frequently occurring anxiety disorder (McManus et al., 2016) but is often missed as a probable diagnosis (Allgulander, 2006). It rarely occurs as a single diagnosis with up to 90 per cent of patients meeting diagnostic criteria for GAD also meeting criteria for one or more other common mental health disorders (CMDs), most often depression, social phobia or panic disorder (Kessler et al., 2005).

Key Point

Core symptoms:

- Excessive anxiety
- Uncontrollable and excessive worry about a number of different situations
- At least three common symptoms present for at least six months.

Common symptoms:

- Restlessness
- Fatigue
- Poor concentration or mind going blank
- Irritability
- Persistent nervousness or feeling on edge
- Muscle tension
- Sleep disturbance.

When reaching a probable diagnosis, however, it is particularly important that worry is recognised as excessive, not limited to situations that would reasonably lead to worry and is disproportionate to the situation(s).

People with GAD may label themselves as having always been a worrier with worries perceived as uncontrollable and leading to significant distress or impairment in functioning.

Worry is often coupled with an intolerance of uncertainty (IoU), but neither worry nor IoU are unique to GAD, being experienced in many other anxiety disorders. As many patients with GAD consider worrying to be a part of their character, they may seek help or are referred to LICBT services after becoming depressed rather than experiences of anxiety. This can lead to GAD being missed in assessments.

Panic Disorder

To meet diagnostic criteria for panic disorder (PD), panic attacks are experienced as spontaneous and not always linked to a single situation in which significant episodes of anxiety have occurred in the past.

Key Point

Core symptoms:

- Frequent unexpected panic attacks or less severe limited symptom attacks
- Occur for at least one month.

Common symptoms:

- Worry about the consequences of the attacks or the occurrence of attacks in future - for example, what they may mean or interpreted as a sign that one is 'going mad'
- Change behaviour in an attempt to mitigate or avoid having further attacks.

When people associate certain experiences with having a panic attack, they may avoid that situation in future or only go through it with support from someone who they believe can help mitigate any consequences. This can become widespread and impair functioning in daily life and be captured as a diagnosis of PD with agoraphobia.

Agoraphobia

Given that the symptoms associated with agoraphobia may present a significant barrier to accessing mainstream service provision, it is rarely seen in mental health services without PD. However, it can be helpful to be aware of the main symptoms of agoraphobia to facilitate a more comprehensive probable diagnosis.

Key Point

Core symptoms:

- Intense fear of places or situations that might lead to a panic attack or where there is no easy way to escape from a situation without causing oneself embarrassment.
- Complete avoidance of the feared situation(s) or only being able to endure them when accompanied by a particular trusted individual.

The key determinants to arriving at the probable diagnosis of agoraphobia without PD is firstly that someone has not had panic attacks in the past, and secondly that the fear they experience relates to incapacitation or humiliation in open or public spaces or situations due to panic-like symptoms (rather than an actual panic attack).

Obsessive Compulsive Disorder (OCD)

OCD is commonly co-morbid with CMDs such as depression, GAD, PTSD and health anxiety, although health anxiety does not include a sense of personal responsibility for the occurrence of feared events. It can also present as co-morbid to conditions such as autistic spectrum disorder (Lenzenweger et al., 2007; Ruscio et al., 2010).

Key Point

Core symptoms:

- Obsessional thoughts: repetitive intrusive thoughts, impulses or images, which are experienced as inappropriate, unpleasant and cause anxiety
- Compulsions: repetitive behaviours or mental acts carried out in response to an obsession or according to some personal rule, experienced as unpleasant and cause anxiety
- *Recognition that these are coming from one's own mind*: rather than being implanted in one's mind by someone or something else
- Attempts to prevent or resist obsessions or compulsions: although over time that resistance may become minimal
- Recognition that obsessions or compulsions are excessive or unreasonable at some point over the course of the disorder.

Common symptoms:

- Thoughts of being responsible for harming others or for the occurrence of unwanted or terrible events.

Specific Phobias

Specific phobias are amongst the most common anxiety disorders with one in eight adults experiencing a phobia at some point in their lives, although many people with these conditions do not seek treatment (Kessler et al., 2005).

Key Point

Core symptoms:

- Persistent fear of a specific situation or object that poses little or no actual danger
- The presence of the phobic situation or object always provokes marked anxiety
- The situation/object is nearly always avoided.

Common symptoms:

- Panic attacks in presence of the phobic situation/object.

Common phobic situations or objects include animals such as spiders, activities such as flying or using a public toilet, experiences such as being in closed spaces or going to the dentist. Specific phobias can also be associated with particular contexts or procedures, such as procedural anxiety related to medical procedures or common events in this context, such as the sight of blood, needles or vomiting.

Diagnosis of CMDs Not Treated with LICBT

There is no NICE evidence base recognised for the treatment of CMDs such as social anxiety disorder, health anxiety and post-traumatic stress disorder. However, it is helpful to be able to recognise the key symptoms associated with these to inform stepping up (Chapter 4).

Social Anxiety Disorder

Social anxiety disorder (social phobia) is a commonly experienced anxiety disorder (Kessler et al., 2005). It is often co-morbid with other CMDs, particularly depression, agoraphobia with or without panic disorder, and alcohol misuse disorders (Kessler et al., 2005).

Key Point

Core symptoms:

- Marked and persistent fear or embarrassment of being ill-judged by others when faced with a social or performance-related situation
- Exposure to the feared performance or social situation will almost certainly lead to marked anxiety and may lead to a panic attack, although situations may be endured with the use of *safety behaviours* that attempt to mitigate the feared outcomes (Clark, 2001).

(Continued)

Common symptoms:

- Avoidance of situations where one could be the focus of attention.

In identifying social anxiety disorder vs depression, LICBT practitioners should consider why someone has withdrawn from social situations and which type of symptoms came first.

Key Point

Differentiating social anxiety disorder and depression

- If fear of judgement from others underlies social withdrawal or preceded low mood, social anxiety disorder diagnosis is likely.
- If a lack of interest or enjoyment in activities, or fatigue that has led to withdrawal from social situations or preceded fear of scrutiny by others, a diagnosis of depression is more likely.

Health anxiety

Health anxiety (hypochondriacal disorder) is relatively rare among anxiety disorders.

Key Point

Core symptoms:

- Persistent preoccupation with the possibility of having one or more serious progressive illnesses
- Preoccupation with normal or common bodily experiences, such as headaches, which are interpreted as signs of severe illness.

Common symptoms:

- Frequent contact with health professionals to request investigations in the belief or conviction that one has a severe and undiagnosed progressive physical illness
- Negative results from such investigations do not lead to prolonged change in belief or behaviour.

Post-Traumatic Stress Disorder (PTSD)

PTSD may develop in response to an event where a person considers themselves or someone close to them to have been at threat of serious harm or death. The traumatic event is considered to be exceptionally threatening or catastrophic and likely to cause distress in almost anyone.

Key Point

Core symptoms:

- Experiencing a traumatic event
- Re-experiencing the traumatic event – having vivid intrusive memories, *flashbacks* or repeated nightmares about the event
- Avoiding or wanting to avoid reminders of the event or things associated with the event.

Common symptoms:

- Difficulty fully recalling some important aspects of the traumatic event
- Increased psychological sensitivity or arousal – difficulty falling or staying asleep, irritability, angry outbursts, concentration difficulties, hypervigilance or easily startled.

Symptoms must have occurred within six months of the traumatic event. Delayed onset PTSD, where symptoms occur beyond six months, is considered a separate diagnosis and is often preceded by other signs of mental distress including alcohol misuse. Experiencing a traumatic event does not necessarily lead to PTSD, and other mental health problems can be more common following traumatic events, including depression, panic disorder, agoraphobia and alcohol misuse (Fear et al., 2010). These are also commonly co-morbid with PTSD (McFarlane and Papay, 1992).

Mixed Anxiety and Depressive Disorder

Across mental health services, significant variation exists in the use of a probable diagnosis of mixed anxiety and depression (MADD).

Key Point

Core symptoms:

- Symptoms of both depression and anxiety are present
- Neither is predominant
- Symptoms are not sufficient to meet diagnostic criteria for a depressive episode or any anxiety disorder.

Reaching this probable diagnosis should rarely be used in mental health services as many service users will come with symptoms sufficient for a diagnosis of depression or at least one anxiety disorder. In these circumstances a probable diagnosis of MADD does not apply.

Validity of Diagnostic Systems

The use of diagnoses in mental health disorders has been the subject of considerable discussion and controversy, not least because diagnostic systems are criticised by some as pathologising distress which might otherwise be considered part of the human condition (Kirschner, 2013). Researchers and clinicians have argued that mental health problems diagnosed by a symptom severity threshold being crossed, particular degree of dysfunction or chronicity of a problem would be better considered dimensionally, with symptoms occurring on one or more continua (Ayuso-Mateos et al., 2010). Specifically, for each group of symptoms used to diagnose mental health problems at present, someone might be considered to be at a certain point on a continuous dimension. This approach would be similar to common conceptualisations of personality where people score at various points on dimensions of extraversion, neuroticism, openness, etc. The pattern of points across various different dimensions might then demarcate the different mental health disorders being experienced.

Multidimensional diagnostic systems such as the Research Domain Criteria (RDoC; Insel et al., 2010) that classify mental disorders based on behavioural phenotypes and biomarkers therefore offer a different way to consider CMDs. By viewing mental disorders on continua, advocates of these systems suggest a more dynamic and flexible method of assessing mental disorders can be created (Insel et al., 2010). This approach may help address questions raised concerning the reliability and validity of diagnoses based on the current categorical diagnostic systems (e.g. Lieblich et al., 2015). Multidimensional approaches could help to resolve the issue of overlap between symptoms of different CMDs – for example, the experience of excessive worry or panic attacks common across many CMDs or the degree of co-morbidity between CMDs (Hirschfeld, 2001; Kessler et al., 2005). Furthermore, they may also help elucidate mechanisms of change and better explain why individuals with the same diagnosis that are given the same treatment can have substantially different treatment outcomes (Insel et al., 2010).

Probable Diagnosis Determining a Problem Statement

To facilitate reaching a probable diagnosis, a probable diagnosis decision support tool adapted from the *IAPT Manual* (NCCMH, 2018) can be helpful.

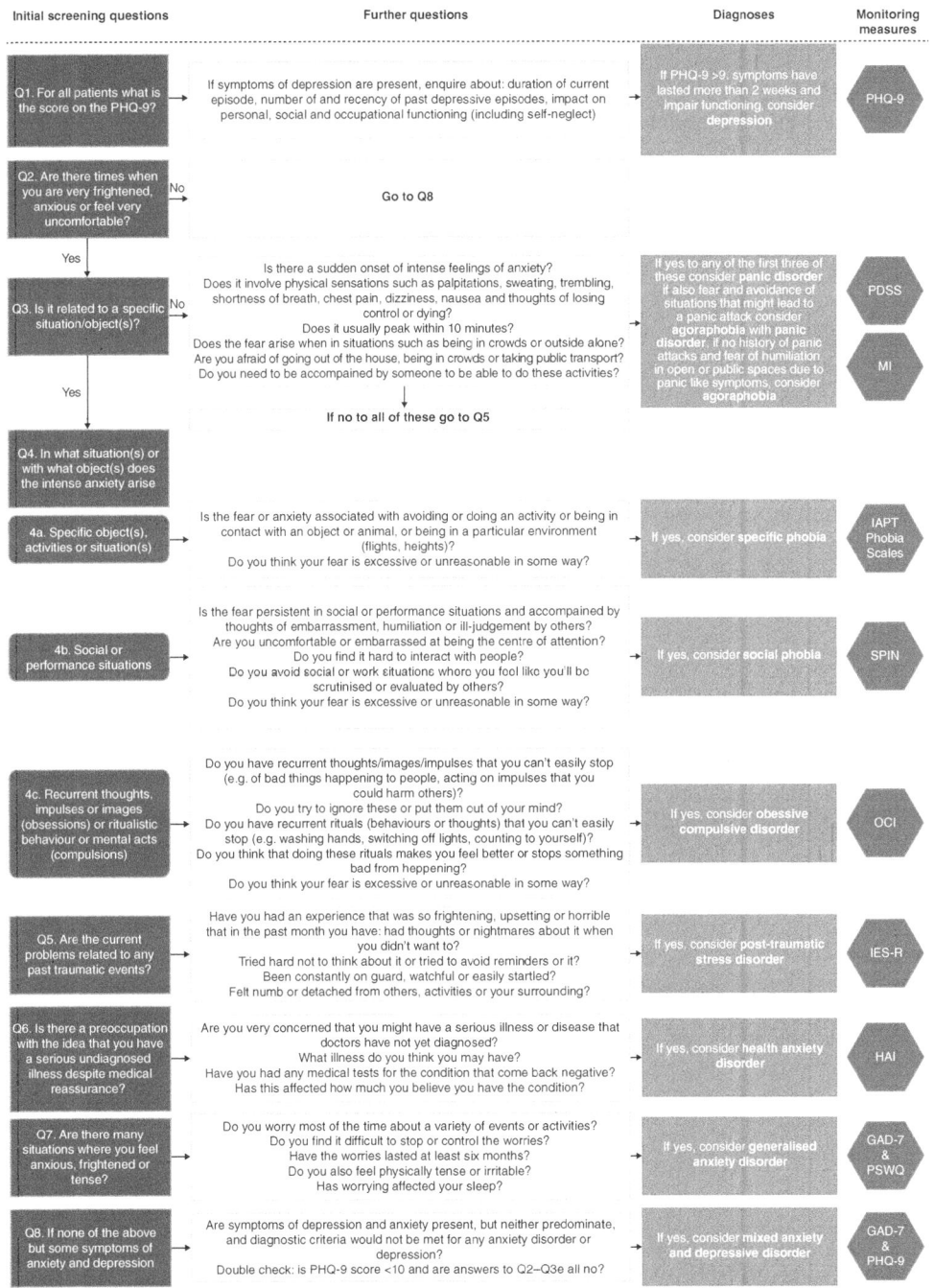

Initial screening questions	Further questions	Diagnoses	Monitoring measures
Q1. For all patients what is the score on the PHQ-9?	If symptoms of depression are present, enquire about: duration of current episode, number of and recency of past depressive episodes, impact on personal, social and occupational functioning (including self-neglect)	If PHQ-9 >9, symptoms have lasted more than 2 weeks and impair functioning, consider **depression**	PHQ-9
Q2. Are there times when you are very frightened, anxious or feel very uncomfortable?	No → Go to Q8		
Q3. Is it related to a specific situation/object(s)? (Yes ↓ / No →)	Is there a sudden onset of intense feelings of anxiety? Does it involve physical sensations such as palpitations, sweating, trembling, shortness of breath, chest pain, dizziness, nausea and thoughts of losing control or dying? Does it usually peak within 10 minutes? Does the fear arise when in situations such as being in crowds or outside alone? Are you afraid of going out of the house, being in crowds or taking public transport? Do you need to be accompanied by someone to be able to do these activities? / If no to all of these go to Q5	If yes to any of the first three of these consider **panic disorder** if also fear and avoidance of situations that might lead to a panic attack consider **agoraphobia with panic disorder**; if no history of panic attacks and fear of humiliation in open or public spaces due to panic like symptoms, consider **agoraphobia**	PDSS / MI
Q4. In what situation(s) or with what object(s) does the intense anxiety arise			
4a. Specific object(s), activities or situation(s)	Is the fear or anxiety associated with avoiding or doing an activity or being in contact with an object or animal, or being in a particular environment (flights, heights)? Do you think your fear is excessive or unreasonable in some way?	If yes, consider **specific phobia**	IAPT Phobia Scales
4b. Social or performance situations	Is the fear persistent in social or performance situations and accompanied by thoughts of embarrassment, humiliation or ill-judgement by others? Are you uncomfortable or embarrassed at being the centre of attention? Do you find it hard to interact with people? Do you avoid social or work situations where you feel like you'll be scrutinised or evaluated by others? Do you think your fear is excessive or unreasonable in some way?	If yes, consider **social phobia**	SPIN
4c. Recurrent thoughts, impulses or images (obsessions) or ritualistic behaviour or mental acts (compulsions)	Do you have recurrent thoughts/images/impulses that you can't easily stop (e.g. of bad things happening to people, acting on impulses that you could harm others)? Do you try to ignore these or put them out of your mind? Do you have recurrent rituals (behaviours or thoughts) that you can't easily stop (e.g. washing hands, switching off lights, counting to yourself)? Do you think that doing these rituals makes you feel better or stops something bad from happening? Do you think your fear is excessive or unreasonable in some way?	If yes, consider **obsessive compulsive disorder**	OCI
Q5. Are the current problems related to any past traumatic events?	Have you had an experience that was so frightening, upsetting or horrible that in the past month you have: had thoughts or nightmares about it when you didn't want to? Tried hard not to think about it or tried to avoid reminders or it? Been constantly on guard, watchful or easily startled? Felt numb or detached from others, activities or your surrounding?	If yes, consider **post-traumatic stress disorder**	IES-R
Q6. Is there a preoccupation with the idea that you have a serious undiagnosed illness despite medical reassurance?	Are you very concerned that you might have a serious illness or disease that doctors have not yet diagnosed? What illness do you think you may have? Have you had any medical tests for the condition that come back negative? Has this affected how much you believe you have the condition?	If yes, consider **health anxiety disorder**	HAI
Q7. Are there many situations where you feel anxious, frightened or tense?	Do you worry most of the time about a variety of events or activities? Do you find it difficult to stop or control the worries? Have the worries lasted at least six months? Do you also feel physically tense or irritable? Has worrying affected your sleep?	If yes, consider **generalised anxiety disorder**	GAD-7 & PSWQ
Q8. If none of the above but some symptoms of anxiety and depression	Are symptoms of depression and anxiety present, but neither predominate, and diagnostic criteria would not be met for any anxiety disorder or depression? Double check: is PHQ-9 score <10 and are answers to Q2–Q3e all no?	If yes, consider **mixed anxiety and depressive disorder**	GAD-7 & PHQ-9

LICBTs are reminded to use the questionnaire measures predominantly as a means to inform discussions in supervision regarding probable diagnoses and appropriate intensity of treatment, and for those diagnoses for which there are NICE evidence-based LICBT treatments, the same measures can be used throughout treatment to monitor progress.

Figure 3.1 Probable diagnosis decision support tool (adapted from NCCMH, 2018)

The case example below can be used to simulate the decision-making processes for arriving at a probable diagnosis.

Clinical Example

Case Example: Sallyanne

Sallyanne is a 52-year-old woman who has three adult children. Her youngest child moved out of the family home after falling pregnant with her first child a year ago. She now lives alone after becoming separated from her husband six months ago. Sallyanne says that she has come for an assessment because she has been feeling incredibly stressed, nervous and tense over the last year. She describes recently feeling increasingly low as she struggles to sleep properly since her husband left, scoring 15 on the PHQ-9. She describes lying awake for hours at night not able to stop herself thinking and worrying about all sorts of things. She also describes herself as not being very good with change. She spent most of the first 15 minutes of the assessment talking about her daughter and new grandson. Sallyanne is very concerned that her daughter does not have the financial wherewithal to support her grandson, and she is concerned with the life he may have. She talks about political concerns, changes to the education system and the struggles local schools are having, the cost of university education and the difficulty young adults have with finding stable work, all of which make her worry for her grandson's future, her daughter's future and the future of generations to come. Sallyanne talks freely about her childhood, which she describes as an unhappy time and reports having been mistreated by her parents, fearing them, being unsure of what they would say or how they would treat her day to day. However, she does not have any unwanted or intrusive thoughts or nightmares about events that occurred.

Based on the case study, the probable diagnosis, treatment decision and justifications are shown in Table 3.1.

Improving Diagnosis Rates

Diagnosis is important for determining appropriate, evidence-based treatments in LICBT services, but in 2018–19 across all IAPT services, only 63.5 per cent of service users who had at least one treatment session had received a probable diagnosis, and the range across all services nationally was between 14 and 99 per cent (NHS Digital, 2019). This suggests that for just over a third of IAPT service users across the country and nearly all of the service users in some services, the clinical problem may not

Table 3.1 Decisions reached following application of probable diagnosis decision support tool

Probable diagnosis	Consider GAD and depression as potential diagnoses. However, as GAD came first and better encapsulates the difficulties Sallyanne describes, GAD should be identified as the probable diagnosis and inform the problem statement.
Recommended treatment	LICBT intervention for GAD and progress monitored throughout treatment
Justifications	
1	Sallyanne scored 15 on PHQ-9, suggestive of moderate depressive symptoms, so consider probable diagnosis of depression.
2	There are times that she feels very frightened, anxious or uncomfortable.
3	Her anxiety is not related to a specific situation or object; it is related to many situations and there is no sudden onset of intense anxiety. When Sallyanne does feel anxious, she does not describe bodily sensations. So, skip Q4 and move straight to Q5.
4	Despite reports of mistreatment in childhood, Sallyanne does not have any intrusive thoughts or nightmares about events that occurred, and whilst thinking about her childhood makes her feel sad and angry, she does not try to avoid thinking about those times and talks about the events freely.
5	There is no suggestion that Sallyanne is preoccupied with the idea she might have an undiagnosed serious health problem.
6	Sallyanne worries frequently about a wide variety of things. She finds it difficult to stop or control worries. This has become worse over the last year since her daughter moved out of the house and she separated from her husband.
7	While Sallyanne reports considerable depressive symptoms, her low mood did not start until after her husband left. That was six months after she noticed a considerable increase in anxiety and worries, and she describes having worries preceding that event that have been keeping her awake, and the anxiety and worry preceded her low mood.
8	She reports symptoms of fatigue, sleep problems, persistent nervousness, muscle tension and describes excessive and uncontrollable worries about many things.

have been adequately identified, which may have resulted in inappropriate treatment being delivered (Clark et al., 2018; Gyani et al., 2011).

The proportion of patients with a recorded probable diagnosis has been found to be associated with the proportion of patients achieving good treatment outcomes – for example, reliable recovery and reliable improvement (Clark et al., 2018). A number of IAPT services have conducted service evaluations to understand the problems associated with a lack of appropriate use of probable diagnosis and clarify ways in which they might improve the use of diagnoses in their services. Such evaluations have shown that most diagnoses are under-identified by LICBTs when comparing rates of probable CMDs to those determined by an established diagnostic screening tool, particularly in relation to PTSD and OCD (Cernis et al., 2016). However, one probable diagnosis may be over-reported by LICBT practitioners. That is MADD, which was determined to be the probable diagnosis none of the time when the Psychiatric Diagnostic Screening Questionnaire (PDSQ) was used (Cernis et al., 2016), however it is quite often used in IAPT services (Table 3.2). To improve the use of

Table 3.2   Prevalence of probable diagnosis in IAPT services 2018–19 (NHS Digital, 2019)

Common mental health disorder	Prevalence (%)
Depression	42
GAD	23
Mixed anxiety and depression	8.4
PTSD	4.3
Social anxiety	2.5
Panic disorder	2.4
OCD	1.9
Health anxiety	1
Specific phobia	0.7
Agoraphobia	0.68

probable diagnoses, some Step 2 services have offered training and consultation about diagnoses to their staff. Others have sent staff reminders when no probable diagnosis has been assigned and a patient has had at least two treatment sessions. This has helped increase the use of diagnoses and also increase the use of the PHQ9 and GAD in relation to MADD (Cernis et al., 2016). The services that have taken action have also had increased rates of good therapy outcomes for their patients (Pimm et al., 2016).

Summary

Making accurate diagnoses and recording them are central to effective interventions by LICBT practitioners. They inform problem statements, goals and treatment plans developed collaboratively with patients, help determine which type of intervention might best be provided and determine the appropriate way to monitor progress throughout treatment. It is therefore important that an assessment is undertaken to ascertain which probable diagnosis best describes the presenting difficulty for all people presenting to LICBT services. To support LICBT practitioners we have suggested the use of a simple screening tool with questions which can be considered for every patient seen by an LICBT practitioner. To use it fully, LICBT practitioners will need adequate training in recognising the common mental disorder diagnoses seen regularly in their services, in monitoring symptoms of these disorders and in communicating outcomes from such monitoring sensitively and usefully to their patients. Enabling LICBT practitioners to effectively determine probable diagnoses is vital in ensuring the effective delivery of appropriate evidence-based interventions and the best possible outcomes for patients.

Assessing Your Understanding

Declarative

Extended Matching Questions

1. Each answer is worth one mark.
2. There are 15 answers.
3. The question is worth 15 marks.
4. There is negative marking.
5. Answer by clearly writing the capital letter associated with each option in the response boxes provided after each question.
6. More response boxes are provided than answers, so you are not required to put an answer in each response box.
7. For each question, only those answers supplied within the appropriate spaces will be marked as correct. If you make an error, put a cross through the space with the answer in it and add a new space with the answer on the appropriate line.

Table 3.3   Theme: Symptoms of common mental health disorders

	Options		
A	Flashbacks of traumatic event	N	Persistent low mood
B	Fear of losing control or going mad	O	Repetitive intrusive thoughts
C	Withdrawal from everyday activities	P	Feeling on edge
D	Lack of energy or fatigue	Q	Poor concentration
E	Ritualistic behaviours	R	Avoidance of reminders of traumatic events
F	Avoidance of feared situations	S	Excessive anxiety
G	Muscle tension	T	Irritability
H	Hyper arousal	U	Fear of ill-judgement from others in social or performance situations
I	Uncontrollable worry	V	Loss of pleasure or interest in usually enjoyable activities
J	Fear of objects which pose little danger	W	Fear of situation where can't escape
K	Fear of being the centre of attention	X	Repetitive intrusive thoughts
L	Hyper-vigilance to normal bodily experiences	Y	Thoughts of responsibility for harm to others/for occurrence of malign events
M	Attempts to prevent or resist unwanted thoughts or feared events	Z	Preoccupation with serious illness

Lead in: Select the 15 most *commonly* identified symptoms associated with each diagnosis. Each option can be used once, more than once, or not at all.

1. Depression

2. GAD

3. OCD

Worth 15 marks

Procedural

Reaching a Probable Diagnosis

Read the case study and use the diagnosis decision support tool to reach the most probable diagnosis and determine the appropriate treatment. Provide a brief justification at each stage of the decision-making process.

Abdul is a 29-year-old man who has been feeling fatigued and had trouble sleeping. He presented to LICBT services for the first time with low mood. About a year ago he was promoted at work and is now responsible for a large team of people and has to pitch ideas to his chief executive and board at weekly meetings. The first time he did this he was acutely anxious. He was worried about messing it up and that both his subordinates and managers would think that he did not deserve his promotion and was not good enough to do the job. On that occasion he felt very hot, his heart was pounding and he could feel himself blushing, which made him much more anxious. He was worried that if the board saw that he was nervous, they would not believe he had confidence in what he was saying. He began breathing more quickly and felt nauseous, and he had to sit down. Abdul says that he struggled to cope with the situation and has since struggled through many similar situations, though the anxiety has been less intense than that first time. He has developed a few strategies to help him deal with these situations like having a bottle of cold water with him and tensing his legs under the desk as hard as possible to distract himself from his fears. All this has, however, been making him feel increasingly low in mood, fatigued and on occasions he has struggled to go in to work.

Complete Table 3.4

Table 3.4 Diagnosis decision support tool

Probable Diagnosis	
Recommended Treatment	
Justifications	
	Worth 15 marks

Answers to **Assessing Your Understanding** questions can be found in the appendix on p. 334.

Further Reading and Resources

Clark, D.M. (2018) Realizing the mass public benefit of evidence-based psychological therapies: the IAPT program. *Annual Review of Clinical Psychology,* 7, 159–83.

Clark, D.M., Canvin, L., Green, J., Layard, R., Pilling, S. and Janecka, M. (2018) Transparency about the outcomes of mental health services (IAPT approach): an analysis of public data. *The Lancet,* 391, 679–86.

Kessler, R.C., Chiu, W.T., Demler, O. and Walters, E.E. (2005) Prevalence, severity, and comorbidity of 12-Month DSM-IV Disorders in the National Comorbidity Survey Replication. *Archives of General Psychiatry,* 62, 617–27.

To access the online resources accompanying this chapter, please visit: https://study.sagepub.com/farrand

4

Clinical Decision-Making in Low-Intensity Cognitive Behavioural Therapy

Integrating Patient Choice, the Practitioner and Evidence Base

Jeffrey McDonnell, Nicola Kirkland-Davis and Rachel Newman

Learning Objectives

By the end of this chapter you should be able to:

- Critically evaluate the fundamental role of decision-making within a stepped care model
- Demonstrate awareness of the main factors informing clinical decision-making within low-intensity cognitive behavioural therapy
- Apply low-intensity clinical-decision principles to ensure fidelity to the evidence base
- Critically evaluate key factors that affect clinical decision-making

---

Background

The quality and cost of a healthcare system is determined by how well decisions are made and implemented by key stakeholders – clinicians, patients and policy-makers (Chapman and Sonnenberg, 2003). Across England, the manner by which clinical decisions are made in healthcare settings is determined by legislative policies (e.g. Department of Health, 2010) whereby low-intensity cognitive behavioural therapy (LICBT) practitioners are expected to be competent across several core characteristics associated with 'shared decision-making' (SDM). These have been specified within the National Curriculum for LICBT practitioners (Richards and Whyte, 2008; University College London, 2015).

Key Point

Characteristics of Shared-Decision Making (Elwyn et al., 2010)

Shared decision-making is an approach in which:

- Both clinician and patient bring their respective expertise to the clinical issue upon which a decision is to be made
- Patient autonomy is respected
- Patient engagement in the decision-making process is promoted
- The decision is reached with reference to reliable research-evidence.

While SDM intends to be based on research evidence, in practice several factors can result in drift from published guidelines and recommendations, rendering decisions less effective, for example when moving a patient between steps of care (Delgadillo et al., 2015).

Key Point

Factors Potentially Causing Drift from the Evidence Base in Decision-Making

- Subjective: beliefs, attitudes and perceptions held by the patient and the clinician.
- Contextual:
  - Service resources
  - Characteristics of workforce – proportion of HICBT and LICBT practitioners
  - Waiting lists.

Within the Improving Access to Psychological Therapies (IAPT) programme across England, ways to address several of the contextual factors have been outlined (National Collaborating Centre for Mental Health; NCCMH, 2018). Subjective factors need ongoing self-monitoring and acknowledgement by practitioners within clinical supervision.

Clinical Decision-Making within Stepped Care

The clinical effectiveness and efficiency of delivering LICBT within Step 2 of a stepped care service delivery model (NICE, 2011b; Chapter 1) is dependent on competency in clinical decision-making which can be considered across 4 key stages. These stages are informed by the core principles of the stepped care model (Bower & Gilbody, 2005; Richards et al. 2010).

Clinical Practice

Principles of the Stepped Care Model Informing Key Decision-Making Stages (Bower & Gilbody, 2005; Richards et al. 2010)

- Offer the least restrictive, evidence-based intervention to patients in the first instance (see Clinical Decisions 1, 2 & 3 sections of this chapter).
- Ensure clinical decision-making supports self-correction within the stepped care model, including stepping a patient up, down or discharging them (see Clinical Decision 4 section of this chapter).
- Risk is managed effectively and with the immediacy required as informed by risk management decision-making protocols during assessment and guided self-help (GSH) sessions (Chapters 2 and 3).

Alongside clinicians, patients and policymakers, within the IAPT programme the case management supervisor also plays a fundamental role in clinical decision-making (Chapter 9; Turpin and Wheeler, 2011). Clinical skills supervision provides an additional space where LICBT practitioners can bring questions regarding clinical decision-making. This further enhances fidelity (Waller, 2009) to appropriate guidance informing service delivery (NCCMH, 2018).

Decision-Making Protocols within Low-Intensity CBT

Working at Step 2 within a stepped care service delivery model (NICE, 2011b; Chapter 1), LICBT practitioners follow service protocols to ensure efficient, effective, safe and acceptable mental health service delivery. It is recommended that these are consulted throughout all decision-making processes (NCCMH, 2018).

Clinical Practice

Common Clinical Decisions within the IAPT Programme and Factors to Consider

- Clinical decision 1: Is a Step 2 or 3 treatment suitable for the patient? Consider:
  - Service inclusion and exclusion criteria
  - Provisional diagnosis
  - Severity
  - Risk
  - Alcohol and drug use.
- Clinical decision 2: Which Step 2 intervention do I offer? Consider:
  - Provisional diagnosis
  - Co-morbidity
  - The role of signposting.
- Clinical decision 3: How should the intervention be delivered?
- Clinical decision 4: Should I discharge or step the patient up?

Decision 1: Is Step 2 or 3 Treatment Suitable for the Patient?

The suitability of a mental health service refers to its capacity to meet the needs of a patient, with need defined as 'the ability to benefit in some way from healthcare' (Stevens and Gabbay, 1991: 20). At referral, suitability of the service to meet patient need must be decided on with initial reference to IAPT inclusion and exclusion criteria (Chapter 1).

Clinical Practice

IAPT Inclusion and Exclusion Criteria

- Inclusion criteria:
  - o Common mental health difficulty such as depression and/or anxiety
  - o Difficulty of mild-moderate (Step 2) to moderate-severe (Step 3) level of severity as determined by standardised, routine outcome measures (ROMs).
- Exclusion criteria:
  - o Failing to meet at least mild severity on ROMs
  - o High level of risk – likelihood of harm to self or others
  - o Severe, complex and enduring mental health problems (e.g. very severe depression, bipolar, psychosis or personality disorder). These will be considered for stepping up to Step 4 secondary care mental health services unless specific IAPT-SMI pathways are in place (Johns et al., 2019).

Following assessment (Chapter 2), the majority of people deemed suitable for IAPT services (Steps 2 and 3) are likely to enter LICBT treatment (Step 2). In some cases, immediate allocation to Step 3 will be indicated; namely by the evidence base, the LICBT practitioner's knowledge of the patient's provisional diagnosis and the availability of treatments at Steps 2 and 3 as outlined in clinical guidelines (see Chapter 3).

Clinical Practice

To Determine the Suitability of Step 2 and 3 Treatments consider:

- Presenting problem/provisional diagnosis: identified through structured interviewing techniques and Routine Outcome Measures (ROM's; Chapter 2).
- Diagnostic criteria: outlined in classification systems, Diagnostic and Statistical Manual of Mental Disorder-V (DSM; APA, 2013); International Classification of Disease-11 (ICD-11; WHO, 2018).
- Step 2 and Step 3 intervention selection criteria outlined in clinical guidelines (NICE, 2011b).

Whilst decision-making may be protocol-driven, it remains important to consider patient-specific factors to maintain a patient-centred approach. If unacknowledged, these factors may result in LICBT treatment being unhelpful or potentially even harmful (Papworth et al., 2015). Maintaining patient-centredness may include adapting practice to accommodate sensory or intellectual disabilities, language, intervention acceptability (Farrand et al., 2019) and existence of co-morbid conditions and/ or symptoms.

Provisional Diagnosis

With the exception of post-traumatic stress disorder (NICE, 2018b) and social anxiety disorder (NICE, 2013), all common mental health difficulties of mild-moderate severity should be initially considered for treatment with LICBT (Table 4.1).

Recommendations are subject to change as the evidence base develops. For example, NICE guidance regarding obsessive-compulsive disorder (OCD; NICE, 2005) was previously only recommended for HICBT treatment at Step 3. However, recent evidence demonstrates that LICBT may confer some benefits for treating OCD including fewer patients needing to be stepped up subsequent to a LICBT intervention (Chapter 14; Lovell et al., 2017).

Severity

Severity generally refers to the number and intensity of symptoms as captured by ROMs. Whilst high baseline/pre-treatment symptom severity may predict limited recovery following an LICBT intervention (Gyani et al., 2013), it does not imply there will be no treatment response (Delgadillo et al., 2017a). For example, for the

Table 4.1 Treatment step for common mental health difficulties

Common mental health problem	Treatment step	
	Step 2	Step 3
Agoraphobia	X	X
Depression	X	X
Generalised anxiety disorder	X	X
Panic disorder	X	X
Post-traumatic stress disorder		X
Obsessive-compulsive disorder	X	X
Social anxiety		X
Specific phobia	X	X

treatment of depression, research has demonstrated that LICBT interventions such as behavioural activation (Chapter 11) can yield clinical effects comparable to components of HICBT interventions (Lorenzo-Luaces and Dobson, 2019). Basing clinical decisions regarding Step allocation on ROM severity alone may therefore not provide a full picture. Rather, adopting a patient-centred approach that considers ROM severity alongside other information may better inform the decision as to step allocation.

Clinical Practice

Wider Information to Consider Alongside ROM Severity (NICE, 2011b, para. 1.4.1)

- Chronicity, history and duration of disorder:
  o Has the patient experienced these symptoms for a long time, or have they presented recently?
  o Is this the patient's first episode or have they had more than one episode in the past?
- Functional impairment and impact: are the symptoms having a substantial impact on patient functioning – for example, in work, school, social, interpersonal domains?
- Treatment history: has the patient been treated for these symptoms before? What was the effectiveness of the treatment received?
- Relevant social or personal factors.
- Co-morbid mental and/or chronic physical health disorders.

For example, following assessment, immediate allocation to Step 3 may be recommended where a condition has been previously treated with LICBT to minimal effect (treatment history) and the patient expresses a preference for another treatment approach (NICE, 2011b).

Risk

Level of risk will impact the decision as to whether LICBT or HICBT is suitable to meet patient need (NICE, 2011b), with risk subsequently assessed at every patient contact and decisions made accordingly (Chapter 6). Where a patient presents at assessment with high risk of suicide, significant self-neglect and/or self-harm or potential to cause harm to others, risk should be managed immediately following the service's risk protocol (Chapter 4). This may result in onward referral to specialist mental health services such as crisis or emergency services.

Alcohol and Drug Use

The NICE guideline for alcohol use disorders (NICE, 2011c) and the *IAPT Drug and Alcohol Positive Practice Guide* (National Treatment Agency for Substance Misuse, 2012) recommend routine assessment of drugs and alcohol with practitioners who are competent to identify harmful drinking. As problematic drinking may not be associated with poorer treatment outcomes such as non-recovery or drop-out (Buckman et al., 2018), it *should not* be treated as an automatic exclusion criterion from working at Step 2 or Step 3 of a stepped care model (National Treatment Agency for Substance Misuse, 2012). Clinical decision-making during assessment should determine patient ability to attend and engage with LICBT treatment alongside the extent of the impact alcohol/drug use is having on their general level of functioning. Appropriate screening tools with cut-offs such as the AUDIT-C (Bush et al., 1998) should be used as part of decision-making to offer treatment to patients using drugs and/or alcohol. In some cases, alcohol and drug use may require the suitability of Step 2 and Step 3 treatment to be reconsidered.

Clinical Practice

Indicators of Unsuitability of Step 2/3 Treatment for Patients Using Alcohol or Drugs

- Meet diagnostic criteria for *dual diagnosis*, where a substance-use disorder is co-morbid with a mental health difficulty, and there may be complex needs.
- Alcohol and/or drug use identified as the primary condition and/or associated with functional impairment which would impact engagement with treatment.

In both instances, recommend treatment for alcohol/drug misuse from specialist services and support referral (NICE, 2011c).

Decision 2: Which LICBT Intervention Do I Offer?

In the first instance, intervention choice will be determined by the provisional diagnosis where the LICBT practitioner will 'match' the patient's presenting problem with the NICE recommended intervention (NICE, 2011b).

Clinical Practice

NICE (2011b) Recommended LICBT Interventions

- Medication management (Chapter 10)
- Behavioural activation (Chapter 11)
- Graded exposure (Chapters 13 and 14)
- Worry management (Chapter 15)
- Problem-solving (Chapter 16)
- Structured exercise (strenuous physical activity) programmes (Chapter 20).

Treatment planning will be further guided by consideration of specific factors associated with the patient's experience, goals and presentation.

Co-morbidity

Co-morbidity occurs when a patient meets criteria (using the DSM-V or ICD-11) for a diagnosis of two or more mental disorders simultaneously (Clark et al., 2017). It is common in mental health populations, with over 70 per cent entering the IAPT programme experiencing two or more mental health difficulties (Hepgul et al., 2016). Where co-morbidity is identified during assessment, the LICBT practitioner is required to use guidelines (e.g. NICE, 2011b) and consult service protocols to determine the main provisional diagnosis before reaching a clinical decision regarding treatment to offer (Table 4.2).

Signposting

For patients experiencing practical and social problems (including housing, debt, and legal issues, lack of social support and/or employment difficulties), signposting

Table 4.2 Decision-making with mental health co-morbidity (see NICE, 2011, para. 1.4.1.5)

Type of mental health co-morbidity	Decision-making guidance
Co-morbidity of disorders, where each set of symptoms meets threshold for clinical case-ness (e.g. depression *and* an anxiety disorder)	Treatment to focus on the specific anxiety disorder
Co-morbidity of symptoms, where *one* set of symptoms meets threshold for case-ness and the other does not (e.g. depression *with* symptoms of anxiety)	Treatment to focus on the disorder which meets the threshold for case-ness
Co-morbidity of symptoms, where *neither* set of symptoms meets threshold for case-ness but nonetheless present and associated with impairment and distress (e.g. mixed anxiety and depression (WHO, 2018)).	Discuss patient preference, focusing on which set of symptoms associates with the greatest level of impairment

to statutory and/or third sector organisations may be an alternative to initiating treatment at Step 2/3. Signposting will also be an essential component of an effective Step 2 LI intervention where involvement of additional support and advocacy services is considered to facilitate and enhance engagement with treatment and its effects (e.g. see Beck et al. 2019). Unemployment has been frequently linked to poorer outcomes in therapy (e.g. see Delgadillo et al., 2016); and within the IAPT programme recognition of the relationship between employment and mental wellbeing has led to the development of employment advisors to support patients seek meaningful employment whilst engaging with their LICBT intervention (Hogarth et al., 2013).

Decision 3: How Should the Intervention Be Delivered?

To improve access and acceptability (Richards, 2010a), LICBT intervention delivery can be supported across a number of different formats (Chapter 7). New technologies, including phone-based apps, are also rapidly developing and being implemented in Step 2/3 settings to augment and support treatment (Bennion et al., 2017). However, more research is needed to determine efficacy prior to full implementation (Leigh and Flatt, 2015).

Despite the potential of telephone- and computerised-CBT to improve access and promote choice for patients, LICBT practitioners may be ambivalent about such formats compared to face-to-face delivery (Meisel et al., 2018). This may be rooted in perceptions that telephone and computerised delivery will have a negative impact on the therapeutic relationship, treatment outcomes and patient levels of satisfaction and perceived acceptability (Turner et al., 2018). However, the evidence base highlights these modalities to be equivalent with respect to dropout and acceptability (Boyden and Dobel-Ober, 2016; Tutty et al., 2010). In some cases, LICBT interventions supported over the telephone have been reported to demonstrate greater effectiveness than face-to-face support (Farrand and Woodford, 2013). Similar findings have been reported for computerised-CBT compared to control conditions with respect to outcomes and acceptability (Andrews et al., 2018). Acceptability of computerised-CBT may be enhanced for those with concerns over confidentiality (Vallury et al., 2015). Given the range of interventions and delivery methods available, a collaborative decision should therefore be reached regarding the most suitable option. The COM-B model (Michie et al., 2011) may aid decision-making, specifically to determine if any factors related to Capability, Opportunity and/ or Motivation are evident that may affect engagement with a specific modality or format (Chapter 8).

Decision 4: Should I Discharge or Step up?

The fundamental role of the self-correcting mechanism within stepped care ensures that minimal response to LICBT treatment results in the patient stepping up to an intervention of greater intensity (Bower and Gilbody, 2005). Monitoring early response to treatment may help determine if a Step 2 intervention is likely to lead to recovery (Delgadillo et al., 2014).

Clinical Practice

Clinical Decision-Making Informed by Number of Treatment Sessions

- Patients demonstrating reliable improvement by their fourth LICBT treatment session have been found to be twice as likely to achieve recovery compared to those who have not (Delgadillo et al., 2014). Therefore providing a minimum of four treatment sessions before reaching a clinical decision as to whether to step up or discharge is supported (except in the case of significant early deterioration).
- As such, where reliable improvement or recovery has not been achieved by the fourth session or there has been little improvement – or worsening of symptoms – by the sixth support session, consider stepping up.
- Providing more than six support sessions has not been found to lead to better outcomes (Delgadillo et al., 2014) therefore prolonging LICBT treatment on the basis of poor treatment response is not recommended except where the patient is beginning to demonstrate significant improvement.
- Where the patient moves below the threshold for case-ness but continues to demonstrate residual symptoms, consider the benefit of additional treatment sessions to ensure symptoms are reduced. This is recommended in acknowledgement of an observed increased likelihood of relapse where there are residual symptoms at the end of treatment (Ali et al., 2017).
- The patient moves below the threshold for caseness with few residual symptoms – discharge them from the service.

Whilst recommendations exist in relation to stepping up, the LICBT practitioner should always work collaboratively with the patient to determine the wider reasons that may have impeded improvement before reaching the decision to step up. This is especially important as these reasons may act to impede engagement with a Step 3 intervention if unchecked. The COM-B model (Chapter 8) is likely to be helpful to explore difficulties for a patient engaging or using the LICBT intervention. In some cases, contextual (e.g. demand and service capacity) and subjective (e.g. therapist and patient characteristics) factors may influence practitioners to hold patients on their caseload instead of discharging or stepping up, for example due to long waiting lists (Delgadillo et al., 2015), contravening available guidelines. Presenting the patient during case-management supervision (Chapter 9) is therefore of fundamental importance in ensuring that clinical decisions to continue treatment are evidence based.

Summary

This chapter has outlined the importance of decision-making for LICBT practitioners working in a stepped care mental health service delivery model. Decision making as to whether Step 2 or Step 3 of a stepped care model are more suitable to meet patient needs have been outlined with respect to exclusion and inclusion criteria and linked to research evidence (NICE, 2011b) and clinical guidelines such as the DSM (APA, 2013) and ICD-11 (WHO, 2018). Finally, the key self-correcting mechanism of stepped care has been highlighted, alongside emerging research on the possible number of sessions and level of patient improvement to inform decision making for stepping up and/or ending treatment.

Assessing Your Understanding

Assessment is based on the case study.

Saoirse is a 53-year-old single parent to Fleur (aged 13) and has also recently become a full-time carer to her mother who has dementia. Since giving up her job as a biomedical researcher she has been feeling down and exhausted, is sleeping poorly and experiencing frequent headaches and back pain. She feels anxious about her future and her own health. She worries about spending money so does not socialise or do things with her daughter and has become isolated from her friends. All her time seems to be spent on household chores, but she struggles to get these done. To relax she sits in front of the TV but struggles to take anything in as she feels overwhelmed and worries about how she will continue to cope. Her thoughts also drift off to what her life used to be like, and whether things can ever change. Although Saoirse's friends invite her out, she often turns them down thinking, 'What do I have to say anyway? All I am is a carer now. What do they understand?' Over time, people have stopped calling her. Saoirse's scores on the PHQ-9 and GAD-7 are 22 and 11 respectively. Saoirse has never had previous treatment. She wants to feel better and get back to how she used to be but can't see how things will change with her mother's poor health.

Declarative

Multiple Choice Questions

1. What would you need to consider when deciding what treatment is indicated and at which step for Saoirse? [Select all that apply]
   (a) Provisional diagnosis
   (b) Practitioner feels confident they can support this patient
   (c) ROM scores
   (d) Service waiting lists for treatment with high-intensity CBT
   (e) The patient requesting a high-intensity intervention
2. Which evidence-based treatment(s) would be most appropriate for Saoirse? [Select all that apply]
   (a) Worry management
   (b) Signposting to community organisations and resources relevant to the patient
   (c) Behavioural activation and worry management combined
   (d) Problem-solving
   (e) Behavioural activation

Procedural

Saoirse has attended four LICBT treatment sessions and noted some improvement in her mood and an increase in her Routine and Necessary activity levels. Her scores are 18 on the PHQ-9 and 10 on the GAD-7. She still reports feeling down and frequently experiences negative thoughts about herself and her future. Saoirse has reported finding it difficult to complete homework tasks (scheduling Pleasurable activities) recently. She'd like to continue seeing you for sessions as she feels you understand her. Taking this information into account, along with the previous information, write down the information you would take to supervision to help decide next steps.

Answers to **Assessing Your Understanding** questions can be found in the appendix on p. 334.

Reflection Point

When considering next steps for Saoirse, what beliefs come to mind?

How might these impact on your decision-making process?

Further Reading and Resources

Bennett-Levy, J., Richards, D.A., Farrand, P., Christensen, H., Griffiths, K.M., Kavanagh, D.J. et al. (eds), (2010) *Oxford Guide to Low Intensity CBT Interventions*. Oxford: Oxford University Press.

National Collaborating Centre for Mental Health (NCCMH) (2018) *The Improving Access to Psychological Therapies Manual*. Available at www.england.nhs.uk/publication/the-improving-access-to-psychological-therapies-manual (accessed 6 October 2019).

National Institute for Health and Care Excellence (NICE) (2011) *Common Mental Health Disorders: Identification and Pathways to Care* (CG123). Available at www.nice.org.uk/guidance/cg123 (accessed 9 October 2019).

To access the online resources accompanying this chapter, please visit: https://study.sagepub.com/farrand

5

Common and Specific Factors

The Importance of What You Do and How You Do It

Zoe Symons

Learning Objectives

By the end of this chapter you should be able to:

- Differentiate between common and specific factors
- Critically evaluate the importance of both common and specific factors in low-intensity cognitive behavioural therapy
- Apply key common factor skills in your low-intensity cognitive behavioural therapy practice
- Recognise examples of good and poor common factor skills

Common and Specific Factors

Common Factors

As the name suggests, common factors are those elements of practice that are common across different therapeutic modalities (Cahill et al., 2008; Richards and Whyte, 2011).

Key Point

Examples of Common Factors

- Practitioner warmth
- Empathy
- Genuineness
- Good therapeutic relationship
- Working collaboratively towards shared goals

A wealth of verbal and non-verbal common factor skills enables low-intensity cognitive behavioural therapy (LICBT) practitioners to develop sound therapeutic relationships (Baguley et al., 2010).

Specific Factors

Specific factors are those elements of practice not common across therapy types and particular to a specific therapeutic modality (Richards and Farrand, 2010; Richards and Whyte, 2011). Examples of LICBT specific factor skills include creating a problem statement and structuring a support session alongside techniques addressed within specific LICBT interventions.

The Importance of Common and Specific Factors

For over 50 years it has been debated whether common or specific factors are more important in bringing about therapeutic change (Mulder et al., 2017). It has long been suggested that common factors may represent active ingredients across therapies (Rosenzweig, 1936) and, in their own right, are sufficient for therapeutic change (Rogers, 1957). CBT, however, also recognises the seminal importance of specific factor CBT techniques in bringing about recovery. Indeed, it was Beck et al. (1979) who described the therapeutic relationship enhanced through common factors as the context within which CBT specific factors can support recovery. The CBT therapeutic alliance has been described as the essential anaesthetic that allows the specific factor surgery to take place (Gaston et al., 1995). Specifically, CBT regards the therapeutic relationship as 'Necessary but not sufficient to produce an optimum therapeutic effect' (Beck et al., 1979: 45).

Evidence Base

Trying to separate out common and specific factors to appreciate their distinct contribution to treatment outcomes and patient experience is a challenge. Consequently, common factors research does not focus on cause and effect but instead considers associations and correlations. This means we cannot say that a positive therapeutic alliance directly leads to patient recovery (Cuijpers et al., 2019b). Instead, research has shown that a good alliance is related to patient recovery (Horvath et al., 2011). This distinction is an important one as, for example, it has been argued that a positive therapeutic alliance may result from, rather than cause, improved outcomes (Mulder et al., 2017).

Bearing in mind the above caveat, what do we know about the impact of common factors in therapy? In CBT, positive patient outcomes are associated with empathy, warmth, genuineness, positive regard and good therapeutic alliance (Keijsers et al., 2000). Attempts to quantify the difference between the influence of common and specific factors on outcomes have resulted in claims that 30 per cent of improvement in psychotherapy can be credited to common factors compared to 15 per cent to specific factors (Lambert, 1992). Whilst these percentages are 'rough estimates of correlates based on impressions from the literature' (Cuijpers et al., 2019b: 209), a meta-analysis of depression treatment using non-directive supportive therapy reported similar estimates (Cuijpers et al., 2012). Authors however noted, that research outcomes appeared to be significantly influenced by researcher allegiance (Cuijpers et al., 2012). It is therefore currently not possible to quantify the exact contribution of specific or common factors to patient outcomes, or indeed to demonstrate that common factors, specific factors or both are responsible for psychotherapy outcomes (Cuijpers et al., 2019b). However, it appears likely that both contribute to the recovery process (Cuijpers et al., 2019b) and best estimates suggest that common factors are important. Indeed the therapeutic relationship has been reported as being at least as important as specific factors in psychotherapy outcomes (Norcross and Lambert, 2019).

On completing CBT treatment, patients consistently rate the therapeutic relationship as being more important than the techniques in helping them overcome their presenting problems (Keijsers et al., 2000). With limited sessions of briefer duration associated with guided self-help, patients continue to identify the common factor input of the self help facilitator as important for their improvement (Richardson and Richards, 2006; Rogers et al., 2004). Furthermore, with specific factors primarily included within the self-help materials (Chapter 1), common factors are potentially of even greater significance with regard to support provided by the LICBT practitioner. In summary, both common *and* specific factor skills are vital for the competent

LICBT practitioner, and trainees should pay attention to both mastering the specific LICBT interventions and developing their common factor qualities and skills.

Common Factors in LICBT

There are a range of key therapist attributes and skills that the LICBT practitioner should look to develop (Baguley et al., 2010; Richards and Whyte, 2011) to best support their patients (Table 5.1).

These will help ensure practitioners respond to patients in ways that demonstrate they care and have a desire to understand their difficulties and offer support.

Table 5.1   Examples of common factor skills

Verbal	Nonverbal
Reflection	Active listening
Summarising	Appropriate eye contact
Verbal empathy	Facial expression
	Posture

(Baguley et al., 2010; Richards and Whyte, 2011)

Practitioner Characteristics

LICBT practitioners bring to their practice key characteristics of warmth, genuineness and empathy.

Warmth

Warmth represents a caring attitude towards patients and having interest in their difficulties, the opposite of being remote or uncaring (Beck et al., 1979). In practice, warmth starts to be demonstrated from the time the patient is greeted during the first session and can set the tone for subsequent support sessions. Making eye contact, tone of voice, manner, the way in which patients are responded to, almost everything done verbally and non-verbally can demonstrate warmth or indifference.

Genuineness

Genuineness is being truthful, real, authentic and meaning what we say! In practice, expressing concern in a manner that says, 'I haven't got time for this' will be recognised by patients and represents a clear barrier to working together. Being yourself is important, and whilst there may be aspirations to become the perfect LICBT practitioner (were one to exist!), it is important not to adopt a façade. Becoming too dependent on scripts or developing a therapy voice may result in a marked incongruence between who the LICBT practitioner actually is and an idealised self.

Empathy

Empathy is sharing and understanding the emotions of another, aiming to see the world from the patient's viewpoint and appreciate emotions linked to their interpretation of their experiences (Beck et al., 1979). When practitioners communicate their empathic understanding, patients feel understood and accepted, which enables patients to continue to share and explore their difficulties, allowing patient and practitioner to develop a shared understanding (Beck et al., 1979). Experiencing empathy for patients can also help the practitioner maintain a non-judgemental attitude (Beck et al., 1979).

Clinical Example

Clinical Demonstration of the Importance of Empathy

Jane had agoraphobia and for five consecutive sessions was seeing David, her LICBT practitioner. David had carefully introduced exposure and habituation, supported Jane to engage with the LICBT materials and start off creating a hierarchy. Together Jane and David developed plans for perfect home practice exposure activities. Yet Jane returned to another session without having completed the home practice plan. David was frustrated, started to think that he may have wasted his time and wondered if Jane really wanted to get better. When David explored Jane's home practice, he took time to understand the challenges Jane encountered and began to appreciate the overwhelming anxiety Jane was experiencing trying to face her fears with the dread of having no escape. David began to appreciate that Jane was highly frustrated with herself and was experiencing guilt, thinking she had wasted his time. Through appreciating Jane's experience, David found that he no longer had this viewpoint; in fact, he came to recognise the courage that even trying to tackle her difficulties had entailed. Through David communicating and demonstrating understanding of the anxiety and frustration, Jane was experiencing and celebrating the courage she had shown, Jane felt understood, less guilty and had greater confidence that David and LICBT may be able to help.

Whilst most practitioners desire to see the world from their patients' perspective and appreciate the value this can bring, being able to empathise and helpfully communicate this empathy to patients involves a series of skills that can be challenging. This subject will therefore be returned to later in this chapter to consider how we verbally communicate empathy.

Nonverbal Skills

A range of nonverbal common factor skills can create a positive environment for the patient to share their story and allow the LICBT practitioner to convey their desire to listen and understand. The SOLER acronym is useful when highlighting the nonverbal skills that help 'visibly tune in' to patients (Egan, 2002: 68).

Clinical Practice

SOLER (Egan, 2002)

- **S**: Squarely face the patient. Orientate posture towards, rather than away, from the patient to demonstrate focus and interest. A slightly angled position may be less threatening than directly facing the patient.
- **O**: Open posture. Uncross arms and legs to portray openness to hear what the patient has to say.
- **L**: Lean in. Leaning forward rather than back portrays interest in what patients have to say.
- **E**: Eye contact. Appropriate eye contact demonstrates interest.
- **R**: Relaxed and natural. Puts the patient at ease.

Egan notes that these guidelines are consistent with North American culture and consideration should be given when working with people from different cultures (Egan, 2002).

Listening Skills

Practitioners should give full attention to the patient's narrative, focusing on what is being said and seeking to understand the patient's experience. They should therefore maintain an awareness of anything that may get in the way of listening, including getting lost trying to find the right response to what the patient is saying, or thinking about the next question to ask. It is preferable to pay full attention to what the patient is saying and then pause to reflect, if needed, before responding (Egan, 2002).

Verbal Skills

Sensitively asking questions conveys the practitioner's keen desire to establish a shared understanding of patient difficulties. Similarly, the way the LICBT practitioner responds to what the patient is saying through the use of empathy, reflection and summaries is hugely important.

Expressing Therapeutic Empathy

Demonstrating therapeutic empathy is the culmination of a process captured in Thwaites and Bennett-Levy's (2007) model of therapeutic empathy.

Key Point

Elements Associated with Therapeutic Empathy (Thwaites and Bennett-Levy, 2007)

- *Empathic attitude/stance*. Desire to help and understand.
- *Empathic attunement*. Following the emotional experience of the patient.
- *Empathic communication skills*. Ability to communicate empathic understanding to the patient.
- *Empathy knowledge*. Knowledge about therapeutic empathy.

Recognising all elements is important given that a focus is often placed primarily on the expression of empathy. In order to ensure expressed empathy is accurate and helpful, benevolent attunement is key.

One helpful practice shown to boost empathic attitude/stance in experienced LICBT practitioners is self-practice/self-reflection (Thwaites et al., 2017). Through experiencing the LICBT interventions and the challenges involved, practitioners can shift their attitude towards patients' experiences. In the previous example with Jane (see p.83), who struggled to complete her home practice exposure tasks, David initially felt frustrated and judged Jane negatively. If David had completed exposure and habituation for himself, however, and appreciated first-hand the challenges of engaging with and experiencing anxiety-inducing exposure tasks, David's initial response to Jane may have been more empathic and compassionate. Role-playing sessions have also been identified as an effective way of developing empathy communication skills (Thwaites and Bennett-Levy, 2007).

Clinical Example

Use of Empathy in Response to Patient Distress

Patient: In that moment, with my heart racing and feeling faint, I think I'm about to die, to collapse, like my whole life's over. It's awful.

LICBT practitioner: That sounds terrifying.

Patient: It is. It's the most frightening experience of my life, I've never known anything like it before. Then, when I'm not actually terrified, I feel really down because it's taking over. I'm doing less and less, I don't exercise any more, I don't see my friends.

LICBT practitioner: So, outside of those frightening episodes it sounds like you feel really low, because of the impact they've had on the rest of your life.

Patient: Yep, terrified or depressed, that's me. I can't remember the last time I had a simple, relaxed day.

LICBT practitioner: It sounds as though things have been difficult for a while.

Patient: They have. I'm worn out, at the end of my tether.

LICBT practitioner: I'd really like to explore this further with you... [assessment continues]

In this example the LICBT practitioner recognises the emotional experience of the patient and through expressing verbal empathy shows that they have listened to and understood the patient's distress. The patient then has the confidence and trust to continue to describe their difficulties, establishing a richer shared understanding prior to funnelling these difficulties further (Chapter 2).

What Empathy is Not!

A common misunderstanding is to confuse empathy with other forms of expressive language. Consequently, the following forms of verbal expression should be avoided.

Clinical Example

Verbal Expressions to Avoid

- 'I understand, I know what you're going through.' This may be ill received and challenged by patients. It is far better to *demonstrate* your understanding with empathy than to *tell* your patient you understand.
- 'Poor you, I'm sorry to hear that.' This may leave the patient feeling *pitied* rather than understood.

Reflection

Reflection is a verbal skill whereby the practitioner reflects back what the patient has said, sometimes simply using the same words, encouraging continued exploration (Miller and Rollnick, 2013).

Clinical Example

Example of Reflection

Patient: Since my children left for university, life just hasn't been the same. All the things I used to do for them. I miss that. I felt useful but now I don't do anything...

LICBT practitioner: You don't do anything. [Repeats the patient's words]

Patient: I don't. I spend so much of the day watching telly, or scrolling mindlessly on my phone. It's such a waste...

LICBT practitioner: A waste.

Patient: Yeah, life is passing me by. I get pretty choked up about it sometimes, it gets me down.

Summarising

Summaries bring together key things that have been discussed and serve a number of functions.

Key Point

Functions of Summaries

- Demonstrate that the practitioner has listened, thought about what has been said, and understood.
- Offer an important opportunity to ensure a shared understanding between practitioner and patient (Westbrook et al., 2007).
  - o   Practitioners offer their understanding and check if it is correct.
- Bring together key discussion points, allowing the patient to hear them back, make sense of their difficulties and develop insight (Westbrook et al., 2007).
- Enable the practitioner to reflect on where they are in a session.
  - o   Allow the practitioner to consider information gathered or given, and outstanding areas to be explored to reach a full and shared understanding (Westbrook et al., 2007).

Whilst summarising has important benefits for both patients and LICBT practitioners, it tends to be underused. It should, however, be recognised as an important verbal skill throughout assessment (Chapter 2) and support sessions (Chapter 6). When adopted, summaries can be employed in two main ways.

Key Point

Types of Summary

- *Capsule summary*: brings together several different things discussed within sections of the LICBT assessment or support session in a briefer format.
- *Full summary*: rounds off a complete section or session – for example, summarising a home practice review.

Rather than generically listing what has been discussed or covered, summaries should bring together the important contents of the area covered (Table 5.2).

At the end of a summary, the patient should be given the opportunity to highlight the extent to which it is consistent with their understanding so that inconsistencies can be addressed. Where relevant, the opportunity to add anything that may have been missed should also be offered.

Table 5.2 Examples of poor and good session summaries

Poor

LICBT practitioner: Today we have discussed your home practice, looked back over the rationale and stages of exposure and habituation, and come up with a new home practice plan for this week.

Good

LICBT practitioner: Today we discussed your home practice and agreed there had been a number of challenges that had left you feeling frustrated as you weren't feeling any improvement in spite of facing your fears and putting all that effort in. We agreed to revisit the rationale and steps of exposure and habituation together and reflected that some of the things on your hierarchy were graded by time. This had meant your anxiety hadn't had time to drop by half in the exposure tasks. We looked at the hierarchy together and started to make some adjustments which you felt able to continue at home so that when you next face your fears you will hopefully experience the drop in anxiety by half and reap the rewards of your hard work. Does this seem consistent with the understanding you have regarding this session?

Working Together

Working with the patient to ensure they are fully engaged in their treatment and working towards shared goals is of significant importance in maintaining the therapeutic alliance (Aspland et al., 2008). LICBT practitioners should therefore guard against being too directive or telling someone what to do (Table 5.3).

The directive approach could have negative consequences for patient engagement and may rupture the working alliance, potentially resulting in treatment drop-out (Safran et al., 2011).

Table 5.3 Examples of good and poor practice in LICBT that may support or inhibit collaborative working

Good practice encouraging and supporting collaboration	Poor practice that may inhibit collaboration
We've got up to 35 minutes for our session together today. Do you have enough time? It will be great if we can explore together how your home practice went, then we can review the intervention we're working on, and together work out a good way forward with the next home practice. How does that sound? Is there anything else you want to make sure we have some time to cover today?	Today we've got 35 minutes and I'll ask you some questions about your home practice, then I'll tell you about the next steps of the intervention, then I'll set a new home practice task.
Having reviewed your problem statement together, do you feel we're still focusing on the right problem in our sessions?	Pressing on with behavioural activation for your depression is definitely going to be a good thing.
Having discussed the principles of behavioural activation together, looking back at last week's home practice, is there anything you'd now do differently?	So, I can see that there have been a number of problems with the way you've used the behavioural activation intervention, you should have...
Can I just check in that we're on the same page with this? What have you taken from this session together?	Does that make sense?
What feels like a good next step for home practice?	So, for home practice I'd like you to...

Challenges to Good Common Factor Skills

'I used to be really empathic, but it seems to have gone!'

When LICBT practitioners focus hard on mastering specific factor skills it is not unusual that such focus has a negative impact on common factor skills. Once mastered the practitioner can once again shift their focus back to the patient, having a positive impact on their common factor skills. However, it is also important to be aware that life or work stresses experienced by practitioners can impact on their empathy (Thwaites and Bennett-Levy, 2007). If LICBT practitioners recognise this, for the benefit of themselves and their patients they should seek support within line management supervision (Chapter 9).

Reflection Point

Consider your use of common factor skills in everyday life and reflect on the extent you believe they are suitable for your clinical practice.

To what extent might your common factor skills vary according to your own emotional state? If you consider that they may vary a lot, what do you believe could be done to ensure they are always appropriate for clinical practice?

Summary

Both common and specific factor skills are vital for the competent LICBT practitioner in assessment and throughout support sessions. It is important to give attention to developing and enhancing specific and common factor skills during training and then throughout practice.

Assessing Your Understanding

Declarative

Extended Matching Question

1. Each answer is worth one mark.
2. There are 12 answers.
3. The question is worth 12 marks.
4. There *is* negative marking.
5. Answer by clearly writing the capital letter associated with each option in the response boxes provided after each question.

6. More response boxes are provided than answers, so you are not required to put an answer in each response box.

7. For each question, only those answers supplied within the appropriate spaces will be marked as correct. If you make an error, put a cross through the space with the answer in it and add a new space with the answer on the appropriate line.

Table 5.4   Theme: True or False?

Options		
A	It is not possible to determine the relative, direct contributions specific and common factors make to treatment outcome at this time	G	In CBT, positive patient outcomes are associated with empathy, warmth, genuineness and good therapeutic alliance
B	'I'm sorry to hear that' is a good example of verbal empathy	H	Empathy can be described as sharing and understanding the emotions of another
C	A good therapeutic alliance is associated with positive patient outcomes	I	Telling a patient what to do for their next home practice is a good way of ensuring they get the most out of their treatment
D	Reflection can involve simply repeating the patient's own words	J	A problem statement is an LICBT specific factor
E	Open posture demonstrates openness to what patients have to say	K	Common factors do not matter in CBT
F	Practitioner empathy can be enhanced by the practitioner trying out LICBT techniques for themselves and reflecting on the experience	L	Summaries can support patients to develop insight into their difficulties

Lead in: Identify true and false statements.

True									
False									

Worth 12 marks

Procedural

Practising Common Factor Skills

- Role play either an LICBT assessment or support session with a peer. Ask a third person to observe and provide feedback on your use of verbal and nonverbal common factor skills and expression of your positive practitioner characteristics such as warmth, genuineness and empathy.
- Utilise your common factor skills in conversation with friends, family and colleagues. Express empathy and use reflection in your conversation. Reflect on the impact such changes have on the conversation.

Answers to **Assessing Your Understanding** questions can be found in the appendix on p. 336.

Further Reading and Resources

Cuijpers, P., Reijnders, M. and Huibers, M.J. (2019) The role of common factors in psychotherapy outcomes. *Annual Review of Clinical Psychology*, 15, 207–31.

Mulder, R., Murray, G. and Rucklidge, J. (2017) Common versus specific factors in psychotherapy: opening the black box. *The Lancet Psychiatry*, 4, 953–62.

Thwaites, R. and Bennett-Levy, J. (2007) Conceptualizing empathy in cognitive behaviour therapy: making the implicit explicit. *Behavioural and Cognitive Psychotherapy*, 35, 591–612.

To access the online resources accompanying this chapter, please visit: https://study.sagepub.com/farrand

6

Supporting Low-Intensity Cognitive Behavioural Therapy Interventions

Teach Me, Don't Tell Me

Katie Lockwood

Learning Objectives

By the end of this chapter you should be able to:

- Demonstrate a critical awareness of the type and role of support in low-intensity CBT
- Critically evaluate the evidence base associated with support for low-intensity CBT interventions
- Demonstrate competency across the six stages associated with the low-intensity CBT support protocol
- Recognise and formulate common difficulties experienced by patients when engaging with low-intensity CBT interventions
- Apply common and specific factors to help patients overcome common difficulties experienced when engaging with a low-intensity CBT intervention

---

Background

Bibliotherapy or written self-help interventions provide patients with a therapeutic approach designed to treat a physical or emotional problem (Glasgow and Rosen, 1978). Self-help represents a health technology (Richards, 2004) and is adopted within the Improving Access to Psychological Therapies (IAPT) programme implemented across England as an evidence-based psychological therapy to meet demands for high-volume and cost-effective treatment for common mental health problems. Interventions centred around the use of CBT self-help materials within the IAPT programme draw on evidence-based CBT protocols and have become commonly classified as low-intensity CBT (LICBT) (Chapter 1; Lucock et al., 2011). LICBT interventions have been classified according to the level of practitioner input provided alongside the self-help material (Glasgow and Rosen, 1978; Farrand and Woodford, 2012).

Key Point

Levels of Practitioner Support Provided for LICBT Interventions

- Self-administered, non-facilitated, pure:
  - No practitioner input, although collection of outcome measures may still occur.
- Minimal contact:
  - The patient is predominantly dependent upon the self-help interventions with limited practitioner input
  - No focus on the process of supporting the intervention process through problem-solving with the patient
  - Practitioner contact takes place during brief meetings or phone calls to review progress.
- Guided self-help (GSH):
  - The practitioner takes a more active role, providing guidance around the process of engaging with self-help interventions
  - When necessary, the practitioner supports problem-solving for difficulties encountered when engaging with the materials
  - Practitioner contact takes place during planned, routine support sessions.

NICE recommendations (NICE, 2009a) stipulate that LICBT interventions should be guided when adopted as a treatment for depression at Step 2 of the stepped care service delivery model (Chapter 1). For generalised anxiety disorder (Chapter 15) and panic disorder, guided and self-administered CBT self-help are identified as treatment options at Step 2 (NICE, 2011b). The required dose of practitioner support is delivered in a variety of formats including face to face, via the telephone and online (Chapter 7), and varies depending on the individual patient (Baguley et al., 2010) as well as the disorder being treated (NICE, 2009a; 2011b). This chapter focuses on the delivery of face-to-face or telephone guided LICBT interventions.

Evidence Base

Systematic reviews indicate support for CBT self-help interventions to be significantly more effective than when self-administered (Andersson and Cuipers, 2009; Gellatly et al., 2007) and propose that engagement with self-help interventions may be enhanced through a supportive positive therapeutic relationship (Khan, Bower and Rogers, 2007). The level of support required for CBT self-help interventions may, however, vary depending on the disorder being treated. Minimal contact is reported to be more effective in the treatment of depression than both guided support and when the intervention is self-administered (Farrand and Woodford, 2012). The effectiveness of support type also varies across support modality with guided and minimal contact more effective when delivered on the telephone rather than face to face. Given significant interactions between support type, support modality and disorders, however, the need for additional research examining the optimal level and modality of support for different common mental health disorders is proposed (Farrand and Woodford, 2012). This includes examining differences between guided and minimal contact, given no clear advantage for guided has been identified (Farrand and Woodford, 2012). Complexity may also account for other studies that report no additional benefit of guided as opposed to self-administered self-help (Gould and Clum, 1993).

Structuring a Course of Treatment

NICE guidelines recommend that the number of support sessions offered is dependent upon the type and severity of the disorder (NICE, 2009a, 2011a) with the range offered reflecting the necessity for support to accommodate the specific needs of patients (Kenwright et al., 2008). Six to eight support sessions are recommended for mild to moderate depression, whereas the recommended dose is between five and seven sessions for generalised anxiety disorder (NICE, 2009a, 2011a). The IAPT Manual (NCCMH, 2018) specifies that the number of sessions provided should not, however, be arbitrarily restricted but determined during case-management supervision (Chapter 9) to ensure that the patient is appropriately stepped up or discharged where necessary. When working with Step 2 LICBT, it is especially important always to recognise that some patients will recover with fewer sessions than otherwise considered optimal (NCCMH, 2018). Services routinely offering a NICE recommended dose of GSH have been reported to achieve better patient outcomes (NCCMH, 2018). The recommended time frame over which support sessions take place is also disorder dependent (NICE, 2009a; 2011b) but usually LICBT support sessions will take place weekly.

Focus of Support Sessions

The principle that the patient has potential to be the most effective manager of their own recovery is fundamental to LICBT (Baguley et al., 2010). Practitioners delivering LICBT should therefore aim to support the patient to realise their potential through the utilisation of well-chosen, evidence-based self-help materials. In order to maintain an LI focus, the chosen self-help materials should support the application of a single-strand CBT intervention (Chapter 1), through which behaviours or, to a lesser extent, cognitions are the key target of change (Baguley et al., 2010). The structure and components of LICBT support sessions emphasise the role of the LICBT practitioner as teacher and supporter (Williams and Morrison, 2010) to provide support around three areas associated with the LICBT clinical method.

Key Point

Types of Support in the LICBT Clinical Method

- Specific factor skills:
  - Enable patients to address and problem-solve difficulties arising with the specific use of the LICBT intervention or technique adopted.
- Common factor skills:
  - Maintain engagement with the LICBT intervention through the cultivation of a sound therapeutic relationship (Chapter 5).
- COM-B (**C**apability **O**pportunity **M**otivation – **B**ehaviour) framework:
  - Supportive framework to routinely apply to patient difficulties where behaviour change or practical barriers are problematic (Chapter 8; Michie et al., 2011).

It is to be expected that many patients will become stuck at different stages in treatment and will require support to overcome any difficulties. On occasions where the patient experiences difficulties, however, the LICBT practitioner should maintain a single-strand approach and not give up on a particular intervention prematurely or be tempted to drift (Waller, 2009) into adopting a medium-intensity approach where low and high intensity become merged (Telford and Wilson, 2010).

Unlike HICBT, the focus of LICBT is to support the patient to work through CBT self-help interventions between sessions rather than to deliver CBT within sessions (Chapter 1; Lucock et al., 2007). Following assessment therefore (Chapter 2), the emphasis within support sessions should be to enable the patient to use the LICBT intervention on their own between sessions (Bendelin et al., 2011; Kazantzis et al., 2005; Khan et al., 2007). The LICBT practitioner is only accessible for the duration of the course of treatment. However, the CBT self-help interventions can be accessed beyond the course of treatment if required. This approach aims to maximise the dose of treatment received with the minimum need for practitioner support (Chapter 1). This contrasts with HICBT, where although between-session home practice is set, the emphasis is on the HICBT therapist using information gathered through home practice to deliver CBT, with treatment generally ending at the final treatment session.

Structure of Individual Support Sessions

Informed by the clinical method specified for subsequent contacts (Richards and Whyte, 2011), LICBT support sessions typically last 20–35 minutes and are delivered using a specific structure with six separate but interdependent stages. The length of support sessions has been reported to vary between services, however.

Clinical Practice

Support Session Structure

- Stage 1: Introduction
- Stage 2: Information gathering: general
- Stage 3: Information gathering: intervention
- Stage 4: Information giving
- Stage 5: Shared decision-making
- Stage 6: Ending.

Although it can be tempting to merge or go forwards and backwards between components constituting each stage, this should be avoided. Each support stage depends heavily upon the information gathered or shared understanding reached in the previous stage. As much as is possible, the stages should therefore be kept distinct. Adhering strictly to this structure enables the practitioner to maintain focus on the LICBT single-strand intervention (Baguley et al., 2010), work more effectively within the constraints of briefer support session times and avoid therapeutic drift (Waller, 2009).

Stage 1: Introduction

The introduction to each support session should orientate the patient to the session and serves to set expectations, ensuring session structure and timing are better maintained.

Clinical Practice

Introduction to Support Session

- Remind the patient of your full and preferred name at the start of the support session. This may be particularly important in earlier support sessions or where the patient is experiencing memory difficulties.
- Provide an overview of the purpose of each support session by outlining the session structure to enable the patient to know what to expect.
- Let the patient know how long the session will last and confirm patient availability for this length of time.

Stage 2: Information-Gathering: General

Following orientation to the session, there are several areas of general information-gathering that should be undertaken within each support session.

Clinical Practice

General Information-Gathering Areas

- Review the problem statement
- Review engagement with other interventions or treatments
- Routine outcome measures
- Review risk.

It is important always to follow up on these areas at each session as they could inform the support or action that may be needed and will be discussed in case management supervision (Chapter 9).

Review the Problem Statement

At the end of the initial assessment, the LICBT practitioner supports the patient in co-creating a problem statement (Chapter 2). A key purpose of the problem statement is to enable the practitioner and patient to routinely review whether the appropriate problem is still being addressed during subsequent support sessions.

Clinical Practice

Structure When Reviewing Problem Statement

- Clarify patient understanding regarding the purpose of the problem statement within each support session.
- Offer choice as to whether the patient or practitioner reads out the problem statement.
- Collaboratively review the problem described to identify if it has changed in any way.
- Explore any changes through *funnelling* (Chapter 5).
- If symptoms of the main presenting problem have deteriorated or improved, the problem statement should not be altered. It should represent a baseline captured during the initial assessment.
- Ask the patient if the problem statement still represents the main problem to focus on.
- Support the patient to develop a new problem statement (Chapter 2) and consider reviewing it in case management supervision (Chapter 9) if the focus has significantly changed – for example, to a different mental health disorder.
- Review patient goals.

Review Engagement with Other Interventions or Treatments

Changes regarding engagement with other psychological, physical health interventions, alternative therapies or medication have the potential to impact patient progress since the last session. Where changes have occurred since the last support session, *funnelling* (Chapter 2) should be adopted to review further. If medication has been changed or started, review this in sufficient detail to support clinical decisions regarding whether any subsequent action is needed (Chapter 4) and raise during case management supervision (Chapter 9).

Routine Outcome Measures

During every support session the practitioner should collect Routine Outcome Measures (ROMs). Before collection, the practitioner should clarify that the patient remembers the purpose of completing the ROMs and how to complete them. Scores and what they suggest should always be fed back for each questionnaire, with the patient given an opportunity to consider whether this reflects their recent experience. Scores from previous sessions should also be fed back and the patient encouraged to highlight what this means with respect to progress and consider whether this also reflects their experience. Any indication from the patient that symptoms are improving or deteriorating should be explored with common factor skills adopted as necessary (Chapter 5).

Risk Review

During every support session the patient should be reminded of the purpose of the risk review. Information gathered during the previous session about every area of risk initially gathered during the assessment session – suicide, self-harm, risk to others, risk from others, self-neglect, dependants, neglect of others (Chapter 2) should be clearly and separately fed back to the patient (Clinical Example: Example 1).

Clinical Practice

Essential Areas of Risk to Review at Every Support Session

- Risk of suicide:
  - Thoughts
  - Plans
  - Actions
  - Protective factors
- Risk of self-harm:
  - Thoughts
  - Actions
- Risk of harm from others
- Risk of harm to others
- Self-neglect
- Dependants
- Neglect of others.

Clinical Example

Example 1: A Section of a Risk Review Undertaken during a Support Session

Practitioner: Last time you told me that you have had no recent thoughts to end your life, made no recent plans to end your life, and have taken no recent action towards ending your life. Have any of these areas changed in any way?

Patient: No, none of these areas have changed.

Practitioner: And you told me last time that if you were to experience thoughts of ending your life, you wouldn't act on these thoughts because you wouldn't want to leave your children or your partner behind and you wouldn't want them to be affected. Has this changed in any way?

Patient: No, that's still the same.

Practitioner: And last session, you told me that you had no thoughts about harming yourself and that you hadn't done anything recently to harm yourself in any way. Has that changed at all?

Patient: No, it hasn't.

(*Important*: This example represents a review of risk of suicide and self-harm only and not the other essential areas of risk to review at *every* treatment session)

In the event of any reported change, the practitioner should use funnelling skills (Chapter 2) to explore changes in sufficient depth. The practitioner should also check patient responses for consistency with any specific risk items included within questionnaires (e.g. Question 9 on the Patient Health Questionnaire, PHQ-9). The practitioner should feed back whether there appears to be consistency and the patient should be given an opportunity to comment on whether this interpretation is accurate or otherwise. Finally, a summary of risk information gathered should be fed back and accuracy clarified with the patient.

Stage 3: Information-Gathering: Intervention

Stage 3 aims to identify how successfully the patient is engaging with the LICBT intervention so far, and whether this engagement has been of benefit in addressing any feature of the main presenting problem and patient goals. Any barriers or difficulties to successful engagement need to be accurately identified at this point in order to enable the practitioner to support the patient effectively to address and resolve these difficulties in the subsequent information giving stage. Before exploring engagement with and experience of the home practice between sessions, it is important to clarify patient understanding of the agreed home practice plan established within the previous session. Gaining an appreciation of the plan from the patient's perspective ensures that there is a shared understanding of the plan. Where differences exist, the LICBT practitioner should communicate their own understanding and seek to understand the source of confusion from the patient's perspective, without assigning blame. The practitioner should also identify whether the patient has experienced barriers engaging with the home practice plan. The practitioner should use funnelling to explore any barriers to engagement in enough detail to understand what the barrier was and how it prevented the patient from completing home practice. It is helpful at this stage to use the COM-B framework to inform the questions asked (Chapter 8; Michie et al., 2011).

Clinical Example

Example 2: Identifying Barriers Engaging with the Home Practice Plan

Practitioner: Did anything get in the way of following the plan recorded in the diary?

Patient: I didn't manage everything we planned, but I did try.

Practitioner: Well done for trying. I guess it must have been quite frustrating not being able to do everything you'd planned. Could you tell me a bit more about what got in the way of the things you didn't manage?

Patient: My daughter wasn't very well at the start of the week, so I ended up having to take care of her. I did do things towards the end of the week and at the weekend.

Practitioner: So, it sounds like your opportunity to complete the activities planned was reduced because looking after your daughter took priority, but you had the opportunity to engage with the plan towards the end of the week? Did anything else affect your opportunity to engage with the plan?

Patient: No, I understood it all and knew what I was meant to do.

Practitioner: And how motivated were you to follow the plan?

Patient: I really wanted to complete everything and for it to work and I'm glad I managed to carry on with the plan. I'm not sure I feel any better for it though.

Practitioner: So, on a scale from 0–10, where was your motivation at the start of the week?

Patient: Quite high, maybe 8/10 but then it dropped off when things got more difficult. It probably went down to about a 5/10 and I'd say I'm still there at about 5/10.

Practitioner: That's not surprising given you've had a lot to contend with. It's really great you managed to keep going with the plan. Is there anything you think may help pick your motivation back up to where it was again?

Patient: I think I just need a reminder of why I'm doing this and put last week behind me.

Practitioner: That sounds like it would be really helpful. We can definitely try to achieve that in our session today.

The practitioner should ask the patient about their use of the LICBT self-help materials. If the patient has not already done so, the practitioner should ask for all relevant worksheets to be positioned to enable them to be explored together. It is helpful to ask the patient to talk through section by section how they used each worksheet and what they recorded. Due to time constraints, if the patient has completed several worksheets or completed worksheets in great detail, it can be helpful to begin by asking questions which allow an overview of what they have done to be gained. More specific questions that address important details and examples should follow. Questions posed should enable the practitioner to gain a clear appreciation of the patient's application of specific factors during each stage of the intervention (Table 6.1).

It is also important to recognise, acknowledge and verbally reinforce progress that has been made in terms of successful engagement with the intervention and improvement. Any remaining difficulties, not adequately addressed during the COM-B analysis, should also be identified at this stage and explored using funnelling (Table 6.1).

Table 6.1 Examples of questions and prompts adopted during information-gathering for a behavioural activation session

Questions/prompts addressing intervention use	Questions/prompts exploring success or difficulty using intervention
How did you get on following the plan?	What went well/ didn't go so well?
Talk me through your week.	What got in the way of this activity?
Tell me about the morning on this day.	Any thoughts/feelings/ behaviours?
How did you put this plan together?	What did you do instead/to cope?
What category did this activity come from?	What are your reflections on how this week has gone
Where on the hierarchy is this activity from?	overall?
Tell me more about why you decided to plan a more difficult activity here.	Were there any particularly good/bad days?
	What do you think made the difference?
How long did you do this activity for?	How did you feel after you completed this activity?
Was anybody with you when you did this activity?	How did you feel when you decided not to do this
Where were you when doing this activity?	activity?
What did this activity involve?	What do you think about the spread of activities across
Is this an activity you have done in the past?	the week?
Are you engaging in the activity in the same way that you used to?	What do you think about the mixture of activities across the week?

Stage 4: Information-Giving

The main purpose is to support the patient to build the knowledge and competence required to successfully engage with the LICBT intervention. The intention here is to promote recovery that can be sustained independently beyond support sessions. It is good practice to explain this intention through inclusion of a bridging statement linking this section to the previous one.

Clinical Example

Example 3: Bridging Statement

I've got a good understanding of how you've used the intervention since the last session, what's worked well for you and what's been difficult. I think it would be really helpful for us to think about why we're using this treatment and how and why we use each of the steps. This will help us to figure out what you could do differently to overcome the difficulties you've told me about and make a sensible plan to keep things moving forward. I'll check along the way what your understanding is so we can both be really confident that this is something you are able to use independently in the future if you experience the same difficulties again. Does that sound OK?

Key Point

Information-Giving Clinical Competencies

- Structuring information giving
- Checking understanding and giving accurate information
- Addressing difficulties.

Structuring Information-Giving

It is helpful to begin by revisiting the patient's understanding of why the specific LICBT intervention has been chosen to treat the main presenting problem (Kennerley et al., 2016) – for example, by highlighting the theoretical rationale for behavioural activation (Chapter 11) as a treatment for depression. It may be helpful to also revisit the completed CBT model that was used at assessment to capture the presenting problem (Chapter 2). When understanding has been demonstrated, the practitioner should check the patient's understanding of the rationale (Why?) and implementation method (How?) for each of the intervention stages engaged with so far. It is not necessary to check full understanding of stages which have not yet been undertaken by the patient. However, it is helpful to give some information about future stages in order to put the current ones into context. At the end of Stage 4, if a new stage is being introduced in the session, the practitioner should teach the patient about this stage and then check their understanding.

Checking Understanding and Giving Information

It is only necessary to give information about the whys and hows of the intervention and stages if the patient is unable to demonstrate this understanding when prompted, as this indicates a gap in understanding that needs to be filled. After asking a specific open question to check for understanding, if the patient indicates no recollection, it is good practice to use a more specific prompt before giving any information. It is good practice to give small chunks of information before asking the patient to reflect back their understanding (Chapter 5). Lengthier explanations may be difficult to absorb and the patient may only feed back their understanding of some of the later points covered by the practitioner.

Clinical Example

Example 4: Checking Understanding and Giving Information during Stage 4 of a Behavioural Activation Session

> Practitioner: Would you be able to tell me about your understanding of why we are using behavioural activation to treat depression?
> Patient: I'm not sure I really remember.
> Practitioner: Do you remember the vicious cycle of depression?
> Patient: Oh yes, that diagram we looked at, where it goes round and round because I've stopped doing things.
> Practitioner: Yes, well remembered. Do you remember the different areas we included in the vicious cycle?

Addressing Difficulties

During Stage 3, any challenges encountered with engaging or undertaking the intervention stages should have been identified and explored. When the why or how regarding each stage of the intervention is being discussed, it is essential that the practitioner provides an opportunity for the patient to reflect upon their use of each stage. Only if the patient is struggling with any of the intervention stages should the practitioner provide support around the specific factors found challenging, in order to enable the patient to move forward in their understanding.

Clinical Example

Example 5: Support Provided to Address Patient Difficulties with Specific Factors associated with Behavioural Activation

Practitioner: Can you remember what we said about the purpose of the hierarchy?

Patient: To make sure I start with easier tasks and work up to the more difficult ones?

Practitioner: Exactly, and do you remember why we do that?

Patient: So I'm more likely to stick to the plan and not feel overwhelmed.

Practitioner: Yes, that's right and if we think about the plan you made for last week, what are your thoughts about how you used the hierarchy to plan activities into the BA diary?

Patient: Well, in the last session we planned in the three easier tasks but I really needed to clean the house because it's such a mess, so I thought I should add that task in as well.

Practitioner: And cleaning the house was one of your more difficult tasks, is that right?

Patient: Yes, but it needs to be done. When it came to actually doing it, I just didn't have the energy. Like I said earlier, I did manage the dishes but nothing else.

Practitioner: You set yourself a challenging task to clean the whole house and I imagine you had a reason for classifying it as one of the 'most difficult'. It sounds like cleaning the house is really important to you. Is there another way we could approach this task?

Patient: Perhaps I could just do a smaller task each week to work towards getting the whole house cleaned? I've already managed the dishes, so maybe I could build this in as a routine activity and next time plan to vacuum the lounge as well?

Practitioner: That sounds really sensible. Would you do these two tasks at separate times?

Patient: I think on different days. The books says it's helpful to spread activities out.

Practitioner: Yes, I'd agree with that. Shall we add vacuuming the lounge to your hierarchy?

Patient: Yes, I think that can go in the 'easiest' section and perhaps I can add some other individual household tasks into the 'easiest' and 'medium difficulty' sections as well.

Informed by their knowledge of the intervention, at all times the practitioner should aim to facilitate an interactive discussion to guide the patient to reach their own understanding and solutions (Beck et al., 1979). This is in contrast to the practitioner immediately problem-solving for the patient or directing them as to what to do.

Stage 5: Shared Decision-Making

To facilitate the best chance of moving forward to reach recovery, the patient should be supported to generate a shared home practice plan consistent with the specific factors associated with the LICBT intervention adopted. Based on discussions during information giving, it can be good practice to ask the patient what they think would be the best way forward. The plan should seek to address any difficulties that were experienced when undertaking the previous home practice and incorporate the patient's developed or renewed understanding of the intervention. Applying the COM-B framework (Chapter 8; Michie et al., 2011) is helpful at this point so that practitioner and patient can address any anticipated barriers to the proposed plan. Additionally, in keeping with the assessment (Chapter 2) consideration should be paid to ensure goals set as part of the home practice plan meet the criteria to be SMART goals (Chapter 2). Patients should be encouraged to record the home practice plan in detail with a written (or other) record of the plan supporting between-session engagement. The importance of engagement with home practice should be reiterated (Bendelin et al., 2011; Kazantzis et al., 2005).

Reflection Point

Reflect on how you will maintain a collaborative approach throughout LICBT support sessions and what challenges you may face.

Stage 6: Ending

Towards the end of each support session the practitioner should summarise the session in a manner that captures the content of the session and is tailored to the patient. The patient should be asked to feed back their understanding of the between-session home practice plan to be completed prior to the next support session. Any gaps in understanding should be identified by the practitioner and discussed with the patient until both agree. Once the plan is firmly in place, a shared decision should be reached regarding the date, time, modality and, if relevant, location of the next support session.

Relapse Prevention

Once treatment goals and recovery have been achieved (Chapter 4), relapse prevention should always be sufficiently covered before ending treatment (Kenwright, 2010).

It is important to be honest with the patient about the possibility of relapse. The steps involved in relapse prevention should usually be introduced during the penultimate treatment session, with the patient encouraged to complete these steps for home practice.

Clinical Practice

Steps within a Relapse Prevention Technique

- Identify early warning signs.
- Recognise what worked well so that it can be implemented again.
- Anticipate high-risk situations that may be encountered.
- Recognise what would be done in high-risk situations.

You may wish to support the patient to develop a staying well plan, with worksheets to support this provided individually (Worksheet 6.1) or included as part of an LICBT intervention.

Worksheet 6.1 Example of a relapse prevention worksheet

What activities helped me feel better?			
What skills have I learnt?			
What helped me put these activities, skills and techniques into practice?			
Potential triggers for feeling worse			
My warning signs:			
My physical feelings	My thoughts	My emotions	My behaviours
How will I manage potential triggers?			
What will I do if I feel worse again?			

In the final session it is important to fully review the completed Staying Well plan, offer any additional guidance needed and make any necessary alterations. It is important to tailor these discussions to the patient's experiences. Some patients may have achieved considerable improvements whilst others will need some guidance on how to continue implementing the LICBT intervention after sessions have ended. If insufficient recovery is achieved, stepping up for more intensive treatment can be considered in case management supervision (Chapter 9). Ensure that this is acknowledged and that the patient is informed of the next steps.

Common Challenges

A number of common challenges may be experienced supporting LICBT that can be addressed by employing a range of specific and common factors (Table 6.2).

Table 6.2 Common challenges supporting LICBT interventions

Common challenges	Specific and common factors to address challenges
Patient wants to discuss home practice or recent experiences during information gathering: general	Be transparent about structure, purpose and time available. Use common factor skills so the patient knows that you are interested and keen to understand and help. Let the patient know there will be time to talk about home practice in more depth.
Unsure if enough information has been gathered around home practice and, if appropriate, to move on to information giving	Consider whether you are clearly aware how the patient has used the intervention and what the experience was like for them. Ensure you have established whether patient engagement is consistent with specific factors to benefit from the intervention.
The patient has not completed home practice or forgotten to bring completed materials to the session	Use COM-B to establish factors preventing completion and use this to inform shared decision-making. Reiterate the importance of engaging with home practice, ensuring the message does not appear critical or blaming. If the worksheet has been forgotten, support the patient to recreate the completed worksheet in the session.
The patient confirms they have understood the information but struggles to feed back	Phrase the question differently, for example, 'I just want to make sure I've explained the intervention in a clear way to you. If not, I can go through it again.'
The patient chooses a home practice plan that does not adhere to the LICBT intervention protocol	Start by asking the patient if they can see any problems with the plan given what they know about the intervention. If unable to identify any issue, be transparent about your concerns and explain that the evidence suggests the intervention is followed in a particular way to promote recovery.
Unable to manage time constraints effectively	Be transparent about time constraints at the start and, where necessary, throughout a session. This enables the patient to take joint responsibility for how session time is used.

It is important to appreciate that every support session should be tailored to the individual patient, the intervention being used and treatment stage. Whilst maintaining fidelity to the evidence base, practitioners must learn to adapt every session to this unique set of circumstances.

Summary

This chapter has focused on the specific factors and competencies needed within support sessions to support patients to engage with LICBT interventions between sessions. The purpose, structure and content of LICBT support sessions has been described. Common challenges experienced when supporting LICBT interventions have been highlighted alongside potential solutions. This chapter should be used to inform the standardised support structure for the intervention-focused chapters (Part II).

Assessing Your Understanding

Declarative

Extended Matching Questions

1. Each answer is worth one mark.
2. There are 18 answers.
3. Answer by clearly writing the capital letter associated with each option in the response boxes provided after each question.
4. More response boxes are provided than answers, so you are not required to put an answer in each response box.

Table 6.3   Theme: Support Stages

A	COM-B analysis	I	Use cognitive restructuring to support patient use of behavioural activation
B	Clarify patient understanding of the home practice plan	J	Fill in the gaps in patient understanding of specific factors
C	Update patient formulation	K	Explain the next step in the LICBT intervention
D	Support the patient to practise mindfulness exercises	L	Elicit the patient's ideas about implementation of next steps
E	Review the problem statement	M	Address difficulties with previous home practice
F	Collect routine outcome measures (ROMs)	N	Explore use of LICBT materials
G	Introduce the idea of within session behavioural experiments	O	Use of common factors
H	Bridging statement	P	Update the problem statement to reflect any improvements in symptoms

Lead in: For each of the four sections of an LICBT support session select the *most likely option(s)* you would associate with each section. Each option can be used once, more than once or not at all.

1. Information gathering: general							
2. Information gathering: intervention							
3. Information giving							
4. Shared decision-making							

Worth 18 marks

Procedural

Using a Patient Example and associated worksheets included in one of the chapters (11–17) in Part II, role play an LICBT support session with a peer. Ask a third person to observe and provide feedback regarding your fidelity to the support session structure. When competency has been developed in adhering to the session structure, focus on factors specific to each LICBT intervention and use of common factors to support patient engagement.

> Answers to **Assessing Your Understanding** questions can be found in the appendix on p. 335.

Further Reading and Resources

Baguley, C., Farrand, P., Hope, R., Leibowitz, J., Lovell, K., Lucock, M., et al. (2010) *Good Practice Guidance on the Use of Self-help Materials within IAPT Services*. Technical Report. Available at http://eprints.hud.ac.uk/id/eprint/9017/1/goodpracticelucock. pdf (last accessed 28 March 2020).

Williams, C., and Martinez, R. (2008) Increasing access to CBT: stepped care and CBT self-help models in practice. *Behavioural and Cognitive Psychotherapy*, 36, 675–83.

 To access the online resources accompanying this chapter, please visit: https://study.sagepub.com/farrand

7

Identifying the Best Match between Delivery Modality and Learning Style

Change is the End Result of All True Learning

Chris Williams and Paul Farrand

Learning Objectives

By the end of this chapter you should be able to:

- Critically evaluate the importance of gaining an understanding of patient learning to enhance support for low-intensity CBT interventions
- Have an appreciation of the different modalities through which LICBT can be delivered
- Critically evaluate the strengths and weakness of each modality
- Develop competency in recognising the preferred learning style of the patient to inform collaborative decision-making surrounding delivery modality
- Appreciate characteristics of written LICBT interventions to inform the most acceptable match to the learning style of the patient

---

Background

Low-intensity cognitive behaviour therapy (LICBT) interventions aim to communicate key elements of CBT using a format the patient can engage in and apply (Chapter 1). By definition people using a low-intensity (LI) intervention receive less support time with the low-intensity CBT (LICBT) practitioner or person providing support than someone receiving high-intensity CBT (HICBT). It is therefore LICBT interventions that are directly responsible for communicating the key elements of CBT that could simply not be delivered by a therapist in shorter 20–35-minute support sessions (Chapter 6). Key elements of the CBT model are therefore communicated largely through the completion of accompanying materials (e.g. books, worksheets, video, online delivered in a variety of ways). The emphasis in LICBT is therefore placed on supporting the patient to use resources to help them learn the new skills associated with CBT in a way they can remember and implement. Considered this way, CBT represents a challenge of adult (or young people) teaching and learning as much as delivering psychotherapy (Williams and Morrison, 2010). This has significant implications for the types of teaching resources used – for example, textbook, video/DVD, online, audio – and the content of materials to ensure they suit and engage the user.

Teaching Resources

A variety of resources are available to supplement teaching and aid learning with some resources large and detailed, and others short and focused. Resources may be interactive (e.g. self-test or worksheet components in a textbook or online course) or simply information provided through non-interactive didactic teaching. Likewise, some courses are content heavy, whereas others will have presented the subject in more varied ways by adopting case studies, using multimedia or class debates. The key point is that people learn in different ways and have different preferences regarding resources to aid that learning and this should be considered when supporting LICBT.

Modality Supporting the Delivery of Low-Intensity CBT

Preferences a patient has towards learning, alongside the best way to support the patient to engage with an LICBT intervention are important considerations for the LICBT practitioner. Meeting patients' learning preferences is possible in LICBT by matching the patient to the best modality – written, computerised, audio – through which LICBT interventions can be delivered (Martinez and Williams, 2010). Adopting the best modality to deliver LICBT interventions has the potential to blend different teaching resources and tools and maximise engagement.

Written CBT Self-Help Interventions

The invention of the printing press by William Caxton helped revolutionise society and over time books themselves became a form of technology and agent of social change. One of the strongest arguments supporting the use of written LICBT self-help interventions for depression and anxiety is that they are well evaluated and are effective (Cuijpers et al., 2019a). Additionally, an infrastructure to access books through bookshops and libraries, alongside Books on Prescription (Farrand, 2005; Frude, 2004) and schemes such as Reading Well is available (Robinson, 2018). Representing a health technology, bibliotherapy in the form of CBT self-help interventions is therefore the most common LICBT format. Delivering LICBT through written interventions presents a number of advantages and disadvantages to the LICBT practitioner and patient (Table 7.1).

Table 7.1   Advantages and disadvantages of written LICBT interventions (Martinez and Williams, 2010)

Advantages	Disadvantages
Clear structure and content that ideally suits the CBT approach	Not everyone likes using written materials
Good evidence base	Good evidence-base but may not be acceptable to everyone
Demonstrates to the patient they are not alone, normalising their experience	Discovering more information about a condition may make the patient initially feel worse
Existing distribution infrastructure (e.g. book prescription schemes, libraries, bookshops, free online availability, e-book purchase structures) improves access	Can place financial costs or travel demands on the patient whilst copyright restrictions may restrict general use by mental health teams
Familiar and easy for the LICBT practitioner to explain to the patient	Familiarity may result in the patient dismissing intervention as being inferior
Can be written in a manner to reduce reading age and improve usability	Most CBT books have reading age above the general population average (Martinez et al., 2008)
Can be well written, readable and use short sentences	Interventions can be perceived to be patronising when written using easy to read language and simple terms
Capable of employing technical terms that can be revisited several times	Potential for information overload, which is especially hard for patients with depression or who struggle to read to engage with
Language translations can be made available	Translations are often done by publishers with no author input and no clear process for cultural adaptation or sign-off for changes
Libraries of worksheets for between-session directed learning activities can be made freely available	Most written interventions are not accompanied by free worksheets available for download
Large stocks of interventions are commonly available	Materials may not be updated – as a result an intervention fails to maintain consistency with the evidence base and goes out of date quickly
A growing number of celebrity authors can raise the profile of written CBT self-help interventions and mental health	CBT self-help interventions are becoming increasingly written by non-accredited, perhaps celebrity, authors reducing quality

Computerised/Internet CBT Self-Help Interventions

Computers can be seen as another way of supporting the delivery of LICBT interventions through apps or the internet. The principles of deciding who might benefit from computerised (cCBT) or internet (iCBT) based CBT programmes, introducing and supporting use, and addressing difficulties patients might have using the programme and keeping them engaged between support sessions are similar whether LICBT is delivered electronically or as written interventions (Chapter 6). Currently most cCBT programmes rely on text, video and audio supplemented by the administration of online questionnaires to enable the patient, and if supported, the LICBT practitioner to monitor progress and reach clinical decisions (Chapter 4). Similar to written interventions, cCBT programmes present the LICBT practitioner and patient with advantages and disadvantages (Table 7.2), although both approaches are only suitable for patients who are able to read effectively enough to navigate through and understand content.

Limitations of cCBT

Like many written interventions, several cCBT approaches use traditional CBT language requiring higher reading ages and this consequently excludes many users (Martinez et al., 2008). Additionally, many early cCBT packages copied the structure of HICBT and consisted of up to hour-long treatment sessions supporting the delivery of CBT as a multi-strand intervention usually requiring over eight treatment sessions (Chapter 1). Such an approach presents something of a paradox, however, regarding the way users of online packages expect to work online. Modern commercial teaching content in fields outside of cCBT tends to last between 5 and 20 minutes. This contrasts with longer sessions seen in many cCBT packages. However, this has not been adequately researched, and perhaps the most important issue is that content should be relevant, engaging and helpful. It is also not known if outcomes are better when they are highly interactive. There are often user expectations that cCBT packages will match the convenience of attractive non-CBT websites such as the ability to type directly into worksheets online or via a phone.

Audio CBT Self-Help Interventions and Resources

An increasing range of LICBT intervention and resources are also available as audiobooks and online downloads (from Spotify, Amazon Music and Amazon Audible) amongst others.

Table 7.2   Advantages and disadvantages of computerised LICBT programmes

Advantages	Disadvantages
CBT has a structure and teaching content that makes it appropriate for delivery online	Very large variations in delivery of cCBT through different programmes requires detailed knowledge of each package to be gained before adoption for use
Availability of evidence-based programmes	Many evidence-based cCBT programmes developed as a result of research-funded RCTs over the last ten years are no longer available after the initial research funding ends
Many programmes are available for free	Given the expense of maintaining programmes, those originally free to use often become subscription based over time. An app can disappear quickly if an operating system update occurs and the developer cannot afford to update it
Websites can add multiple interactive features (mood ratings, making and reviewing plans, keeping a diary, text reminders, etc.)	It is unclear if adding interaction or 'exciting' ways of delivery actually improves outcomes. Supporting cCBT interventions continues to be the most important predictor of outcome
Language translations may be available	Language translations may or may not be available or well done. When produced, they are often only distributed in the country linked to the translated language with translated worksheets separately available
Corporate/company ownership means websites can be delivered over time and continue to be available	Sites and courses can be closed down quickly if failing to return on investment
Data security and protection	iCBT and apps vary in quality and design with regard to security. Issues can include data vulnerability, poor handling of sensitive data, poor GDPR compliance, a lack of intrusion testing and inconsistent encryption
cCBT packages are typically designed for desktop use	Most current users use smartphones/tablets that may not render content appropriately. Few use a Mobile First design.
Websites and apps can use the most up-to-date communication and social media tools	In healthcare settings, older browsers used on NHS machines may not work and prevent newer sites running
Practitioners can support people as they use the programmes at home	Many NHS Trusts prevent staff from emailing patients and do not allow patients to use NHS computers
Live video chat between the LICBT practitioner and patient offers a truly flexible real-time live support option	Video chat applications may store data in the USA and keep copies of the video chats for a time. This currently breaches many NHS data storage rules
Personalisation of content should be easy to program as long as content has been created	Few programs provide even simple personalisation – e.g. choice of female or male narrator, regional accents, or bespoke content for someone with co-morbidities such as long-term physical illness

Key Point

Advantages of Audiobooks and Downloads

- Easily downloaded at little extra cost to the service or patient or can be included in some subscriptions (e.g. Amazon Prime)
- Highly accessible and can be made available on mobile phones
- Can improve access for patients who have difficulty reading
- Downloads can be recorded and available as audio CD at low cost
- Recordings can be made of the practitioner's own voice talking through a relaxation or mindfulness session.

Whilst audiobooks of many CBT and mindfulness books are available, the LICBT practitioner should give some consideration to their suitability for the patient before recommending them. Many audiobooks were first written as books and were not adapted to suit an audio format. Additionally, whilst audiobooks may be preferred as a way to receive content, interaction with worksheets to plan LICBT techniques or monitor progress is a fundamental feature of CBT (Chapter 1). As such, if audiobooks are chosen then the LICBT practitioner should consider ways to support the patient to engage with the accompanying worksheets both within and between sessions. In addition to audiobooks, many online audio resources and downloads are available that can be used to complement appropriate single-strand LICBT techniques.

Key Point

Examples of online and audio resources

- Amazon Alexa has helpful resources to aid sleep – e.g. white noise, babbling brook, wind or sea sounds
- Spotify – relaxing music to aid winding down
- Living Life to the Full (www.llttf.com) – CBT for mindfulness practice such as relaxation, body scan or compassion/ forgiveness exercises.

Matching Learning Style to LICBT Modality

Some patients like to read books, others prefer not to, whilst others may struggle with reading but be better accommodated through online CBT programmes or audiobooks.

Reflection Point

Reflect upon ways that you prefer to learn and match them to the range of delivery modalities and LICBT resources available.

Similar preferences can apply regarding the preference for face-to-face or telephone support. A number of initial questions can begin to inform the best match between the LICBT delivery modality and the patient's learning style.

Clinical Example

Useful Initial Questions to Match Learning Style to Modality

- Do you ever read newspapers, magazines or books?
  - This determines patients' attitudes towards reading and their ability to read. If a patient indicates that they read, ask them what sort of things they enjoy as this can help inform decisions about the best LICBT resources to recommend with respect to reading age, presentation of content, etc.
- Do you have web access or use the web often for information or communication?
  - If they answer yes, ask them what they use and why. This can inform concerning preferences for the way information is presented and may highlight a preference for material delivered in a multimedia format or presented interactively.

Informed by preferences indicated by responses to each of the questions, the LICBT practitioner can introduce the range of LICBT modalities available.

Clinical Example

Example Dialogue to Introduce LICBT Modality

Using low-intensity CBT, we will be working together to help you tackle the difficulties we've talked about in the assessment. Between sessions you will be asked to complete some planned directed learning activities to help you learn and try out new skills. Delivery of these activities is available through workbooks, an online computer programme or audiobook supplemented by worksheets. Because you told me you like information delivered through [Daily Mirror/Telegraph/Sun/Times Newspaper, BBC Online News, academic texts, audiobooks, radio], it may be that [written/cCBT/ audio] best meets your preferences. However, the choice of the way you would like to work through low-intensity CBT is up to you. Do you have any questions about any approaches, or would you like to see brief examples of each?

The aim of asking these questions is for the LICBT practitioner to move away from fully describing all the different modalities available and instead focus on recommending just one or two individualised recommendations based on their clinical and learning assessments. On occasions it can be helpful to provide examples of cCBT programmes, such as showing a short piece of video of the programme content and how it can be used.

Choosing Written LICBT Intervention

If a written LICBT intervention is most appropriate, significant variation exists in the way written materials are presented (Martinez et al., 2008) and these should be considered before recommending a specific written intervention.

Key Point

Different Ways Written Materials Are Presented

- Writing style
  - Academic or informal and conversational
  - Active or passive voice.
- Reading age
  - Lower reading age with simpler and shorter sentences
  - Higher reading age with use of technical terms, often presented within longer sentences
  - Consideration should normally be given to recommending written LICBT interventions with a low reading age. On occasions, however, the patient may consider these to be patronising and a written intervention with a higher reading age could be considered.
- Interactivity
  - A fundamental characteristic of CBT is that the patient is active between sessions, engaging with worksheets and undertaking activities. Written resources, however, vary in the extent to which they support interactivity. On these occasions, the extent to which they actually reflect a CBT approach should be considered
  - Interactive: Sections of text describing the presenting difficulty and specific factors associated with the LICBT intervention alongside worksheets associated with the *here and now* CBT model (Chapter 1) and LICBT intervention
  - Highly interactive: Use of text response boxes, tick boxes throughout the text in addition to wider sections of text and specific LICBT worksheets.
- Presentation
  - Large sections of white space compared to more dense presentation of text
  - Use of illustrations to supplement text.

Given large variations in the way written LICBT interventions are presented, it can be helpful for LICBT practitioners to have small extracts from a range of relevant interventions to provide the patient with examples to inform their choice and ensure the best match.

Summary

LICBT interventions are best seen as teaching resources with an aim to help patients become their own therapist and better manage their wellbeing. As with any learning resources, those that communicate well are the most effective and maintain engagement when they match the learning preferences of the patient. The match between the patient's preferred learning style and way in which the LICBT intervention is presented can be enhanced through careful consideration of the modality in which the intervention is presented. Identifying patient learning style during assessment will help to best match them with the most acceptable modality delivering the LICBT intervention with potential to enhance engagement, reduce drop-out and improve outcomes.

Assessing Your Understanding

Declarative

Multiple Choice Questions

1. Which of the following represent *advantages* of written CBT LICBT interventions? [Select all that apply]
    (a) They are always regularly revised
    (b) Mostly written in a way to match the reading age of the general population
    (c) Help to normalise the experience of the patient
    (d) Content is available for repeated consultation
    (e) Translation into different languages is commonly done by authors
2. Which of the following are *true* with respect to computerised/internet based LICBT interventions? [Select all that apply]
    (a) Free to use programmes often become fee-paying over time
    (b) Websites and apps need to be commonly updated to continue working
    (c) Almost all NHS services allow staff to email patients to provide support
    (d) Video chat applications never store data
    (e) Personalisation of content to match patient demographics is commonly done

3. Which of the following are *true* with respect to written LICBT interventions? [Select all that apply]
    (a) Reading age is consistent with that for the majority of the population
    (b) The potential for interventions to be patronising should still be a consideration even when reading age is consistent with that for the majority of the population
    (c) To improve accessibility for the patient they are never written adopting a more academic writing style
    (d) Readers always prefer case-based examples
    (e) Published books can be easily photocopied and given freely to patients

Procedural

- Work with a colleague to role play identifying their learning style and match this to the best modality of presentation and learning resources. Reflect upon any challenges you experienced.
- Identify the range of LICBT resources available to you across presentation modalities and familiarise yourself with the ways in which they support learning.

    Answers to **Assessing Your Understanding** questions can be found in the appendix on p. 335.

Further Reading and Resources

Martinez, R. and Williams, C. (2010) Matching clients to CBT self-help resources. In J. Bennett-Levy, D. Richards, P. Farrand, H. Christensen, K. Griffiths, D. Kavanagh, B. Klein, M.A. Lau, J. Proudfoot, L. Ritterband, J. White and C. Williams (eds) (2010) *Oxford Guide to Low-Intensity CBT Interventions*. Oxford: Oxford University Press.

Free access CBT psychoeducational leaflets:

- Living Life to the Full (www.llttf.com/resources)
- Northumberland leaflets (https://web.ntw.nhs.uk/selfhelp)
- Royal College of Psychiatrists CBT intervention leaflets (www.rcpsych.ac.uk/mental-health/problems-disorders).

Free access worksheets:

- GetSelfHelp (www.getselfhelp.co.uk)
- Living Life to the Full (www.llttf.com/resources).

Audiobook and audio recording resources (relaxation/mindfulness):
Visit your preference of

- Amazon Music
- Audible
- Living Life to the Full (www.llttf.com/resources)
- Spotify.

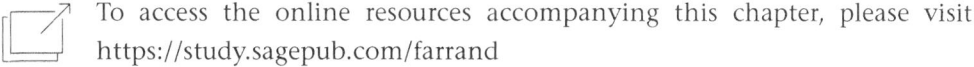 To access the online resources accompanying this chapter, please visit: https://study.sagepub.com/farrand

8

Using Behaviour Change Models to Support Low-Intensity Cognitive Behavioural Therapy Interventions

Enabling Patients to Engage and Make Lasting Change

Paul Chadwick

Learning Objectives

At the end of this chapter readers should be able to:

- Understand and describe the Capability, Opportunity, Motivation – Behaviour (COM-B) model of behaviour and the Behaviour Change Wheel Framework
- Identify opportunities for applying behaviour change principles within low-intensity CBT interventions
- Apply the COM-B model to carry out a behavioural diagnosis to identify barriers to behaviours related to LICBT outcomes
- Apply the COM-B model and Intervention Functions of the Behaviour Change Wheel to identify interventions to change influences on behaviour

Introduction

Recovery from anxiety and depression requires individuals to change their behaviour, with the behaviour changes required multiple and varied. These changes may involve carrying out the behaviours outlined in CBT protocols (e.g. completing activity scheduling diaries or thought records), using CBT self-help resources (e.g. reading and following the guidance in a self-help manual) and taking medication as prescribed. Behaviours may also influence the degree to which patients engage with psychological support (e.g. turning up to appointments). Given the centrality of behaviour to the outcome of all therapeutic interventions it makes sense for low-intensity CBT (LICBT) practitioners to understand what drives behaviour, and how to modify it to maximise wellbeing.

Models, Theories and Frameworks of Behaviour Change

A recent scoping review has identified 83 formal theories of behaviour change that could be applied to low-intensity interventions (Michie et al., 2014). Whilst it is not practical for LICBT practitioners to learn and apply all of these in routine practice, simple and parsimonious models of behaviour are available to guide assessment and intervention. The most common of these is the Capability, Opportunity, Motivation – Behaviour model (COM-B; Michie et al., 2011). COM-B states that there are three necessary conditions for the performance of any behaviour – Capability, Opportunity and Motivation (Michie et al., 2011).

___

Key Point
___

Necessary Conditions for Behaviour

- Capability: The physical and psychological abilities to complete a behaviour
  - Physical
    - Physical skills, strengths and stamina to behave in a certain way (e.g. being fit enough to travel on public transport to get to appointments).
  - Psychological
    - Mental process required to carry out a behaviour, such as knowing what to do and how to do it
    - Ability to engage in the necessary mental (e.g. decision-making) and behavioural regulation (e.g. goal-directed behaviour) processes to perform it.
- Opportunity: Influences on behaviour that are largely external to the individual and are found in the physical and social environment

- ○ Physical
  - □ Resources (e.g. financial) and cues that facilitate or trigger behaviour
  - □ Ways the physical environment may influence behaviour (e.g. set-up of the home or work environment).
- ○ Social
  - □ Ways in which behaviour is shaped by interpersonal influences such as through behavioural norms, peer influences and role models
  - □ Broader aspects such as the linguistic and cultural resources that shape behaviour and its expression.
- Motivation: Conscious and unconscious processes that energise and direct behaviour.
  - ○ Automatic
    - □ Emotional states and reactions (e.g. actual or anticipated feelings of guilt when completing self-monitoring records)
    - □ Drive states such as fatigue, hunger and withdrawal
    - □ Automatic learnt behaviour performed outside of conscious control (e.g. eating in response to stress) that constitute habits.
  - ○ Reflective
    - □ Conscious plans, beliefs, desires and intentions that influence behaviour (e.g. the way an individual's identity and values shape their beliefs and goals)
    - □ Beliefs about the consequences of changing behaviour (e.g. whether it will be harmful or beneficial) or about whether they can make the change (e.g. self-efficacy).

Achieving behaviour change can therefore be considered as opening a COM-Bination lock where all relevant enablers to complete the behaviour need to be in place. If just one of these is not in place, the desired behaviour will not be performed. The COM-B model of behaviour sits at the hub of the Behaviour Change Wheel framework (BCW; Michie et al., 2014), a systematic but pragmatic approach to understanding and changing behaviour in context. The BCW is a synthesis of 19 frameworks of behaviour change identified in a systematic literature review and consists of three layers (Figure 8.1).

Surrounding the COM-B hub is a layer of nine intervention functions that can be used to address deficits in one or more of the three necessary conditions. These intervention functions can then be linked to specific behaviour change techniques (BCTs) that represent the active components of an intervention described in published taxonomies (Michie et al., 2013). Finally, the outer layer of the wheel identifies seven types of policy that can be used to deliver or reinforce the impact of the intervention functions. Although application of the full BCW process is not possible in routine LICBT clinical practice, elements of the approach, particularly the COM-B model, may be helpful when working with patients experiencing difficulties with engagement.

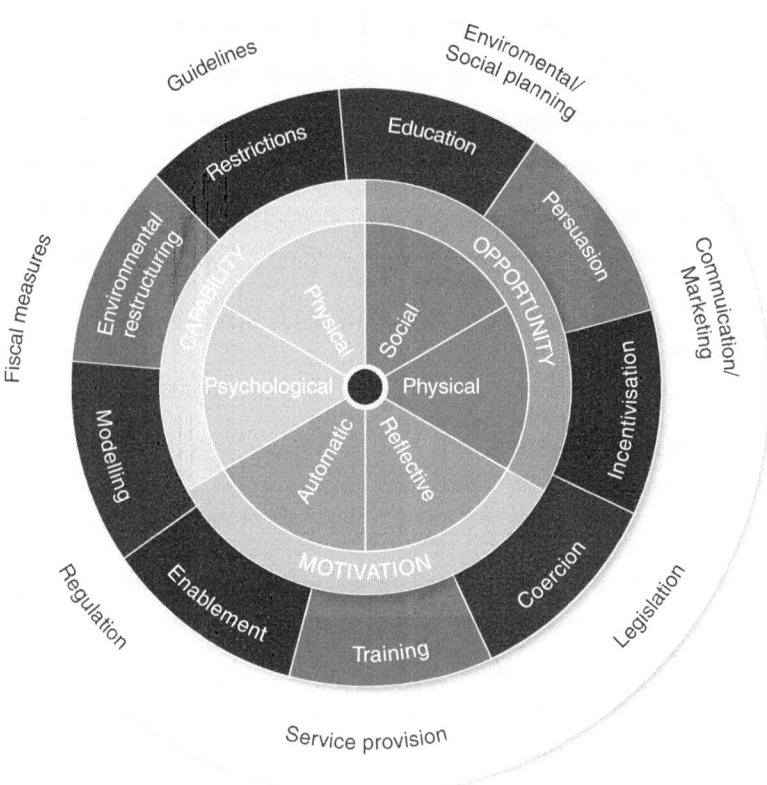

Figure 8.1   The Behaviour Change Wheel

Source: Michie, S., Atkins, L. and West, R. (2014) *The Behaviour Change Wheel: A Guide to Designing Interventions*.
London: Silverback Publishing. www.behaviourchangewheel.com

Reflection Point

Identify a behaviour change you have been struggling to make in your own life related to physical or psychological wellbeing. Use the COM-B model to generate a behavioural diagnosis for
yourself and identify some interventions you could carry out to modify those influences.

Application of COM-B to Support LICBT Interventions

The COM-B model can be applied within support sessions on occasions when the
patient has experienced difficulties engaging with the LICBT intervention between
sessions (Chapter 6). There are three stages in the process of using COM-B to address
difficulties with engagement.

Clinical Practice

Intervention Stages

- *Step 1*: Identify targets for behaviour change
- *Step 2*: Understanding what needs to change – behavioural diagnosis
- *Step 3*: Designing and delivering interventions to modify influences on a behaviour.

Step 1: Identifying Targets for Behaviour Change

Difficulties with engagement present in two forms:

- Problems carrying out a specific therapeutic technique – for example, doing relaxation exercises
- General lack of engagement with the process of therapy itself – for example, repeatedly turning up late to appointments.

The following Clinical Practice box illustrates some of the behaviours that may be targeted as part of engagement.

Clinical Practice

Common Difficulties Faced Engaging with LICBT

- *Specific factors engaging with the intervention between sessions*: for example, scheduling time to use LICBT intervention, completing techniques within the LICBT intervention such as filling out thought records, completing graded exposure tasks, addressing necessary tasks identified in the Behavioural Activation schedule.
- Engaging within-support session: for example, difficulty completing worksheets due to physical difficulties, challenges with English as a second language.
- Attending sessions: for example, turning up at the right time, not being able to access support required to attend.
- Medication: for example, taking medication as prescribed, following dietary guidance to avoid certain foods.

Once difficulties with engagement have been identified, LICBT practitioners can work collaboratively with the patient to identify the behaviours that need to change in order to enhance engagement and improve treatment response. For example, if a patient is struggling to make progress because they are struggling to carry out relaxation exercises between sessions, the practitioner can highlight this and suggest that they work together to identify why this is the case, empathising with challenges experienced (Chapter 5). Reframing difficulties with engagement in terms of behaviours can help avoid the perception of blame. This approach can help maintain a supportive therapeutic alliance and reinforce the benefit of problem-focused support (Chapter 6).

Step 2: Understanding What Needs to Change – Behavioural Diagnosis

This involves understanding why the patient is having difficulty with performing the behaviours that will improve their response to the LICBT intervention. Just as we expect doctors to make a diagnosis of the nature of a medical complaint before recommending or implementing a treatment, LICBT practitioners should seek to understand what might be preventing the patient from using specific therapeutic techniques, or other behaviours getting in the way of engaging with the therapeutic process, before collaboratively initiating a plan to change them. The process of figuring out what it is about the patient or their environment that needs to change for them to do the behaviour is known as the behavioural diagnosis.

Using COM-B to develop a behavioural diagnosis

Behavioural diagnosis involves using the COM-B model to identify what needs to be in place for the patient to perform the behaviour(s) getting in the way of engaging with the therapeutic process. Different constructs fall under each of the three COM-B domains and LICBT practitioners can ask themselves a number of questions to generate hypotheses about the patient's behaviour (Table 8.1).

The three necessary conditions for behaviour – capability, opportunity, motivation – influence each other (Michie et al., 2011). For example, making something easier by increasing capability or opportunity can increase motivation to do it (Figure 8.2).

An effective behavioural diagnosis identifies the different capability, opportunity and motivational influences for a behaviour, also considering how they interact. For example, patients may experience poor motivation to engage with an LICBT intervention because they do not fully understand how to apply the specific factors

Table 8.1 Questions for LICBT practitioners to consider when supporting behavioural diagnosis and formulating areas to explore

Necessary condition	Questions
Capability	Do they know what the desired behaviour is?
	Do they have the strength, stamina, psychomotor skills or dexterity to do the behaviour?
	Do they have the mental skills required?
	a. Memory, attention and decision-making skills?
	b. Numeracy and literacy skills?
	c. Interpersonal skills?
	d. Self-regulation skills?
	Do they understand why it is important for them to do it and how to do it?
Opportunity	Do they have the time, financial or material resources to do the desired behaviour?
	Do they have the social support required?
	Do they have access to credible models for performing the behaviour?
	Do they need more or less exposure to certain physical or social influences in order to change the behaviour?
	What are the linguistic or cultural influences on the performance of the behaviour?
Motivation	What are the person's values and how does this influence the behaviour?
	What do they believe will happen if they perform the behaviour?
	Do they believe they can perform the behaviour (self-efficacy)?
	What is the role of habit and routine in performing the behaviour?
	What emotions are generated by performing the behaviour?

(capability) or have not yet found an easy or practical way to carry out a technique (opportunity). Collaboratively working with the patient to reach a behavioural diagnosis can help improve transparency, increase engagement and empower patients to make change. This will minimise the potential for rupturing the relationship between the LICBT practitioner and patient (Safran and Safran, 2000).

Behavioural diagnosis is an iterative process and it may take several cycles of hypothesis generation and testing to reach an accurate understanding of the

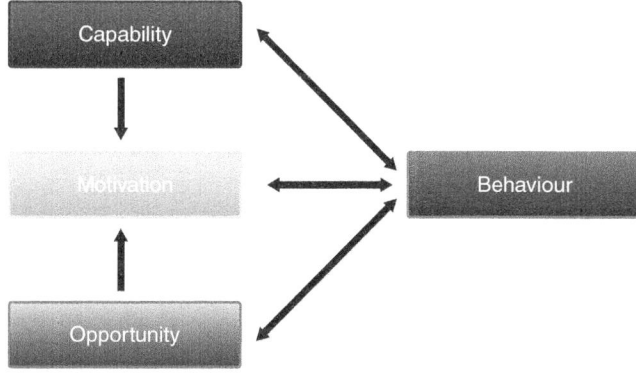

Figure 8.2 The COM-B Model of Behaviour

Source: Michie, S., van Stralen, M.M. and West, R. (2011) The behaviour change wheel: a new method for characterising and designing behaviour change interventions. *Implementation Science*, 6, 42.

influences on behaviours associated with poor engagement. Table 8.2 illustrates how COM-B can be used to develop and test out hypotheses to improve attendance of the patient at LICBT support sessions. LICBT practitioners can also use COM-B as a tool for thinking and reflecting on any challenges faced supporting the patient during clinical skills or case management supervision (Chapter 9).

Step 3: Designing and Delivering Interventions to Modify Influences on a Behaviour

The behavioural diagnosis alerts the LICBT practitioner to factors that may be influencing a patient's behaviour. This is the starting point for thinking about ways to address any difficulties. LICBT practitioners should use a collaborative problem-solving approach with patients to identify ways to overcome difficulties engaging

Table 8.2 Using COM-B to generate hypotheses concerning a patient struggling to attend support sessions and identify strategies

Domain	Hypothesis		Strategy to test hypothesis
Capability	Physical	• Patient experiencing health issues influencing ability to get to the appointment	• Ask the patient if they are having any health problems that are getting in the way of attending
	Psychological	• Patient does not know the quickest route to get to the clinic • Patient does not have the skills to organise their daily routine to create enough time to attend	• Ask the patient to describe their typical journey to the appointment • Ask the patient to describe their typical routine prior to the appointment on days that they are late, and days that they are on time
Opportunity	Physical	• Patient does not have the money or time to get to the appointment	• Ask the patient whether they have enough money to travel to appointments
	Social	• Other people are influencing the patient's ability to get to the appointment	• Ask the patient if other people influence their ability to get to the appointment on time, and if so what they do
Motivation	Reflective	• Patient does not believe that turning up late to support sessions has any consequences • Patient does not believe they have any ability to improve attendance at support sessions	• Ask the patient whether they understand how turning up late influences their ability to benefit from the sessions • Explore the patient's beliefs about whether it is possible to change
	Automatic	• Patient believes that turning up late will help reduce their anxiety	• Ask the patient about any emotional influences on their ability to turn up on time, including exploration of what emotions might be avoided by turning up late

with the LICBT intervention or techniques. Additionally, LICBT practitioners can use information collected during the behavioural diagnosis to modify how they interact with a patient to encourage engagement (see Case Study: Behavioural Activation). In most cases the opportunities for intervention will be obvious and emerge from collaborative discussions between the patient and LICBT practitioner (Table 8.3).

Table 8.3 Examples of adopting COM-B to inform ways of supporting the patient to overcome difficulties engaging with the LICBT intervention

Necessary condition	Ways to overcome difficulty
Capability (Physical)	Remove the physical effort involved in performing a behaviour (e.g. offering telephone appointments)
Capability (Psychological)	*Knowledge/Skills:* Provide information in session – paper or online materials that will support patients develop the required knowledge (e.g. signposting to a website about a particular community group)
	Memory, attention and decision-making skills: Make written or audio recordings of the main action points reached within session for patients with memory or attentional difficulties to inform behaviour between sessions
	Self-regulation skills: Support patients apply the principles of SMART goal-setting, behavioural self-monitoring, problem solving and action-planning, so they are better able to put plans into action
Opportunity (Physical)	*Time:* Use diary scheduling to help patients make time for engaging with the LICBT intervention or specific techniques
	Resources: Provide patients with resources (e.g. online self-help tools, apps) to make it easier to perform the behaviour
	Triggers and cues: Identify triggers or cues that can be placed in the patient's environment to help them perform the behaviour
Opportunity (Social)	*Peer influences:* Identify different sources of social support that may help the patient undertake the behaviour and work with them to identify how to make use of them
	Modelling: Put the patient in touch with support groups or other individuals who successfully perform the behaviour
	Norms: Provide the patient with information about how typical or desirable the behaviour is (e.g. most people who engage in an LICBT intervention do some form of self-monitoring)
	Language and cultural: Put the patient in touch with other people from the same cultural background who have experienced and overcome similar barriers or offer sources of support
Motivation (Reflective)	*Beliefs about consequences:* Construct a behavioural experiment with the client to test the accuracy of any predictions that harm will arise from performing the behaviour
	Beliefs about control: Use graded hierarchies and positive reinforcement to help clients increase their belief that they can perform the behaviour
	Habits and routines: Use positive reinforcement or help the patient overcome sources of negative reinforcement to establish new habits and routines for the desired behaviour
Motivation (Automatic)	*Emotions:* Encourage the patient to use a thought record between sessions to challenge unhelpful thoughts leading to strong emotions that discourage performance of the behaviour

Using BCW Intervention Functions to Modify Influences on Behaviour

LICBT practitioners can also use intervention functions of the BCW to generate ideas to overcome difficulties identified in the behavioural diagnosis. Intervention functions comprise eight distinct ways in which influences on behaviour can be modified (Table 8.4).

Most LICBT interventions will contain techniques for changing behaviour that involve several different intervention functions.

Table 8.4 Identifying intervention functions to generate ideas to support LICBT interventions

Intervention function	Definition	Example
Education	Increasing knowledge and understanding by informing, explaining, showing and providing feedback	Working with the patient within support sessions to check understanding regarding the theoretical basis for the intervention and addressing any misunderstandings or confusion
Persuasion	Using words and images to change the way a patient considers a behaviour to make it more or less attractive	Inviting a patient to reflect on the benefits they may experience as a result of engaging with self-monitoring
Incentivisation	Changing the attractiveness of a behaviour by creating the expectation of a desired outcome or avoidance of an undesired one	Working with the patient to instigate a reward system for engaging with a step in their exposure hierarchy
Training	Increasing the skills needed for a behaviour by providing repeated practice and feedback	Working collaboratively with the patient within session to start a thought record
Restriction	Constraining performance of a behaviour by setting rules	Asking the patient to form a rule to help them complete the behaviour (e.g. no television until at least one thought record has been completed)
Environmental restructuring	Constraining or promoting behaviour by shaping the physical or social environment	Working with the patient to set an alert on their phone to perform self-monitoring tasks
Modelling	Showing examples of the behaviour for people to imitate	Sharing anonymised stories of how other patients have overcome barriers completing necessary activities identified during behavioural activation
Enablement	Providing support to improve ability to change in a variety of ways not covered by other intervention types	Providing the patient access to an online platform which makes it easier to complete self-monitoring tasks

Key Point

Intervention Functions Associated with Behavioural Activation (BA)

- Education: teaching the theoretical basis and intervention principles
- Training: giving feedback to the patient on their attempts to categorise routine, pleasurable and necessary activities and add activities to the diary
- Enablement: providing access to resources that make it easier to schedule activities.

If supported within a group setting intervention functions may also include:

- Modelling: encouraging group members to share experiences
- Incentivisation: creating conditions for positive reinforcement in the form of praise between group members.

The use of intervention functions to address barriers engaging with a LICBT intervention is illustrated in the case study that highlights application with a patient experiencing barriers completing a BA schedule (Chapter 11).

Clinical Example

Case Study: Behavioural Activation

Lucas had been attending support sessions with Beth, his LICBT practitioner, to deal with depression. He struggled to appreciate the BA theoretical rationale or understand how to complete the stages of the LICBT BA intervention and so made little effort to engage with the intervention between sessions. Applying the COM-B model to this behaviour, Beth was able to elicit the fact that Lucas felt stupid for not being able to grasp the theoretical rationale (*automatic motivation* – negative emotions) and was avoiding engaging with the intervention for fear that Beth would judge him (*reflective motivation* – beliefs about consequences). Using this understanding, Beth was able to reassure Lucas that she was not judging him (*persuasion*), explain that many patients experience similar difficulties (*modelling*), and suggested that they spend time in the following support session starting each stage of the intervention together (*training*) for Lucas to continue with the intervention between sessions. Within subsequent support sessions Beth took care to ensure that she always verbally praised any attempt by Lucas to complete activities included within his BA schedule (*incentivisation*).

Working with Multiple Influences on Behaviour

On occasions where there are multiple influences on the target behaviour, LICBT practitioners should consider the potential interactions between different influences when planning interventions. Ways to effectively work with behaviours where there are multiple influences at play is illustrated in the case study that highlights application with a patient experiencing barriers completing exposure therapy (Chapter 13).

Clinical Example

Case Study: Exposure Therapy

Ashanti attended LICBT support sessions to address her fear of driving over bridges. With the help of her LICBT practitioner Anika, she constructed an exposure hierarchy by repeatedly turning up to sessions without starting the process. Using the COM-B model Anika was able to identify two influences on Ashanti's lack of engagement with the exposure protocol. Ashanti stated that the long diversions she takes to avoid driving over bridges means that she has little time to start work on the exposure hierarchy (*physical opportunity* – time). After some exploration she also revealed that she had a very low belief that the exposure technique would actually work for her (*automatic motivation* – beliefs about consequences). Anika took the case to her clinical supervisor to help her think about which COM-B influence to tackle first. In this case they considered that it would be more effective to tackle the *motivational* influence before addressing the *physical opportunity* influence. This could be achieved by reviewing Ashanti's understanding of the theoretical rationale for exposure therapy (*education*) using brief motivational interviewing techniques within the support session to help address her belief that exposure would be ineffective. Once Ashanti appreciates the theoretical rationale and has a stronger belief in the benefits of exposure, she is more likely to accept this as a useful treatment option and engage with it. Anika and her supervisor reflected that addressing the time influence (*physical opportunity*) without first addressing unhelpful beliefs in the effectiveness of exposure (*automatic motivation*) would be unlikely to lead to change.

Summary

Adopting LICBT to manage or recover from a common mental health difficulty always involves some degree of behaviour change in the patient. The COM-B model (Michie et al., 2011) and the Behaviour Change Wheel framework (Michie et al., 2014) offer LICBT practitioners and supervisors a systematic way of understanding the drivers underlying the behaviours that facilitate engagement with LICBT or that get in the way of recovery. These models and frameworks can also be used to generate solutions to any barriers that are uncovered.

Assessing Your Understanding

Declarative

Classify the following influences on medication-taking behaviour in terms of whether they primarily operate through capability, opportunity or motivation.

1. Having a feeling of shame about having a mental health problem
2. Having a messy and chaotic living space
3. Memory problems relating to symptoms of depression
4. Partner is scornful about taking medication
5. Belief that psychoactive medications are toxic to the body
6. Symptoms of peripheral neuropathy in the fingertips which makes opening medication blister packs painful and fiddly

Procedural

Pick a recent LICBT support session where you have been working on an issue relating to engagement with a patient.

a) Reflect on the questions you used to understand their behaviour and classify them according to the COM-B model.
b) Use the information in the chapter to generate a bank of questions that you could ask patients in order to help you carry out a behavioural diagnosis in future sessions.

Repeat this exercise for situations where patients do not carry out between-session tasks.

> Answers to Assessing Your Understanding questions can be found in the appendix on p. 335.

Further Reading and Resources

Behaviour Change Wheel (www.behaviourchangewheel.com).

Michie, S., van Stralen, M. and West, R. (2011) The Behaviour Change Wheel: a new method for characterising and designing behaviour change interventions. *Implementation Science*, 6, 42.

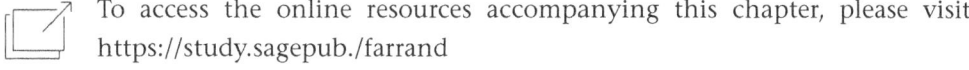 To access the online resources accompanying this chapter, please visit: https://study.sagepub./farrand

9

Supervision in Low-Intensity CBT
Fundamental to the Clinical Method

Faye Small

Learning Objectives

By the end of this chapter LICBT practitioners and supervisors should be able to:

- Appreciate the purpose of supervision for low-intensity practitioners
- Demonstrate an awareness regarding the function of supervision in low-intensity CBT
- Critically evaluate differences between case management and clinical skills supervision
- Critically evaluate the fundamental role of case management supervision in the low-intensity clinical method
- Develop competency in the delivery of case management and clinical skills supervision

Background

Although different definitions of supervision are evident across all psychological therapies (Milne, 2009; Scaife, 2001), supporting the development of new skills and increasing the likelihood of achieving the best outcomes for patients are common aims (Binnie, 2011; Turpin and Wheeler, 2011). To achieve these aims, supervision of clinical practice seeks to deliver on three main objectives (Inskipp and Proctor, 1993).

Key Point

Supervision Objectives

- *Formative*: Facilitation of learning and development around practitioners' delivery of patient work.
- *Normative*: Ensuring adherence to professional and ethical standards. This is inclusive of the supervisor overseeing overall responsibility for patient care in addition to supporting the practitioner adhere to organisational requirements such as length of sessions and number of patient contacts. It is also helpful to agree on an ethical framework to adhere to.
- *Restorative*: Facilitation and support of emotional processing. This can be focused on emotional content within patient work, organisational stressors and personal difficulties that may impact on a practitioner's work. The restorative function acknowledges the emotional impact on the individual and the potential impact upon their patient work. A trusting relationship is essential to support this function (Scaife, 2001).

As highlighted, supervision remains fundamental to the clinical method of all psychological therapies. However, with a focused training curriculum, a workforce that often has less experience on entry into training, combined with high-volume working, makes supervision especially important for the low-intensity CBT (LICBT) workforce (Chapter 1; Shepherd and Rosario, 2008).

Supervision in Low-Intensity CBT

In traditional models of supervision all three objectives are achieved within clinical skills (CS) supervision. However, to optimise patient outcomes in LICBT, CS supervision is provided alongside case management (CM) supervision to achieve five main objectives (Turpin and Wheeler, 2011). Engagement with both forms of supervision is more likely to enhance the effectiveness of LICBT practitioners and achieve better patient outcomes (Bower et al., 2006; Green et al., 2014).

Key Point

LICBT Supervision Objectives (Turpin and Wheeler, 2011)

- *Fidelity to the evidence base*: Ensures interventions are delivered in line with NICE guidance.
- *Case management and collaborative care*: Review of all cases on caseload to facilitate regular liaison with other healthcare professionals.

- *Clinical governance*: Ensures adherence to service governance structures, protocols, fidelity to risk management protocols and appropriate ethical guidelines.
- *Continued personal and professional development*: Facilitates skills development and access to ongoing training.
- *Supports staff and prevents burnout*: Provides support for personal and professional difficulties.

To achieve these supervision objectives, the supervisory alliance remains key to effective supervision (Ladany et al., 1999; Ramos-Sanchez et al., 2002) and is associated with lower levels of practitioner burnout alongside higher levels of wellbeing (Livni et al., 2012).

Case Management

CM supervision was originally developed as part of the Pathways trial to provide a model of supervision to support a collaborative care case manager (Katon et al., 2004). This represented a new role undertaken by registered nurses working within a stepped care (Chapter 1) service delivery model for patients with diabetes and co-morbid depression. Positive outcomes from this trial informed implementation of collaborative care and CM supervision into the Doncaster demonstration site established as part of the Improving Access to Psychological Therapies (IAPT) programme (Richards and Suckling, 2008). Recognising this unique form of supervision has led to a dedicated supervisory competence framework for LICBT CM supervisors (Roth and Pilling, 2008).

Key Point

Characteristics of CM Supervision Implemented within the IAPT Programme (Turpin and Wheeler, 2011)

- Weekly, individual, hour-long, service-led review of cases on an LICBT practitioner caseload undertaken by a CM supervisor
- Cases pre-selected using defined selection criteria (Richards et al., 2008)
- Balances patient need with available resources
- Undertaken by a member of the healthcare workforce trained to deliver CM supervision with knowledge and competency in LICBT.

As implemented within the IAPT programme, CM supervision is therefore 'central to the effectiveness of LICBT within the IAPT model' (Richards, 2010a: 129). It enables the LICBT workforce to carry patient caseloads comprising 45+ active cases at any time (Richards and Whyte, 2008) whilst achieving better patient outcomes (Firth et al., 2015). Without CM supervision the high-volume nature of LICBT working would be unlikely to be as effective (Pullen and Loudon, 2006). Challenges have been recognised, however, regarding difficulties the CM supervisor may face when juggling potentially conflicting service and patient demands (Applebaum and Austin, 1990).

Clinical Skills

A number of different models exist regarding CS supervision (Milne, 2009). Within LICBT however, the main function of CS supervision is to complement CM supervision to support the 'development and maintenance of competence in low-intensity methods' (Turpin and Wheeler, 2011: 6).

Key Point

Characteristics of CS supervision implemented within the IAPT programme (Turpin and Wheeler, 2011)

- Minimum of one hour per fortnight
- Delivered on a one-to-one basis or as part of a group to manage service resource considerations
- Literature differs around the ideal size of a group varying from 3–12 practitioners (Proctor and Inskipp, 2001) to a maximum of six (Vec et al., 2014).

In doing so, as with HICBT, it is important that CS supervision reflects the LICBT clinical method (Corrie and Lane, 2015; Liese and Beck, 1997), which may be different to traditional forms of CS supervision. It is also important that CS supervision places a specific focus on avoiding 'therapeutic drift' (Waller, 2009) from the LICBT clinical method into non-evidence based 'medium intensity CBT' (Chapter 1).

Enhancing the Delivery of Clinical Skills Supervision

To help address limited guidance regarding features of CS supervision, the Declarative-Procedural-Reflective (DPR; Bennett-Levy, 2006) model of therapist skills development has been adopted as a useful framework. For practitioners new to the role, especially if they have had less experience on entry into training, using the DPR systems can provide a useful structure for CS supervision to support the ongoing development of competence in the LICBT clinical method.

Table 9.1 Examples of ways the DPR model can be used to inform clinical skills supervision

System	Focus for supervision	Question type	Example low-intensity question	Potential learning strategies
Declarative	Knowledge gaps – e.g. how to apply an intervention	Information questions (Who? What? Why?)	Which disorder-specific measure should I use? What is negative reinforcement?	Reading, lectures, didactic/modelling, case studies
Procedural	Procedural gaps – e.g. how to apply the intervention to a patient who does not fit the usual conventions	Learning questions (How could I?)	How can I explain habituation to a patient? My patient has chronic fatigue, how can I apply behavioural activation?	Practice, experiential training, role play, experiential/ modelling
Reflective	Reflective challenges – e.g. emotional processing of cases or the need to develop skills further	Feedback questions (How did I do? Was it OK?)	My patient was talking about something I found very upsetting. My patient was really talkative and I ran over time. How can I manage this differently?	Reflective attitude, reflective practice, reflective/Socratic supervision, reflective writing/ reading

Using the DPR model to structure CS supervision may also provide a 'safe space' through the reflective system for the LICBT workforce to address professional or personal challenges and the potential for burnout (Painter, 2018; Steel et al., 2015). This would address one of the main concerns directed at supervision of the LICBT workforce that highlights a perceived lack of emotional support facilitated through supervision (Painter, 2018; Rizq et al., 2010). Potentially such concerns arise from a misunderstanding of LICBT supervision whereby CM supervision is considered to be a stand-alone supervision model, rather than being recognised as performing different functions alongside CS supervision.

Specific Factors

Case Management Supervision

The predominant characteristic of CM supervision that facilitates the delivery of collaborative care within the IAPT programme is the use of pre-defined selection criteria to identify cases for supervision (Richards et al., 2008). Where cases meet multiple criteria, they should be categorised by importance.

Reflection Question

Reflect upon some of the challenges you may face when taking cases to case management supervision. How might you address these challenges? What support could you access?

Clinical Practice

Patient Selection Criteria for Case Management Supervision

- New to caseload
- Presenting with high risk
- Presenting with high scores (suggested as a score of 15 and above on the PHQ-9 (Kroenke et al., 2001)) and/or GAD-7 (Spitzer et al., 2006)
- Scheduled review (usually every fourth contact)
- Did not attend a scheduled appointment (DNA)
- Further support where practitioners can discuss patients who do not fit into any of the other pre-determined categories.

Once patient cases have been selected according to these criteria, CM supervision follows four main stages. Given the level of detail discussed in the presentation of each case, preparation for CM supervision is key and the use of patient selection criteria essential to effectively progress through each of these stages.

Clinical Practice

Stages Involved in CM Supervision

- *Stage 1:* Check for burnout
- *Stage 2:* Introduce caseload
- *Stage 3:* Individual case discussion
- *Stage 4:* Summary and action planning.

Stage 1: Check for Burnout

The first stage of CM supervision requires the practitioner to introduce the size of their overall caseload to raise discussion around caseload manageability (Richards et al., 2008; Roth and Pilling, 2008). This enables the CM supervisor to monitor potential indicators of practitioner burnout when working with high-volume caseloads. The LICBT workforce are, however, also able to raise issues that may lead to burnout within CS supervision.

Stage 2: Introduce Caseload

To manage the time available, the supervisee introduces the number of cases they are bringing to supervision and specifies the criteria by which cases have been selected. Whilst all selected cases should be overviewed within the time available, on occasions this may not be possible and prioritisation is required. When necessary, cases presented as meeting the high-risk criteria should be prioritised for discussion first.

Stage 3: Individual Case Discussion

The supervisee presents each case, providing a detailed account of information gathered from their work with the patient from assessment through treatment sessions (Table 9.2).

During initial case presentation the CM supervisor's role is to 'be alert to missing information' (Richards, 2010b: 133). They should therefore avoid interrupting the supervisee with questions about decision-making regarding the case as it is common that information they wish to ask about will shortly be presented. Case discussion should enable the CM supervisor to monitor the supervisee's clinical practice or allow the supervisee to ask questions. However, the expectation should be that the supervisee is able to reach clinical decisions themselves rather than the CM supervisor acting as an expert. Presentation and discussion of each case should be concluded within three to four minutes, making it reasonable to review up to 20 cases in an hour.

Stage 4: Summary and Action Planning

Brief discussion around each case is followed by the supervisee providing a summary and specifying an explicit action plan. Whilst the action plan may be as simple as continuing with the work already in place, specifying it serves to close off the particular case discussion and move to the next case. CM supervision is often where learning needs are identified (Richards, 2010b). Case discussions that appear more complex or require additional declarative or procedural skills development should be put on the agenda for a subsequent CS supervision session.

Clinical Skills Supervision

Consistent with HICBT, little specific guidance exists regarding the essential features of LICBT CS supervision (Corrie and Lane, 2015). However, several features have been found to be especially suitable to inform CS supervision for the LICBT workforce.

Table 9.2 Information for presentation of patient cases (based on Richards et al., 2010b)

Information to present for *all* patients taken to supervision
Category
Age
Gender
Main problem statement
Risk status
Onset and duration of problem
Previous episodes/past treatment
Current data set scores
Co-morbidity
Cultural, language, disability considerations
Employment status
Treatment from GP/other workers
COM-B considerations/barriers to treatment
Patient's goals
Low-intensity actions already taken
Low-intensity treatment plan
Additional information for patients where there is a four-weekly review, risk, high scores or further support
Reason for supervision
Intervention summary
Number and duration of contacts
Patient engagement
Patient response to treatment
Continuation scores
Treatment plan
Action plan
Additional information for patients who have not attended
Reason for supervision
Summary of progress before non-contact
Number of contact attempts made
Number and methods of contact attempted

Case Presentation

Presenting a case succinctly within CS supervision provides the supervisee with more time and opportunity to work on the supervision questions presented. This can be aided for the LICBT practitioner by using information previously gathered (Table 9.2) that provides important detail about a case without needing further lengthy discussion. Where necessary, additional relevant information may also be discussed to provide appropriate depth, but with recognition that case presentation should be succinct (Gordon, 2012).

Supervision Questions

The use of supervision questions relating to information (Who? What? Why?), learning (How could I?) and feedback (How did I do? Was it OK?) are essential to help supervisees make the most out of CS supervision (Gordon, 2012). These questions can be used to address features associated with each of the DPR systems (Table 9.1) associated with practitioner development (Bennett-Levy, 2006). Usually having less experience early in practice, it may be necessary to support the LICBT practitioner to develop well-formulated supervision questions and create a clear action plan when the supervision question has been addressed.

Agenda Items

As in all forms of CS supervision, the supervisee is encouraged to reflect on their practice and identify questions concerning practice to inform the agenda for the next CS supervision session. Questions serving as agenda items can be related to any aspect of practice. In LICBT, however, they may commonly arise from case discussions during CM supervision where the CM supervisor has identified issues related to clinical decision-making or patient treatment (Richards, 2010b). On these occasions it can be helpful for the CS supervisor to use supervision questions to identify the appropriate DPR system (Bennett-Levy, 2006) and learning strategy (Table 9.1) to enhance practitioner development. Active learning strategies are of most benefit to facilitate fidelity to the LICBT clinical model (Bearman et al., 2017; Gordon, 2012) where the development of procedural or reflective systems becomes the focus of supervision.

Enhancing the Reflective System

On occasions when the reflective system is identified as the focus of supervision, it is especially important for the CS supervisor to encourage reflective practice to enhance the development of clinical skills (Schön, 1983). This can represent a challenge in LICBT, however, as reflective practice is a skill that novice practitioners often find challenging early in training and practice (Farrand et al., 2016). Based on a model of reflective practice (Rolfe et al., 2001), an approach to support the development of reflective practice in the LICBT workforce during CS supervision has been developed to address this challenge (Worksheet 9.1).

Worksheet 9.1 Reflection record for use in clinical skills supervision (Farrand et al., 2016a)

Reflection record		
Name of PWP:	Name of supervisor:	Date of next clinical skills supervision:
To be completed before clinical skills supervision		
Section 1: Description and context of event		
Section 2: What is the problem/difficulty? What was I trying to achieve? What actions did I take? What were the consequences?		
Section 3: So... What does this tell me/teach me? What did I base my actions on? What other knowledge can I bring to the situation (literature)?		
Supervision question:		
To be completed at clinical skills supervision		
Section 4: Now what do I need to do differently to do things better?		
Section 5: Action plan... What practical steps can I take to achieve the above?		

In this approach a reflection record is used to support practitioners reflect during CS supervision when presenting a case (Farrand et al., 2016).

Clinical Practice

Using a Reflection Record to Support CS Supervision for the LICBT Workforce

- *Prior to supervision*: Based around their clinical practice, the supervisee completes sections 1–3 enabling them to generate a specific question to serve as the basis of CS supervision.
- *During the supervision session*: Case discussion with the CS supervisor supports the supervisee identify the steps they need to take to address the question and the steps are made explicit in section 4.
- *At the end of the supervision session*: The CS supervisor helps the supervisee summarise their reflective cycle and identify a series of explicit practical steps needed to address the problem or difficulty.

In addition to addressing supervision questions associated with clinical practice, the reflection record is also able to provide a focus on practitioner well-being to identify sources of available support, promote resiliency and prevent burnout.

Consideration of Supervision for the LICBT Workforce

As a consequence of the LICBT workforce often having lower levels of experience on entry into training and clinical practice, consideration should be given to the level of disclosure the supervisee may be willing to share within the supervisory relationship. Research has highlighted features of clinical practice that supervisees do and do not share with their supervisor (Gunn and Pistole, 2012; Ladany et al., 1996; Yourman, 2003). With respect to the LICBT practitioner with lower levels of experience concerns regarding disclosure can be particularly salient for individual cases representing diversity with respect to cultural norms including personal, family, social and spiritual values or presenting with risk. The practitioner may be less likely to present these cases for further support in CM supervision or formulate a CS supervision question about them for fear of negative evaluation by the supervisor. The supervisor should therefore be vigilant for signs of non-disclosure associated with all patient cases. This is especially important given that practitioner effectiveness is associated with their willingness to disclose within supervision (Green et al., 2014; Ladany et al., 1996).

Summary

Supervision for LICBT practitioners is an essential component to support effectiveness regarding the delivery of supported self-help within a stepped care framework (Richards, 2010b). CM supervision facilitates high-volume working by supporting the delivery of service protocols and ensuring patient progress and safety (Pullen and Loudon, 2006). CS supervision addresses the potential for practitioner burnout, the support of skills development and reflective practice for novice practitioners. However, to support better patient outcomes, CM and CS supervision cannot be delivered in isolation; the combination of both types of supervision is crucial to the success of the low-intensity CBT clinical method.

Assessing Your Understanding

Declarative

Extended Matching Question

1. Each answer is worth one mark.
2. There are 15 answers.
3. The question is worth 15 marks.
4. There *is* negative marking.
5. Answer by clearly writing the capital letter associated with each option in the response boxes provided after each question.
6. More response boxes are provided than answers, so you are not required to put an answer in each response box.
7. For each question, only those answers supplied within the appropriate spaces will be marked as correct. If you make an error, put a cross through the space with the answer in it and add a new space with the answer on the appropriate line.

Table 9.3 Theme: Selecting cases for clinical case management supervision

Options	
A Depression, on caseload for 2 weeks, little risk, last session disclosed childhood abuse. Entry: PHQ-9=19, GAD-7=13; Recent: PHQ-9=11, GAD-7=10	**N** Depression, on caseload for 2 weeks, little risk. Entry: PHQ-9=13, GAD-7=10; Recent: PHQ-9=17, GAD-7=6
B Agoraphobia, on caseload for 3 weeks, little risk. Entry: PHQ-9=15, GAD-7=19; Recent: PHQ-9=11, GAD-7=13	**O** Depression, on caseload for 2 weeks, little risk, some difficulties engaging with materials. PHQ-9=15, GAD-7=10; Recent: PHQ-9=13, GAD-7=8
C Depression, on caseload for 6 weeks, little risk. Entry: PHQ-9=21, GAD-7=3; Recent: PHQ-9=14, GAD-7=5	**P** Depression, on caseload for 5 weeks, little risk, started to talk about difficulty sleeping and bad nightmares. Entry: PHQ-9=16, GAD-7=10; Recent: PHQ-9=11, GAD-7=14
D GP referral for a new patient, during assessment patient highlighted an 8-year history of OCD. Entry: PHQ-9=10, GAD-7=14	**Q** Agoraphobia, on caseload for 3 weeks, little risk. Entry: PHQ-9= 8, GAD-7=16; Recent: PHQ-9=5, GAD-7=7
E Depression, new referral, appointment arranged, not yet seen.	**R** Panic disorder, new referral. Entry: PHQ-9=4, GAD-7=7
F Depression, on caseload for 6 weeks, little risk. Entry: PHQ-9=21, GAD-7=17; Recent: PHQ-9=25, GAD-7=20	**S** Specific phobia, on caseload for 4 weeks, little risk. Entry: PHQ-9= 8, GAD-7=9; Recent: PHQ-9=5, GAD-7=6
G Referred with depression, assessment completed and two treatment sessions arranged but never seen for treatment after missing both appointments. Entry: PHQ-9=16, GAD-7=10	**T** Depression, on caseload for 6 weeks, started to talk about suicide plan. Entry: PHQ-9=19, GAD-7=10; Recent: PHQ-9=6, GAD-7=7

Table 9.3 (Continued)

Options		

H Panic disorder, on caseload for 7 weeks, little risk. Entry: PHQ-9=14, GAD-7=16; Recent: PHQ-9=6, GAD-7=5

U Depression, on caseload for 3 weeks, little risk, engaging well. Entry: PHQ-9=18, GAD-7=4; Recent: PHQ-9=11, GAD-7=3

I Depression, on caseload for 6 weeks, little risk, current session appeared unrealistically positive. Entry: PHQ-9=23, GAD-7=12; Recent: PHQ-9=0, GAD-7=12

V GP referral for a new patient highlighting symptoms of generalised anxiety disorder for many years. Assessment session booked for next week.

J Depression, on caseload for 5 weeks, little risk. Entry: PHQ-9=17, GAD-7=13; Recent: PHQ-9=17, GAD-7=13

W GAD, on caseload for 3 weeks, little risk. Entry: PHQ-9=8, GAD-7=19; Recent: PHQ-9=6, GAD-7=13

K GAD, on caseload for 2 weeks, little risk. Entry: PHQ-9= 9, GAD-7=17; Recent: PHQ-9=6, GAD-7=11

X Panic disorder, on caseload for 2 weeks, little risk, missed last session. Entry: PHQ-9=6, GAD-7=11; Recent: PHQ-9=7, GAD-7=11

L Referred with panic disorder, appointment made for next week.

Y Panic disorder, on caseload for 2 weeks, little risk. Entry: PHQ-9=7, GAD-7=20; Recent: PHQ-9=4, GAD-7=14

M Agoraphobia, on caseload for 4 weeks, little risk. Entry: PHQ-9=7, GAD-7=21; Recent: PHQ-9=12, GAD-7=14

Z GAD, new referral, no risk. Entry: PHQ-9=7, GAD-7=14

Lead in: For the patients outlined in Table 9.3, select which of the categories is the best fit for case management supervision. Each patient presentation can be used once, or not at all.

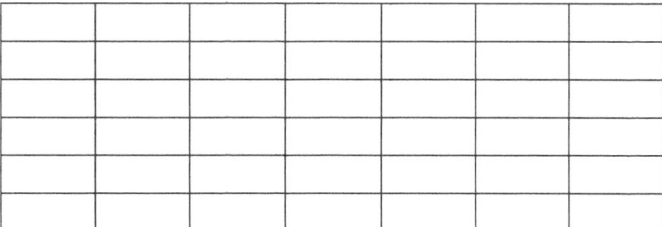

1. New to caseload

2. Presenting with high risk

3. Presenting with high scores

4. Scheduled review

5. DNA

6. Further support

Worth 15 marks

Procedural

Practise preparing the following cases for supervision using the proforma in Table 9.2 (see p. 146).

Patient 1 – Scheduled Review

You have seen Paul (43) for an assessment and three treatment sessions. He presented at assessment with depression although admitted he found it quite difficult to talk about everything. He had been experiencing symptoms of depression for about six months, having never experienced any mental health problems in the past. He wondered if his lack of energy might be a barrier but felt he had adequate opportunity to engage and was motivated to start work (7/10 at assessment). There were no co-morbidities or cultural/language/disability considerations. Paul reported low energy, disrupted sleep, thoughts of hopelessness, lack of enjoyment and a reduction in his activity level. He has managed to remain at work through his depression and feels his boss has been supportive. Paul had spoken to his GP who had suggested contacting IAPT and then coming back if he wanted to discuss medication. Paul said at assessment that he had stopped showering and shaving daily and now only did this two or three times a week when his wife nagged him to. There was no other risk stated and Paul did not feel his reduced showering was detrimental to his health.

PHQ-9=18, 15, 11, 10; GAD7=10, 8, 5, 5

Problem statement: My main problem is feeling low and having no energy. I feel tired most of the time. I am not sleeping well and have stopped enjoying things like going to football. I am also putting off jobs I need to do around the house. I sometimes think that everything is hopeless and that I can't be bothered. This is having an impact on lots of areas of my life.

Goals:

- Start going to football with friends once a month again.
- Organise the bookcase in the spare room before my sister comes to stay in three months.
- Shower at least every other day.

You agreed to work on BA. Paul has engaged well and is making good progress towards his goals. He had some difficulty at first (planned in too much and then wasn't able to complete the plan and felt bad about himself). However, since then he has seemed to get the hang of scheduling activities in and feels pleased with how the intervention is going.

Patient 2 – High Score

Maria (18) lives at home with her three younger brothers (aged 11, 15 and 16) and her mum who has diabetes. Maria does a lot around the house as her mum struggles. Maria has noticed feeling increasingly tense and is getting a lot of headaches. She is currently studying for her A-levels and is hoping to go to university.

Maria worries about her mum and her mum's health. Although her mum has been living with diabetes for a long time Maria worries that something might go wrong with the insulin. Maria worries about her A-levels. Her mum wants her to go to a 'good' university and Maria is worried she might disappoint her. She worries about what she will do if she doesn't get into university but also about how she will cope if she does. Maria reports 'small, stupid' worries too – for example, she worries about whether she has got enough chicken out of the freezer for dinner, she worries about forgetting to put the bins out, she worries about forgetting to take library books back and racking up big fines, and whether she is going mad because of all the worries. Maria has no risk of harm to herself or others and does not feel at risk of harm. She is not neglecting herself. She feels that her mother and brothers are dependent on her and worries she is not doing a good job (although identifies that actually she is doing everything she is supposed to and everyone seems OK).

> PHQ-9=(Assessment 9), 8, 8; GAD-7=(Assessment 20), 21, 21
> COM-B: Worries that treatment will give her something new to worry about and worries that she will not have enough time to engage, although she really does want to 'get her head straight'.
> Goals: Get on top of my worrying! Be able to relax and enjoy things again without worrying all the time. Be able to concentrate on studying for my A levels.
> *Problem statement*: My main problem is worrying, all the time! I feel tense and am getting headaches, I am having difficulty concentrating and am not studying or seeing friends as much as I would like. I worry about my A-levels, my mum, my brothers and lots of other little things. This is impacting my college work and my social life.

You have seen Maria for two treatment sessions and agreed to start worry management. At her third appointment she said her anxiety feels worse.

Answers to Assessing Your Understanding questions can be found in the appendix on p. 336.

Further Reading and Resources

Richards, D.A. (2010) Supervising low-intensity workers in high volume clinical environments. In J. Bennett-Levy, D.A. Richards, P. Farrand, H. Christensen, K.M. Griffiths, D.J. Kavanagh, et al. (eds), *Oxford Guide to Low Intensity CBT Interventions*. Oxford: Oxford University Press. pp. 129–36

Richards, D.A., Chellingsworth, M., Hope, R., Turpin, G. and Whyte, M. (2008) *Reach Out: National Programme Supervisor Materials to Support the Delivery of Training for Psychological Wellbeing Practitioners Delivering Low-Intensity Interventions*. London: Rethink.

Roth, A.D. and Pilling, S. (2008) *A Competence Framework for the Supervision of Psychological Therapies*. University College London.

Turpin, G. and Wheeler, S. (2011) *IAPT Supervision Guidance*. London: Department of Health IAPT Programme. Available at https://webarchive.nationalarchives.gov.uk/20160302160224/http://www.iapt.nhs.uk/silo/files/iapt-supervision-guidance-revised-march-2011.pdf (accessed 25 May 2019).

To access the online resources accompanying this chapter, please visit: https://study.sagepub.com/farrand

10

Medication for Common Mental Health Problems

Extending the Evidence-Based Treatment Toolkit

Alje van Hoorn, Paul Farrand and Chris Dickens

Learning Objectives

By the end of this chapter you should be able to:

- Demonstrate awareness of NICE guidance on medication for depression and anxiety
- Demonstrate an understanding of types of antidepressants and anxiolytics
- Critically evaluate theories accounting for ways in which antidepressants work
- Apply specific factors to gather information on medications as part of a low-intensity cognitive behavioural therapy assessment and during subsequent support sessions
- Apply specific factors to address anxiolytic taking in patients engaging with exposure therapy
- Apply service-level protocols to address common medical and unwanted side effects where concerns arise regarding medication taking

---

Background

Depression and anxiety are among the most common conditions seen by doctors in the UK. Consequently, medications (i.e. the prescribed drugs) used to treat depression and anxiety are among the most commonly prescribed of all drugs. In 2016, prescriptions for 64.7 million items of antidepressants were dispensed in England, an increase of more than 6 per cent from the previous year and more than double the number of prescriptions ten years earlier. Up-to-date figures for anxiolytics are more difficult to find, although between 2008 and 2012 approximately 11 million prescriptions were made annually for benzodiazepines (e.g. diazepam, temazepam, lorazepam). Since these drugs are prescribed so frequently, it is inevitable that any practitioner supporting low-intensity CBT (LICBT) interventions will encounter patients who are taking antidepressants and/or anxiolytic medications.

This chapter will present basic information on the use of the most common medications for people who suffer from anxiety and depression, what they do and what they are prescribed for. This will enable the LICBT practitioner to recognise problems, appreciate how they can affect the delivery of LICBT interventions and facilitate effective management. It is not intended to be a fully comprehensive account and will not turn you into experts on medication for these conditions.

Reflection Point

Reflect upon your personal attitude towards medication for depression and anxiety, considering ways it may influence your practice.

NICE Guidance on Medication for Depression and Anxiety

Whilst the LICBT practitioner will never be required to prescribe medication, understanding NICE guidance in this area can help support the quality of referrals made to medical professionals when considered helpful.

Depression

At Step 3 of the stepped care model (Chapter 1), the National Institute for Health and Care Excellence (NICE) recommends combining antidepressant medication with an evidence-based high-intensity psychological intervention (CBT or interpersonal therapy) for moderate to severe depression (NICE, 2018a).

Key Point

Specific recommendations for depression

The recommendations include:

- A selective serotonin reuptake inhibitor (SSRI) is the first-choice medication, given the effectiveness and relative safety of these drugs.
- If there is no (or minimal) response after three or four weeks of treatment the options are to increase the dose or switch to a different antidepressant.
- Given the risk of new or worsening suicidal thoughts, follow up a week after prescribing antidepressants and frequently thereafter for those under 30 or considered to be at suicide risk.
- Patients who benefit from antidepressant medication should continue for at least six months after symptoms resolve.
- If medication is ineffective or unsuitable, recommend CBT or mindfulness-based cognitive therapy for relapse prevention.

Anxiety

Unlike NICE guidance concerning antidepressants, guidance related to the prescribing of anxiolytics varies across specific anxiety disorders and therefore general recommendations for anxiolytics are not made. In complex and refractory cases, medication can be considered for use alongside a high-intensity evidence-based psychological therapy (NICE, 2011a).

Key Point

Specific recommendations for anxiety disorders

The recommendations include:

- If a person with GAD chooses or requires a drug treatment, an SSRI should be offered – usually sertraline as first line. If sertraline is ineffective, an alternative SSRI or a serotonin–noradrenaline reuptake inhibitor (SNRI) could be offered (NICE, 2011a).
- Benzodiazepines should only be offered to people with GAD for short-term treatment in crisis, in line with the guidance in the British National Formulary (BNF, 2020).
- Antidepressants should be the only pharmacological intervention used in the longer-term management of panic disorder, either SSRIs or tricyclic antidepressants (NICE, 2011b).
- Benzodiazepines, sedating antihistamines and antipsychotic medications should not be prescribed for panic disorder (NICE, 2011b).

(Continued)

- As for people with depression, those with anxiety disorders who are under 30 years of age and/or have suicidal ideation should be warned that these drugs can be associated with increased suicidal thinking and increased risk of self-harm. They should then be reviewed after one week and frequently thereafter until the risk is no longer clinically significant.
- If drug treatment is effective for GAD or panic disorder then treatment should be continued for 6 to 12 months, because the risk of relapse is high (NICE, 2011a).

Addressing Medication in LICBT

An LICBT practitioner has *no role* in prescribing antidepressants and anxiolytic medications. However, given that these medications are commonly prescribed it is inevitable that patients who are taking them will be encountered. In the vast majority of cases they will not be causing patients any problems and will not complicate treatment. However, during assessment and subsequent support sessions the role of the LICBT practitioner is to recognise any medications the patient may be taking, appreciate attitudes towards medication and have an awareness regarding the main considerations associated with their use. At times the patient may present in a manner that could indicate difficulties with medication and the LICBT practitioner should always be aware of this possibility.

Assessment and Subsequent Contacts

As part of the 'Other important information' section of the assessment session (Chapter 2), information should be gathered about the use of medications and attitudes towards taking them. A range of considerations exist around the use of medications, some of which may be reported within the problem statement or as a symptom of the presenting problem. If any considerations regarding medications are reported at assessment, it is helpful to raise these during information-giving and, when appropriate and safe to do so, to provide the patient with useful information regarding their use. Where possible, options could then be raised during shared decision-making and any decisions reached followed up during subsequent contacts and raised during case management supervision (Chapter 9).

Recognising Concerns with Medication Taking

In the course of assessing or supporting a patient, the LICBT practitioner may become aware of concerns associated with their use of medications. These may be related

Table 10.1 Action to take where concerns arise regarding medication taking

Consideration	Action
Mild medical side effects that do not cause the patient significant problems are commonly experienced by people taking medications, with the benefits perceived to outweigh the adverse effects	If medical side effects are unexpected, distressing for the patient, increasing in intensity or severe, discuss the issue with the patient and encourage them to make an appointment to see the prescriber or another appropriately qualified member of the MDT. As determined by the service protocol adopted, the LICBT practitioner should also contact the prescriber/MDT member, citing the medical side effects being experienced and their severity
Medical side effects recognised during risk assessment as potentially associated with a recent or distant overdose could constitute a medical emergency	Follow high-risk service protocols and consider contacting a doctor for an opinion regarding whether an immediate medical assessment is required
Problems taking medications as prescribed	Unless reported as causing medical side effects, raise directly with the patient, the prescriber or appropriate member of the collaborative care team
Unwanted effects identified – evident in the presenting symptoms or problem statement	Highlight these to the patient as potentially being related to the medication they are on and encourage them to raise with the prescriber

to problems with medication taking, concerns regarding medical side effects and/ or their impact on the patient. If identified, the practitioner should encourage the patient to discuss problems or concerns with the prescriber or another appropriately qualified member of the multidisciplinary team (MDT; e.g. a nurse) as they may require some additional support, education, a change in dose or change in prescribed drug. Depending on the nature of the concern, liaise as appropriate with wider professionals within the collaborative-care team.

In all cases, the ways in which concerns about medication-taking were addressed should be raised during case management supervision, and at times it may be helpful to add this to an agenda for clinical skills supervision (Chapter 9).

Depression and Antidepressants

Antidepressants are prescribed to reduce the severity of symptoms, the length of depressive episodes and prevent relapse once symptoms have gone away. There are a number of different types of antidepressant, with different chemical structures targeting different chemical messengers in the brain, but all go under the umbrella term 'antidepressant'. Other drugs may improve specific symptoms of depression (e.g. by improving sleep or appetite), but if these do not shorten depressive episodes they are not regarded as antidepressants. Confusion arises because, as well as treating depression, antidepressants can also be useful at relieving the symptoms of anxiety. Furthermore, antidepressants can sometimes be used to treat conditions that are completely different to depression, such as to relieve chronic pain.

Antidepressants consist of a large number of different chemical compounds and share characteristics in that they change the levels of neurotransmitters important in determining who gets depression (particularly serotonin and/or noradrenaline). These drugs were first discovered by accident in the 1950s following the observation that a new anti-tuberculosis treatment had the unusual side effect of stimulating mood, appetite and sleep. In research trials, this new drug was found to improve symptoms in about 75 per cent of people with depression (Yeragani et al., 2011). Early antidepressant drugs were unpleasant to take with many side effects and were very dangerous in cases of overdose. Successive generations of antidepressant drugs have, however, become better tolerated and safer.

Types of Antidepressant

There are a large number of classes of antidepressant drugs with differing modes of action. In general, the choice of drug will be dictated by effectiveness, tolerability, safety and sometimes the presence of beneficial effects not directly related to the primary purpose of the drug (e.g. promoting sleep).

Key Point

Common Classes of Antidepressants Involved in Treating Depression

- Selective serotonin reuptake inhibitors (SSRIs)
- Serotonin norepinephrine reuptake inhibitors (SNRIs)
- Noradrenergic and specific serotonergic antidepressants (NaSSAs)
- Tricyclic antidepressants (TCAs)
- Monoamine oxidase inhibitors (MAOIs).

Choice of drug will usually be based on patient preference in consultation with the prescribing doctor and clinical guidelines with consideration of cost-effectiveness. However, the most commonly used group of antidepressants are the SSRIs.

Key Point

Common Types of SSRI

- Citalopram
- Escitalopram
- Fluoxetine
- Fluvoxamine
- Paroxetine
- Sertraline.

SSRIs are generally considered the first line of drug treatment for depression because they are usually well tolerated, have fewer side effects and are relatively safe in overdose (Cipriani et al., 2018). They target the serotonin systems in the brain, increasing the availability of this neurotransmitter.

Duration of Treatment

Generally, antidepressants take some time to work, around one to two weeks. Relapse after stopping antidepressants is common, and a single episode of depression should usually be treated for at least six months after symptoms have remitted. In those at risk of relapse, for example in people who have experienced multiple episodes of depression in the past, treatment should usually continue for at least two years.

Effectiveness

Most classes of antidepressant have broadly similar effectiveness, with 50–60 per cent of patients showing meaningful improvements in depression (Cleare et al., 2015), response rates about the same as CBT. However, relapse rates for people taking antidepressants are high, with around half of treatment responders relapsing within six months if antidepressants are discontinued following initial response (Sim et al., 2016).

Combined with CBT

The British Association of Psychopharmacology suggests that antidepressants may enhance CBT (Baldwin et al., 2014). Evidence from studies that combine psychological and drug treatment for depression indicate that combined treatment (psychological treatment plus antidepressants) has greater short-term effects than using either psychological treatment or antidepressants separately (Cuijpers et al., 2014; Cuijpers et al., 2009b). Whilst the additional acute treatment effect of combining treatment is small compared to single treatments alone, benefits of combining antidepressants and psychological treatment may go beyond the treatment effects. Specifically, there is evidence that combined treatments may reduce discontinuation of antidepressant treatment, which may lead to better long-term outcomes (Hollon et al., 2014; NICE, 2009a; Pampallona et al., 2004).

How Do Antidepressants Work?

Despite being some of the most commonly prescribed drugs, somewhat surprisingly, it is uncertain how antidepressants work. Various theories have been proposed to explain their beneficial effects on depression.

Monoamine Theory of Depression

Early observations identifying that antidepressants increased the availability of certain neurotransmitters, alongside recognition that drugs reducing their availability increased the likelihood of depression, led to the development of the monoamine theory of depression. This theory postulated that depression arises from a deficiency in the monoamines – serotonin, noradrenaline (also called norepinephrine) and dopamine. Whilst this theory has been important in the development of further antidepressant drugs, it tells us nothing about what neurotransmitters do in the brain that leads them to cause depression when levels are reduced or result in the remission of depression when levels are increased.

Effects of Antidepressants on Cognition

Antidepressant drugs change the way people process information relevant to their emotional state that can result in positive biases in the way information is processed. For example, among non-depressed individuals, a single dose of an SSRI antidepressant has been associated with subjects perceiving ambiguous facial expressions as happy (Harmer et al., 2003). On the other hand, amongst older depressed individuals, treatment with citalopram improved accuracy of recognition of happy faces within seven days and improvement predicting emotion at 56 days (Shiroma et al., 2014). Additionally, repeated administration of an SSRI led to increased memory of positive personally relevant information, reduced processing of threatening stimuli, increased problem-solving and reduced submissive behaviour (Harmer et al., 2004; Knutson et al., 1998; Tse and Bond, 2002). Acute and short-term effects of antidepressants have, however, been less studied in depressed individuals, although results appear to be consistent with findings in non-depressed volunteers (Harmer et al., 2009).

Cognitive Neuropsychological Model of Depression

Arising from observations that antidepressants change the way people process information, the cognitive neuropsychological model of depression states that negative biases in the processing of emotionally relevant information (emotional processing) have a central role in causing and maintaining depression (Roiser et al., 2012). Negative emotional processing bias leads to the development of dysfunctional negative schemata, which in turn leads to learned states of anhedonia and dysphoria that characterise depression. The model proposes that antidepressants improve depression by increasing levels of key brain monoamines that correct negative emotional processing biases that maintain depression. This has helped to develop an understanding of key processes that interact to result in the development and maintenance of depression (Figure 10.1).

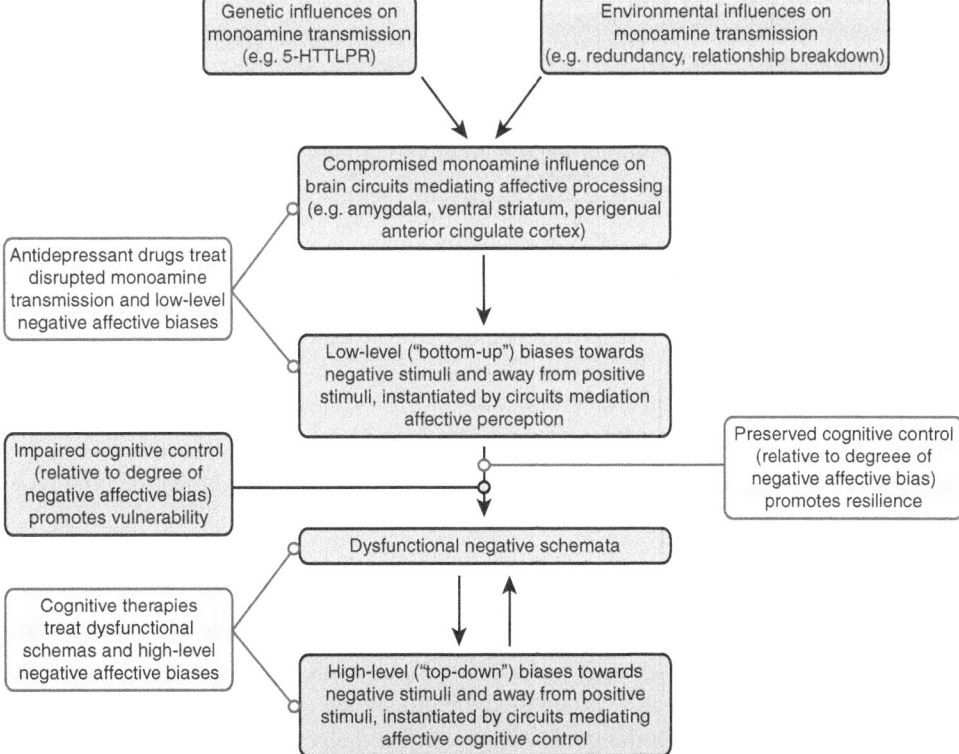

Figure 10.1 Cognitive neuropsychological model of depression (Reprinted by permission from Springer Nature: Neuropsychopharmacology - Cognitive Mechanisms of Treatment in Depression by Roiser et al., 2011)

Importantly, the cognitive neuropsychological model of depression presents a unified explanation highlighting how, and why, psychological treatments and antidepressant treatments may be complementary.

For example, LICBT interventions such as behavioural activation (Chapter 11), which act to increase rewarding experiences, may be further enhanced via the positive effect of antidepressants on information processing biases (Figure 10.2).

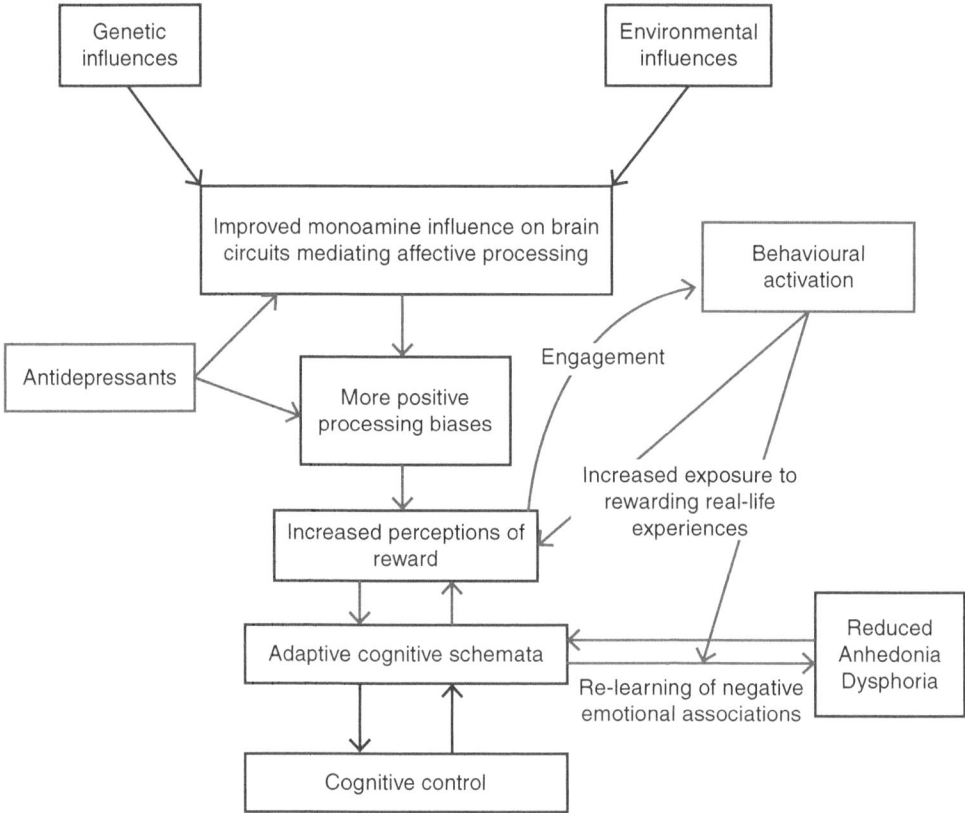

Figure 10.2 Proposed mechanisms of action of antidepressants and behavioural activation on the cognitive neuropsychological model of depression

Clinical Considerations

Suicide Risk with SSRI and SNRI

There is some research evidence for a small but significant increase in suicidal thinking in the early stages of antidepressant treatment (NICE, 2009a). Meta-analyses of completed trials of antidepressants have revealed possible evidence of increased suicidal/self-harming behaviour with SSRIs compared to placebo (Fergusson et al., 2005; Gunnell et al., 2006). This effect was most obvious amongst individuals 18 years old and younger, with the risk diminishing after the age of 30 years (Martinez et al., 2005). As a consequence of this possible increase in risk, medical professionals are advised that when prescribing antidepressants to someone with increased risk of suicide or someone who is aged less than 30 years of age, they should normally be reviewed after one week and frequently after that until the risk of suicide and self-harm is insignificant.

From the perspective of the LICBT practitioner, when asking about medications being taken, if the patient indicates that they have recently started taking an antidepressant, the LICBT practitioner should ask about any changes in suicidal thinking/self-harming behaviour and explore risk of future suicide/self-harm thoroughly during the risk assessment undertaken. If risk has become an increasing concern it should be addressed as part of clinical decision-making (Chapter 4) with service protocols followed.

Overdose

In the course of assessing or treating patients, the LICBT practitioner may become aware that the patient has accidentally or deliberately taken an overdose of medication. Taking more antidepressants than prescribed can result in serious side effects and even death. Risks associated with overdose are not the same across all drugs with SSRIs being the safest and SNRIs and venlafaxine moderately toxic. Particularly dangerous in overdose, however, are monoamine oxidase inhibitors (MAOI) and due to their cardiac effects, older tricyclic antidepressants like amitriptyline. If the overdose is more recent, the symptoms and signs of overdose may be apparent within LICBT sessions from the way the patient is behaving, appearing drowsy or slurring their words and the LICBT practitioner should remain vigilant for these signs.

Anxiety on Initiation

SSRIs and SNRIs can both cause anxiety after the drug is started. This is usually worst in the days immediately following initiation of the drug and can settle, but it may be problematic and could potentially cause patients to discontinue psychological treatment. Anticipating these side effects during information giving and ensuring the patient is aware that they may be experienced, but are often temporary, may help continued engagement.

Sexual Dysfunction

This is a common side effect, particularly with SSRI antidepressants where patients may report a loss of sex drive and difficulties with sexual performance. Regrettably this area is too often ignored by clinicians prescribing the drugs, perhaps because they find raising this topic difficult or because of a mistaken belief that people with depression do not have sex given that loss of libido may represent a symptom of depression. During assessment, recognising such difficulties whilst giving information that sexual function will return to normal when the drug is discontinued may be helpful. Otherwise, if the patient highlights this as having a significant impact, referring them back to the prescriber to consider alternative antidepressants may improve adherence.

Discontinuation Syndrome

If stopped suddenly, a number of antidepressants can cause unpleasant symptoms. Gradual withdrawal over four weeks minimises discomfort for the majority of individuals (NICE, 2009a). Whilst symptoms are usually mild and settle rapidly, for some patients they can be highly unpleasant.

Key Point

Common Physical Symptoms Associated with Antidepressant Discontinuation

- Dizziness
- Numbness
- Tingling
- Gastrointestinal disturbances
- Headaches
- Sweating
- Anxiety
- Sleep disturbances.

The occurrence of discontinuation syndrome may contribute to incorrect beliefs that antidepressants are addictive, which patients commonly cite as a reason for not wanting to take them. Attitudes towards the use of medications should be explored during information gathering and information giving and if the patient expresses concerns about addiction and antidepressant medication information to challenge this belief should be provided.

Clinical Example

In the Session

Some people can experience unpleasant symptoms if they stop their antidepressants too quickly. Although these symptoms that occur when antidepressants are stopped can sometimes be quite unpleasant, slow withdrawal of the medication over four weeks, or occasionally even more, can make these symptoms manageable for the majority of people. Antidepressants are not addictive, however. Drugs that are addictive are usually associated with tolerance, which is when people need to take increasing doses of the drug to get the same effect, and are associated with craving or drug-seeking behaviour, which antidepressants are not.

If after information giving surrounding addiction and discontinuation syndrome the patient is interested in further exploring antidepressant medication as a treatment choice, making an appointment with the GP for further discussion could be suggested.

Bleeding

Blood platelets are the components of the blood responsible for normal blood clotting after injury or simply during normal wear and tear. Normal platelet function is altered by drugs that act on the serotonin system, with the result that patients may experience bleeding, particularly from the gut. Unless patients are taking other medications that increase the risk of bleeding, this is usually not a problem. However, the LICBT practitioner should refer the patient to the prescriber if bleeding is reported during support sessions.

Anxiety and Anxiolytics

Like antidepressants, anxiolytics consist of a broad range of chemical compounds with differing mechanisms of action. They relieve symptoms of anxiety by either reducing levels of psychological arousal or lessening the physical effects of anxiety. Specifically, anxiolytics target the symptoms of anxiety but do not shorten an often chronic course. To optimise the effects and minimise unnecessary doses, patients may be able to determine when they take anxiolytic medication (i.e. take as required).

However, complete cessation or sudden reduction of anxiolytics taken regularly for a long time is not advisable. It can result in a marked rebounding of physical and psychological symptoms of anxiety, and can also cause other potentially serious medical problems, such as epileptic seizures. Because depression and anxiety frequently occur together, it is not uncommon to see patients prescribed an anxiolytic alongside an antidepressant.

Types of Anxiolytic

Whilst a range of anxiolytics are available for the treatment of anxiety, benzodiazepines are the most commonly prescribed.

Benzodiazepines

Gamma aminobutyric acid (GABA) is one of the most important inhibitory neurotransmitters in the brain, reducing activity in specific brain circuits involved in anxiety. The effect of GABA can be enhanced through benzodiazepines providing rapid relief from anxiety within hours, with the duration of effect varying across the different types available. Prolonged use of benzodiazepines is, however, recognised to cause dependence so recommendations advise use for short-term crisis management only and that the treatment dose and duration are kept to a minimum. Additionally, for some anxiety problems such as panic disorder, their use is contraindicated. In addition to controlling anxiety, benzodiazepines can also be used to aid sleep, for sedation, to treat seizures and alcohol withdrawal, and as muscle relaxants. Whilst not being a treatment for depression, they are sometimes prescribed alongside an SSRI to alleviate any anxiety that occurs with the initiation of an SSRI.

Key Point

Common Types of Benzodiazepines for Treating Anxiety

- Chlordiazepoxide: sometimes known as librium
- Diazepam
- Lorazepam
- Nitrazepam: sometimes known as Mogadon
- Oxazepam
- Triazolam.

Clinical Considerations

Dependence

Benzodiazepines can cause dependence and are therefore prescribed at the lowest possible dose for a very short timeframe (BNF, 2020). As with other drugs that control unpleasant symptoms – pain killers, drugs promoting sleep – they do not change the course of the underlying problem, and difficulty discontinuing anxiolytic medications can be experienced because anxiety symptoms can often recur quickly. Under these circumstances there is a risk that people may end up taking these medications for many years.

Withdrawal Effects

Anxiolytics generally work by reducing arousal in the central nervous system and therefore sudden withdrawal can result in rebound activation. In its mildest form this can take the form of rebound anxiety, poor sleep, loss of appetite, tremor and perspiration. However, on a small number of occasions abrupt anxiolytic withdrawal can result in epileptic seizures, which themselves can be fatal. Withdrawal effects usually come on within a day of discontinuing short-acting drugs and within weeks for long acting drugs, and may last for weeks or months. Under the direction of a medical practitioner, slowly withdrawing the drugs, sometimes over months, can reduce the severity of withdrawal effects.

Impact on Exposure-Based LICBT Interventions

From a theoretical perspective, if an LICBT treatment involves exposing the patient to a trigger that provokes anxiety in order to facilitate habituation (Chapter 13), taking anxiolytic medication to suppress symptoms of anxiety is likely to hinder treatment success. This perspective is supported by research proposing that certain types of anxiolytic medication may interfere with fear extinction (Corcoran et al., 2015). Consequently, if the patient is taking anxiolytic medication to manage anxiety, the LICBT practitioner should provide encouragement to stop or reduce medication taken prior to exposure therapy. However, this could be a significant challenge when the patient expresses strong beliefs that they can only cope when taking the medication. Removal of the drug may be perceived as being too threatening, or the resulting increase in anxiety following discontinuation may discourage engagement with exposure therapy. In such cases it may be helpful to explain the theoretical rationale for exposure therapy (Chapter 13) within the context of taking anxiolytic medication.

Clinical Practice

Reducing Anxiolytic Medication During Exposure Therapy

Step 1: Provide the theoretical rationale for exposure and habituation to patients.

Step 2: Discuss with the patient the levels of anxiety being experienced despite medication.

Step 3: Re-emphasise the need to experience anxiety by exposure to the trigger.

Step 4: Explain how quickly after being taken benzodiazepines work to provide rapid relief from anxiety and minimise physical symptoms associated with anxiety.

Step 5: Demonstrate that whilst taking benzodiazepines helps to reduce anxiety in the short term, by staying on them they will never habituate to the anxiety caused by the trigger and the cause of the underlying problem may never be addressed.

Step 6: Explain the exposure hierarchy and how it may be possible to reduce the dose of benzodiazepine as fear begins to drop when progressing up the hierarchy. This would result in complete withdrawal being reached towards the top of the hierarchy (Chapter 13).

Step 7: With patient agreement, talk to the prescriber for advice on a controlled reduction of the benzodiazepine to allow the patient to experience a little more anxiety to facilitate their completion of the exposure hierarchy.

Step 8: If the patient is not willing to consider reducing their benzodiazepine as part of their exposure hierarchy, consider pressing on with exposure and observing what happens to anxiety when they are exposed to the trigger.

Although concerns about the effects of anxiolytics on psychological treatment can be understood from a theoretical perspective, definitive trials addressing this question have not been undertaken.

Overdose

As with antidepressants, all anxiolytics can be dangerous in overdose, with patients experiencing significant side effects, potentially even death. Such effects can be significantly worse if anxiolytics are combined with other sedative medications. If there is any suggestion that the patient may have overdosed, follow service protocols for high-risk patients and seek an adequate risk assessment.

Summary

Across England, drug treatments for depression and anxiety are frequently prescribed, making it inevitable that LICBT practitioners will encounter patients who are taking antidepressants and/or anxiolytics. The LICBT clinical method requires practitioners to gather information around medication taking during assessment (Chapter 2) and subsequent sessions (Chapter 6), have knowledge regarding unwanted and medical side effects, and follow appropriate protocols, all of which are addressed in this chapter. Many considerations faced by the LICBT practitioner with regard to medication are faced by all members of the healthcare team and in the event of concern the patient should be referred to the prescriber. As predicted by the cognitive neuropsychological model, antidepressants may even enhance effectiveness of psychological treatments for depression, although from a theoretical perspective, anxiolytics may interfere with exposure-based interventions. In most cases, however, the belief that commonly prescribed antidepressants and anxiolytics will not interfere with LICBT interventions remains.

Assessing Your Understanding

Declarative

Multiple Choice Questions

1. Which of the following are benzodiazepine medications? [Select all that apply]
   (a) Chlordiazepoxide
   (b) Meladomam
   (c) Oxazepam
   (d) Polatopam
   (e) Triazolam
2. Which of the following are specific serotonin reuptake inhibitors (SSRIs)? [Select all that apply]
   (a) Amatriptoline
   (b) Estilopine
   (c) Fluvoxamine
   (d) Gabapentine
   (e) Sertaline

3. Which of the following are associated with the cognitive neuropsychological model of depression? [Select all that apply]
   (a) Antidepressants improve depression by having a direct positive effect on brain monoamines
   (b) Fluzosamine impacts on negative schemata by enhancing neurotransmitters
   (c) The model can help predict specific LICBT techniques that may be augmented by antidepressant treatment
   (d) The model helps to account for the combined effect of neurotransmitters and LICBT techniques on the brain
   (e) Cognitive restructuring initiates changes in information processing associated with depression, with an SSRI used to support relapse prevention

Procedural

Self-Practice/Self-Reflection

- Role play a case where you have been working with a patient with agoraphobia and have chosen to support exposure therapy but during assessment you have identified that the patient is currently taking diazepam to manage their anxiety. Reflect upon any challenges you experienced.
- Role play a situation where during assessment you recognise that the patient is taking citalopram for low mood and has highlighted that poor sexual function is having a significant impact on his relationship. Reflect upon any challenges you experienced.

Answers to **Assessing Your Understanding** questions can be found in the appendix on p. 336.

Further Reading and Resources

Joint Formulary Committee (2020) *British National Formulary* (79). London: Pharmaceutical Press.

Stahl, S.M. and Muntner, N. (2013) *Stahl's Essential Psychopharmacology: Neuroscientific Basis and Practical Application*. Cambridge: Cambridge University Press.

Taylor, D., Barnes, T.E. and Young, A. (2018) *The Maudsley Prescribing Guidelines in Psychiatry*. Chichester: Wiley.

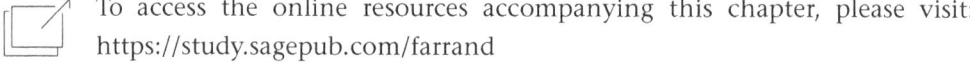 To access the online resources accompanying this chapter, please visit: https://study.sagepub.com/farrand

Part II
Supporting Low-Intensity Interventions

11

Behavioural Activation

Working Outside In, Rather Than Inside Out

Paul Farrand

Learning Objectives

By the end of this chapter you should be able to:

- Critically appraise the theoretical rationale informing the behavioural activation model used in low-intensity cognitive behavioural therapy
- Demonstrate an understanding of the specific factors associated with the low-intensity model of behavioural activation
- Apply specific factors associated with supporting a patient engage with low-intensity interventions based on behavioural activation for the treatment of depression
- Formulate common difficulties experienced by patients when engaging with low-intensity behavioural activation and demonstrate appropriate decision-making to guide the patient to overcome these

---

Intervention Description

Whilst largely considered a component intervention within high-intensity cognitive behavioural therapy (HICBT; Beck et al., 1987), behavioural activation (BA) is increasingly recognised as a treatment in its own right (Martell et al., 2001). The BA model employed within low-intensity CBT (LICBT) was developed by David Richards (2010c) and implemented within the Improving Access to Psychological Therapies (IAPT) programme. The intervention is particularly informed by the clinical protocols serving as the foundation of previous models of BA (Hopko et al., 2003; Martell et al. 2001). It shares several features with other BA interventions (e.g. Jacobson et al., 2001; Lewinsohn, 1975) recommended by the National Institute for Health and Care Excellence (NICE, 2018a) and employed within high-intensity CBT (HICBT). Common across all models is a focus on treating depression *outside in*, focusing on sources of reinforcement in the environment and their subsequent impact on behaviour (Jacobson et al., 2001). This contrasts to approaches such as cognitive restructuring (Chapter 12) more commonly associated with cognitive therapy that seek to work *inside out* by recognising and challenging unhelpful thinking styles.

Evidence Base

BA has a large evidence base with a recent systematic review identifying 26 randomised controlled trials (RCTs; Ekers et al., 2014). This review concluded that BA represents an effective treatment for depression with outcomes at least as effective as anti-depressant medication with no difference in effect between populations including general adult, post-natal, older adults and students. Studies have also determined BA to be as effective as HICBT and more effective than other psychological therapies (Ekers et al., 2008). Additionally, a Phase III RCT demonstrated that BA delivered by a practitioner from the mental health workforce, such as a psychological wellbeing practitioner (PWP), is as effective as HICBT (Richards et al., 2016). This finding is especially impressive given the cost savings associated with employing and training a practitioner compared to a high-intensity therapist (Chapter 1). Cost savings identify BA as being 21 per cent cheaper than CBT to deliver by clinical services with no increased patient use of other healthcare services. Importantly, BA is equally as acceptable to patients as CBT (Finning et al., 2017), including within specific populations such as armed forces veterans (Farrand et al., 2019a).

Theoretical Rationale

BA is based on the theory that behaviours that lead to depression are learned through contingencies existent within the environment that serve as sources of reinforcement (Hopko et al., 2015). Adopting this rationale, depressive behaviour results from lower levels of exposure or avoidance of sources of positive reinforcement, activities constituting life-routines and necessary activities. This is maintained through sources of negative reinforcement, such as a patient experiencing relief by not engaging with a physically strenuous task, feeling physically less tired after going to bed early in the evening or avoiding social situations thinking friends will find them dull. Over time this can help establish a downward spiral of depression, as in the case of Sam (Figure 11.1).

Problem statement: My main problem is feeling tired and low, from the time I wake up in the morning to going to bed at night. As a result, I've started to do less and less, and given up my weekly gym class as I feel too tired. I also no longer see my friends as much as I used to. I guess they'll find me a bit dull now as I'm not as much fun as I used to be. As a result, I'm home alone much more, find myself going to bed earlier in the evening after work, not yet completed direct debits to pay overdue bills and eating more as I think it makes me feel a little more content – for a short time at least.

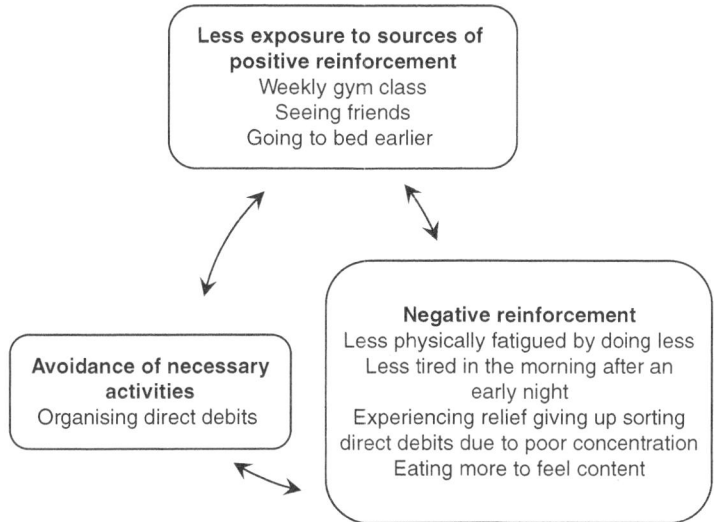

Figure 11.1 Sam's problem statement and downward spiral of depression

BA is targeted at supporting a patient to re-engage with activities previously found rewarding, or believed to be rewarding in the future, in addition to tasks that previously gave their lives a routine whilst reducing the deleterious impact of negative reinforcement. The focus on addressing sources of positive and negative reinforcement distinguishes BA from activity scheduling, which has an emphasis on enhancing opportunities for positive reinforcement (Richards, 2010c). It is not uncommon to struggle to appreciate the difference between negative reinforcement and punishment. Theoretically, negative reinforcement results in a behaviour such as avoiding socialising with friends being increased, whereas punishment, such as a school child being put into detention for talking in class, decreases a behaviour (Skinner, 1969).

Application of Behavioural Activation

Unlike other LICBT interventions (Part II), the evidence-based application of BA for common mental health problems is restricted to the treatment of depression.

However, the BA model within LICBT (Richards, 2010c) has been used in combination with physical activity promotion for the treatment of depression (Chapter 20; Farrand et al., 2014). Combining BA within an individual or group-based structured physical activity programme for the treatment of depression offers a way to combine two evidence-based treatments for depression (NICE, 2018a) into a single approach for LICBT delivery.

Specific Factors: Supporting Behavioural Activation

Informed by the theoretical rationale supporting the foundation of BA, the LICBT BA model was first reported within clinical training support materials (Richards and Whyte, 2011). Consistent with the LICBT focus on single-strand interventions (Chapter 1), the LICBT BA model is an independent intervention (Richards, 2010). To help people with depression increasingly re-engage with activities, this BA model follows a six-stage protocol.

Clinical Practice

Intervention Stages

- *Stage 1*: Explain BA
  - o   Step 1a: Keep a BA diary (when necessary)
- *Stage 2*: Identify routine, pleasurable and necessary activities
- *Stage 3*: Grade activities in terms of how difficult they are to achieve at present
- *Stage 4*: Schedule activities into the behavioural activation schedule
- *Stage 5*: Patient follows schedule
- *Stage 6*: Review progress.

Stage 1: Explain BA

As with all LICBT interventions, in session it is important to explain BA to patients in a manner that enables them to appreciate the underpinning theory supporting the LICBT BA model and highlighting the evidence base supporting adoption.

Clinical Example

In Session

Based on our understanding that the difficulties you're currently experiencing are associated with depression, the recommended evidence-based treatment I can support is behavioural activation, or BA for short. This approach helps people with depression re-engage with activities they previously found pleasurable and those that formed part of their life routine. If needed, it can also help people complete necessary activities, because although these can be a real struggle, they do help us avoid what could be significant consequences. With my support helping you work through the BA intervention, this approach will help you build activities up from where you are now to where you want to be, but at a pace and in steps acceptable to you. Re-engaging once again with activities you find enjoyable or formed part of your life routine can help improve your current low mood and reduce other symptoms associated with depression.

However, to enhance common factors and promote engagement (Chapter 5), it is important to ensure that the explanation is tailored to the specific patient as based on features of the referral and/or appreciation of the patient gained during assessment (Chapter 2).

Reflection Point

Reflect upon ways you could adapt your explanation of behavioural activation for different groups of patients representing diversity with respect to cultural norms including personal, family, social and spiritual values or presenting with risk.

Once the theoretical basis for the LICBT BA model (Richards, 2010c) is explained, it is helpful to use common factors (Chapter 5) to gain an appreciation of patient understanding. If after providing the opportunity to ask questions it appears that understanding is adequate then introduce Stage 2 if the patient is willing to continue. If the patient is struggling to appreciate the main rationale behind BA but appears interested in the BA approach moving to Step 1a may be helpful. Additionally, Step 1a may be a helpful adaptation on occasions where the patient is unaware of the impact that physical limitations associated with physical health difficulties or older age may have upon increased activity (Chapter 19). Appreciating any limitations may help to inform within session support for the intervention (Chapter 6).

Step 1a: Keeping a BA Diary

Based upon knowledge of the patient gained during assessment or from features of the referral, consider benefits that may arise from introducing the use of *Behavioural Activation Schedule* (Worksheet 11.1) as a diary to record activity prior to the next support session. At the next support session this could serve as a baseline to work from and help support an explanation of BA before moving to Stage 2.

Worksheet 11.1   Behavioural activation schedule

		Write below the day of the week you want to start your schedule						
Morning	What							
	Where							
	Who							
	When							
	What							
	Where							
	Who							
	When							
Afternoon	What							
	Where							
	Who							
	When							
	What							
	Where							
	Who							
	When							
Evening	What							
	Where							
	Who							
	When							
	What							
	Where							
	Who							
	When							
Comments								

Whilst bearing similarities to forms of diary or schedule used in other BA or activity scheduling approaches, the Behavioural activation schedule comprises boxes to record details of each activity for the morning, afternoon and evening for each day following the previous assessment or support session. Having this detail is especially important if used to schedule activity (Stage 4). If initially adopting this as a diary to enable patients to record their activity prior to the next support session, however, completing details beyond *what* the activity undertaken was, is less important. However, if patients are able to complete some of the other detail requested, it can be very helpful. This schedule differs slightly from that employed within the original clinical support materials (Richards and Whyte, 2011), with days of the week not specified in advance. This enables a shared decision to be reached with the patient regarding when to start the schedule.

Stage 2: Identify Routine, Pleasurable and Necessary Activities

The next stage of the LICBT BA model (Richards, 2010c) is for the patient to categorise activities. They will be encouraged to identify the range of activities they currently do less of, avoid or in some cases engage in more frequently and categorise them as *routine*, *pleasurable* or *necessary*, as outlined in the 'Key Point'.

Key Point

Specific Factor Knowledge

Routine	Activities regularly undertaken that form part of a person's life routine, giving their life structure and making them feel comfortable in their surroundings. Such activities may include tasks such as cooking, taking the dogs for walks, driving the kids to school, going to work. Routine activities may also represent daily routines that can be disrupted, such as having a shower, going to bed or waking up.
Pleasurable	Activities that bring pleasure and may include seeing friends for a pint, clothes shopping, reading, playing sports. Of all the three categories, this one is likely to vary the most between patients.
Necessary	Activities that are often very important to complete given their potential to have a significant negative impact on a person's life if not completed, such as paying bills, delivering to work deadlines, taking prescribed medications.

The patient is encouraged to use the Classifying activity worksheet (Worksheet 11.2) to write each activity in the appropriate column. It is worthwhile checking the worksheet in the following support session to identify the inclusion of potentially unhelpful or harmful activities. Additionally, deadlines for necessary activities should be considered with respect to impending or exceeded deadline dates.

Worksheet 11.2　Example of a classifying activity worksheet

Classifying activity worksheet			
Think about activities you now do less of, avoid or engage in more frequently and write these below in one of the following categories.			
Routine Activities that form part of your daily life routine – e.g. cooking, walking the dogs, going to work, having a shower	**Pleasurable** Activities you enjoy doing – e.g. seeing friends, clothes shopping, sports. This varies a lot from person to person	**Necessary** Activities that are important to achieve given their potential, if not completed, to have a negative impact on your life – e.g. paying bills, taking medication, working to deadlines	**Deadlines** For each necessary activity, provide the date by which it needs to be completed
Walk the dog	Meet Dave and Sal for Euchre	Sort direct debits	This Tuesday
Shower	Work out in gym	Take warfarin	Every day
Get out of bed	Tinker with my car	Get bus pass sorted	Friday 8 May
Buy a newspaper at local shop	Read newspaper		
Part-time job			
Sort bins			

Unhelpful Activities Being Engaged in or Necessary Activities Not Completed

Where unhelpful or potentially harmful routine or pleasurable activities are being undertaken or necessary activities have not been completed, a decision should be made regarding the best way to proceed with treatment (Chapter 6). Whilst the patient may continue to be supported to work through the BA protocol, a shared decision should be reached about ways to address these activities, with consideration given to signposting opportunities or additional support available within your service. It may also be helpful to raise this at the following supervision session (Chapter 9) to ensure appropriate advice or service protocols have been followed.

Reflecting an ideographic BA model (Jacobson et al., 2001), it is important to ensure that support enables the patient to identify activities they believe they will find pleasurable and positively reinforcing rather than being determined in advance. The influence such activities have on mood should then be reviewed as part of Stage 6.

Stage 3: Grade Activities in Terms of How Difficult They Are to Achieve at Present

The focus in Stage 3 is to grade the routine, pleasurable and necessary activities according to difficulty. The patient is encouraged to consult their Classifying activity worksheet (Worksheet 11.2) and grade each activity into least difficult, medium difficulty and most difficult, depending upon how difficult they are to complete at present (Worksheet 11.3).

Worksheet 11.3 Example of an activity grading worksheet

Activity grading worksheet		
Consider how difficult you would currently find engaging with each activity identified on the Classifying activity worksheet and write your answers in the appropriate column		
Least difficult	Medium difficulty	Most difficult
Get out of bed	Shower	Get to part-time job
Walk the dog	Sort bins	Work out in gym
Buy newspaper	Euchre with Dave and Sal	Sort direct debits
Take warfarin	Read newspaper	
Tinker with car	Get bus pass sorted	

Especially for patients with moderate to severe levels of depression (see Chapter 3) and currently engaging in very little activity, the idea of engaging in any additional activity may seem difficult to comprehend. In these circumstances, confirm that activities graded as medium difficulty to most difficult represent those they are seeking to work towards and are best considered treatment goals. Reaffirm that as far as possible the intervention will start with routine and pleasurable activities graded as least difficult.

Use empathy at this point to ensure that the patient appreciates that you recognise they may struggle with the idea of completing any activities given their depression (Chapter 5). Check with the patient that difficulties graded as least difficult do not represent too big a step. If they do, consider working with the patient to identify less difficult activities or consider ways to make them more manageable by breaking them down further or other ways to encourage behaviour change (Chapter 8).

Stage 4: Schedule Activities into the Behavioural Activation Schedule

Towards the end of the assessment session it is of immense benefit to support the patient to schedule the number of activities into their Behavioural activation schedule they believe they can manage to engage with before the next support session.

This helps to engage the patient with treatment as soon as possible and encourages them to complete the schedule between sessions. These rules should be followed when supporting the patient to schedule their own activities (Table 11.1).

Table 11.1 Rules to support scheduling of activities within the Behavioural activation schedule

Rules	Rationale
Initially support the patient schedule activities graded as least difficult	Re-engaging in activity is difficult with depression, therefore choosing activities identified as least difficult represents those most likely to be achieved. However, even with these activities the patient may initially find them difficult to achieve
The patient should schedule as many, or as few, activities they feel they can engage with before the next support session	Based on identified activities, only the patient is aware of the number of activities they feel they can achieve during the following week. However, be vigilant to over-ambition when a patient who is currently doing very little wants to fill their schedule
Scheduled activities should be selected from both the routine and pleasurable categories, avoiding an over-emphasis on either category	A well-balanced weekly routine drawing on routine and pleasurable activities often results in the highest sense of enjoyment, satisfaction and fulfilment associated with the highest level of wellbeing
Activities should be scheduled across the week to avoid prolonged periods of little or excessive activity	Spacing scheduled activities across the week will better ensure positive reinforcement arising from completed activities if received all week
Consideration should be given to the completion of any necessary activities identified	Although often difficult to achieve, necessary activities frequently have significant consequences if not completed within a certain time frame

When scheduling activities, it is helpful for the patient to include details to assist activity planning (Table 11.2). Providing this detail may be considered a form of enablement (Michie et al., 2011), helping to prompt each activity prior to the following support session.

Table 11.2 Helpful detail for the patient to include when scheduling activity

Question	Example
What the activity being planned constitutes	I'll meet up with friends at the social club for bingo
Where the activity will be undertaken	The social club
When the activity is planned during the day	As usual, at 10.30 in the morning
Who the person or people the activity is planned with, if not alone	The usual gang, Bill, Ashok, Alice and Aileen

An example of a completed Behavioural activation schedule for a patient who had completed three support sessions is shown in Worksheet 11.4.

As can be seen, this patient is building up their activities by drawing on the routine and pleasurable activities graded as least difficult and spreading these out across the week. However, there are two exceptions – 'Get to job' and 'Pay direct debits' – scheduled. Whilst graded as having most difficulty, the practitioner has recognised

Worksheet 11.4 Example of a completed behavioural activation schedule after three support sessions

Write below the day of the week you want to start your schedule

		Thurs	Fri	Sat	Sun	Mon	Tues	Wed
Morning	What	Get out of bed	Get out of bed	Get out of bed	Get out of bed	Get out of bed	Get out of bed	Get out of bed
	Where	Home	Home	Home	Home	Home	Home	Home
	Who	Me	Me	Me	Me	Me	Me	Me
	When	8am	8am	10.30am	11am	9am	8am	9am
	What						Get to Job	
	Where						Butchers	
	Who						Me	
	When						9.30	
Afternoon	What	Buy newspaper		Sort direct debit	Walk dog			
	Where	Shop			Park			
	Who	Me			Me and Jim			
	When	4pm			12.30pm			
	What		Work on car					
	Where		Garage					
	Who		Me					
	When		2pm					
Evening	What	Take warfarin	Take warfarin	Take warfarin	Take warfarin	Take warfarin	Take warfarin	Take warfarin
	Where							
	Who							
	When							
	What			Walk dog				
	Where			Park				
	Who			Me and Debs				
	When			7.30pm				
Comments		Great to get started, not much but did it!	Glad not too much planned but got up and enjoyed tinkering with the car	Great to sort direct debits out, no fun but done, glad Debs helped though	Nice lie in, but got up! Love walking dogs with Jim	Good to have easier day again, but did get up! Bit worried about work	Work was hard, but I stayed most of the day! Feel tad better	Glad of rest today and GP called about warfarin and was so happy I've taken it every day!

that these are necessary activities with imminent deadlines or have potentially important-to-avoid negative impacts. The practitioner employed the COM-B model (Chapter 8) with the patient to problem-solve ways to complete them. The employer was very helpful by agreeing to a gradual return.

Additionally, within the first support session, the practitioner recognised 'Take Warfarin' as another necessary activity not being undertaken although graded least difficult. Using funnelling (Chapter 5), the practitioner recognised that the patient's difficulties with concentration were resulting in problems remembering to take this medication. Whilst the practitioner was unaware of the importance of this medication, liaison with the practice GP indicated it was of utmost importance to take it daily and a further appointment with the GP was made straight away. The practice pharmacist discussed solutions with the patient to support medication taking, and at the following session the practitioner recognised additional benefits to aid patient memory by putting this activity into the Behavioural activation schedule.

Stage 5: Patient Follows Schedule

Once the patient has been encouraged to complete their Behavioural activation schedule between sessions, they should be encouraged to engage with the schedule as soon as possible and complete the activities written down in the schedule before the next within session review. To support the progress review (Stage 6), the patient should be asked to make notes in the Comments box at the bottom of the Behavioural activation schedule. In particular, patients should be asked to record any achievements or difficulties they faced when completing the activities whilst making a note of whether completing the activity made them feel any better or worse.

Stage 6: Review Progress

The aim of the next support session is to review patient progress following completion of the Behavioural activation schedule. In the first support session following assessment, attention should be directed towards ensuring that the patient has written the activities into their schedule and not made any slip-ups (Table 11.3). In the following support sessions, the patient should be encouraged to review progress since the previous session and receive feedback. Feedback should employ common factors skills associated with funnelling to recognise what went well or challenges faced. Empathy should be used where challenges have been encountered (Chapter 5).

When challenges have been met, a good opportunity is provided to reflect back on the rules of scheduling (Table 11.1) and identify common difficulties (Table 11.3). Where helpful, an opportunity is also provided to review *the here and now* formulation (Chapter 2) and identify the impact that difficulties have had across the four

Table 11.3 Common difficulties experienced by patients engaging with behavioural activation

Difficulty	Specific factor to address difficulty
Unable to begin or continue with activities included within the schedule	Consider ways to break larger activities down into more manageable ones or consider the benefits of using the COM-B or SOC models if challenges engaging in the activity are experienced
Trying to do too many difficult activities, resulting in struggles to continue	Avoid 'boom' and 'bust', supporting the patient to increase the number of activities at a rate suitable for them
Mood dropping and difficult to continue engagement with the schedule	Ensure pleasurable and routine activities are spread across the week to ensure reinforcement is received for longer periods of time
Difficulties completing a necessary activity	Recognise and consider signposting opportunities to address necessary activities, paying attention to deadlines as this may indicate the urgency of any further action
Recently acquired problems making it too difficult to undertake previous activities	Consider using the COM-B or SOC model to enable the patient to recognise new ways of achieving the activity or to consider other activities of equal value to them
Cannot think of pleasurable activities as depressed for so long	Support the patient to recognise helpful ways of identifying pleasurable activities. This can sometimes be assisted by focusing on tasks recognised as having 'value' rather than just pleasure
Struggling to categorise routine, pleasurable and necessary activities	When categorising tasks, encourage the patient to think back to a time before they had depression, but most important is achieving a balance across the scheduled activities

systems. To enhance learning, it is important initially to support the patient to identify rules that may not have been followed and correct them, rather than correcting them yourself too early. However, employ a supportive and collaborative approach if the patient is struggling to identify rules (Chapter 5).

When challenges have been faced that have influenced progress, specific factor skills should be employed to inform the changes to the Behavioural activation schedule that are necessary in advance of the next support session (Table 11.1). Where appropriate, adopting the Capability, Opportunity, Motivation - Behaviour (COM-B) (Chapter 8) or Selection, Optimisation, Compensation (SOC) model (Chapter 19) to help address the difficulties experienced may be helpful. Within support sessions it is important to remain responsive to the needs of the patient given that they are likely to progress well between some support sessions but experience setbacks between others. Variable progress, especially early in treatment, is commonly experienced and patients should be supported to view setbacks as learning opportunities.

At the end of the support session a shared decision should be reached with the patient regarding steps to take between support sessions. If the patient has been making good progress, raise the possibility that discharge may be discussed at the next support session. However, in the event of poor progress with treatment having little effect on mood severity, the possibility of stepping up to HICBT should also be raised (Chapter 4). Where appropriate, it should be mentioned that HICBT is available within the same service, specifying the expected waiting time. Informed by service protocols, detail the next steps.

Summary

This chapter has focused on the BA model (Richards, 2010c) forming the seminal treatment option for depression within LICBT. Representing an intervention in its own right, BA has been identified as effective as HICBT and anti-depressant medication, and more effective than other psychological therapies (Ekers et al., 2008). Based on a behavioural model of depression, the focus of BA is on treating depression from the *outside in* whereby the intervention supports the patient identify and engage with sources of reinforcement in the environment (Jacobson et al., 2001). This focus is achieved by supporting the patient follow a six-stage protocol – explain, categorise, grade, schedule, follow, review – forming the basis of the BA model employed in LICBT. Several opportunities are presenting themselves for this basic and straightforward BA model to be employed as part of other evidence-based LICBT interventions, such as physical activity promotion (Farrand et al., 2014), including within a web-based format (Lambert et al., 2018).

Assessing Your Understanding

Declarative

Multiple Choice Questions

1. Which activities form the basis of the behavioural activation model used in low-intensity CBT? (Richards, 2010c) [Select all that apply]
    (a) Kinaesthetic
    (b) Autonomic
    (c) Necessary
    (d) Routine
    (e) Physical
2. Which of the following are common difficulties when scheduling activities into the Behavioural activation schedule? [Select all that apply]
    (a) Scheduling too many activities over too few days
    (b) Identifying activities from across the categories
    (c) On occasions needing to schedule necessary activities even when identified as having most difficulty
    (d) Choosing routine activities graded as having most difficulty before progressing up the hierarchy
    (e) Not remaining exposed to the situation causing fear until the rating has been reduced by at least 50 per cent of that recorded at the start of treatment

3. Which of the following distinguish between activity scheduling and the model of behavioural activation used in low-intensity CBT? [Select all that apply]
   (a) Use of a diary to record activities
   (b) Sole focus on enhancing opportunities for positive reinforcement
   (c) Collaborative working with the patient to schedule activities
   (d) Providing empathy when the patient struggles to complete activities scheduled in their diary
   (e) Ideographic approach to scheduling activities

Procedural

Self-Practice/Self-Reflection

- During the next week, keep a behavioural activation diary for yourself and at the end of the week categorise the activities undertaken and grade them in terms of difficulty. Reflect upon any challenges you experienced.
- Adopt specific factors to develop a Behavioural activation schedule for yourself to follow over the next week. Reflect upon any challenges you experienced.

   Answers to **Assessing Your Understanding** questions can be found in the appendix on p. 336.

Further Reading and Resources

Ekers, D., Webster, L., Van Straten, A., Cuijpers, P., Richards, D.A. and Gilbody, S. (2014) Behavioural activation for depression; an update of meta-analysis of effectiveness and sub group analysis. *PLoS One*, 9: e100100.

Hopko, D.R., Lejuez, C.W., Ruggiero, K.J. and Eifert, G.H. (2003) Contemporary behavioural activation treatments for depression: procedures, principles, and progress. *Clinical Psychology Review*, 23, 699–717.

Richards, D.A. (2010) Behavioural activation. In J. Bennett-Levy, D.A. Richards, P. Farrand, H. Christensen, K.M. Griffiths, D.J. Kavanagh, et al. (eds), *Oxford Guide to Low Intensity CBT Interventions*. Oxford: Oxford University Press. pp. 141–51

   To access the online resources accompanying this chapter, please visit: https://study.sagepub.com/farrand

12

Cognitive Interventions

A Thought is Just a Thought

Simon Grist

Learning Objectives

By the end of this chapter you should be able to:

- Critically appraise the theoretical basis for adopting a low-intensity CBT cognitive-based intervention
- Demonstrate an understanding of specific factors associated with low-intensity cognitive interventions based on cognitive restructuring alone, or combined with behavioural experiments
- Recognise when to move on to behavioural experiments when combined with cognitive restructuring in a single-strand low-intensity cognitive intervention
- Reflect on common difficulties a low-intensity psychological practitioner may face applying low-intensity CBT cognitive interventions and how these may be overcome

---

Intervention Description

Cognitive-based approaches to working with patients are a fundamental tool in the toolkit of the psychological practitioner workforce. As the name suggests, these approaches target patient thoughts or cognitions and represent a key intervention adopted within high-intensity cognitive behavioural therapy (HICBT) as part of a multi-strand approach. Beck and colleagues argue that most affective disorders develop from distorted thinking and ultimately lead to the development and maintenance of mental health difficulties (Beck et al., 1987).

However, within low-intensity CBT (LICBT) this is not to say that all LICBT psychological practitioners should strive to adopt cognitive approaches as the single-strand intervention. Cognitive interventions can be difficult for patients to effectively engage with and this can put pressure on briefer support sessions used in LICBT (Chapter 1). Whilst many mental health difficulties have a cognitive component therefore, especially with LICBT, some are better addressed with behavioural interventions, such as behavioural activation for depression (Chapter 11; Richards, 2010c) and graded exposure therapy for simple phobias (Chapter 13; Rosqvist, 2005). Cognitive interventions are adopted within both low- and high-intensity CBT (HICBT) and whilst sharing some similarities there are also fundamental differences.

Key Point

Differences between Cognitive Interventions

- LICBT only targets negative automatic thoughts associated with the presenting problem in the here and now.
- HICBT cognitive interventions are adopted to target dysfunctional assumptions and core beliefs identified within a longitudinal formulation.
- Within HICBT behavioural experiments (BE) are employed alongside cognitive restructuring (CR) within a multi-strand cognitive approach.
- LICBT cognitive interventions vary between those adopting CR alone, whilst others combine CR with BE within a single-strand cognitive intervention.

Although debate exists as to what differentiates a single from multi-strand approach (Chapter 1), in this chapter it is considered that given the intention of CR with BE is to target 'cognitive or schematic change' (Clark, 2013: 2) the intervention is single strand. LICBT cognitive interventions that adopt CR only (Lovell and Richards, 2012) and combine CR and BE (Farrand et al., 2015) are therefore addressed in this chapter. Training manuals such as *Reach Out* (Richards and Whyte, 2011) laid the foundations for the LICBT cognitive intervention based on CR alone with subsequently written CBT self-help interventions (Farrand et al., 2015) and books (Papworth and Marrinan, 2019) building on this foundation by including BEs.

Evidence Base

Cognitive interventions have a long history and evidence base following their pivotal role within Beck's seminal HICBT protocol (Beck et al., 1987) and manuals such as *Mind Over Mood* (Padesky and Greenberger, 1995). Whilst there is a wealth of evidence for the application of cognitive interventions in HICBT (Beck et al., 1987; Bennett-Levy et al., 2004; Clark, 2013; Leahy and Rego, 2012), the current evidence base within LICBT is limited. However, protocols for the LICBT cognitive interventions are informed by those used with HICBT, with adaptations to facilitate delivery in a time-limited and single-strand intervention.

A number of studies have demonstrated the effectiveness of CR for depression (Fennell, 1989; Miskowiakn et al., 2016; Teasdale and Fennell, 1982), panic disorder (Clark, 1996; Beadel et al., 2016) and post-traumatic stress disorder (Ehlers and Clark, 2000). Additionally, a series of case studies demonstrated that BEs lead to longer time before relapse in interventions using exposure (Craske et al., 2014). However, a systematic review reported limited evidence favouring BEs in the treatment of specific phobias (McMillan and Lee, 2010) with change associated with BE argued to occur through exposure and not by challenging a cognition (Longmore and Worrell, 2007). Cognitive interventions are, however, increasingly adopted for populations (e.g. intellectual disability) previously considered to struggle to access cognitive approaches (Roberts and Kwan, 2017).

Theoretical Rationale

The LICBT cognitive interventions addressed in this chapter enable patients to adopt an objective stance to challenge NATs (negative automatic thoughts) in a balanced and realistic way using CR (Richards and Whyte, 2011) and then use BE to test them out (Farrand et al., 2015). This enables patients to challenge NATs without being influenced by their emotional state and the subsequent bias this can cause (Beck, 1987). The LICBT CR technique adopts a number of verbal strategies (Clark, 2013) written into self-help interventions that help the patient challenge NATs that influence their affective state.

Key Point

Examples of Verbal Techniques Adopted in LICBT CR (Clark, 2013)

- Evidence-gathering
- Cognitive bias identification
- Generate alternatives
- Distancing
- Reframing.

Where the LICBT cognitive intervention combines CR and BE (Farrand et al., 2015) empirical hypothesis testing (Clark, 2013) then generates new 'evidence' that may refute or support the NAT. Whilst 'behavioural' implies a specific focus on changing behaviour, a BE targets a change in cognition identified via CR (Clark, 2013). The change in cognition is therefore generated through experimentation and the development of new evidence to challenge the cognition. Within an LICBT single-strand CR intervention (Farrand et al., 2015), therefore, the BE targets an additional mechanism to that targeted by CR and uses 'evidence' to challenge the level of belief associated with the NAT.

Application of the LICBT Cognitive Intervention

Excluding generalised anxiety disorder (GAD; Chapter 3), the LICBT CR intervention can be adopted for the treatment of all common mental health problems determined by the National Institute for Health and Care Excellence (NICE, 2011b) for LICBT treatment. Choosing an LICBT CR intervention should reflect the patient's assessment and treatment goals (Chapter 2). Unless the patient expresses a preference for cognitive interventions in working on depression, however, behavioural activation is a more suitable alternative (Chapter 11). Within the Improving Access to Psychological Therapies programme (IAPT; Chapter 20; Seward and Clark, 2010) two LICBT cognitive interventions are generally adopted by services.

Key Point

Common LICBT Cognitive Interventions

- Focused solely on CR (Lovell and Richards, 2012) as specified in the original IAPT training curriculum (Richards and Whyte, 2011). This intervention is covered by intervention stages 1 to 4 addressed later in this chapter.
- Combines CR with BE (Farrand et al., 2015). This intervention is covered by intervention stages 1 to 9 addressed later in this chapter.

Neither LICBT CR single-strand approach is currently supported by definitive research. However, BE logically follows on from CR as it aims to generate new evidence to help shift belief in NATs and their emotional content. The key thing to remember is that CR evaluates current evidence supporting NATs whereas BEs generate new evidence for or against it.

Specific Factors: Supporting Cognitive Interventions

Key Point

Intervention Stages

- *Stage 1*: Explain the cognitive intervention adopted
- *Stage 2*: Identify unhelpful NATs
- *Stage 3*: Examine NATs and search for evidence
- *Stage 4*: Use gathered evidence to reconsider thoughts
- *Stage 5*: Review progress with CR.

Where cognitive intervention combines CR with BE:

- *Stage 6*: Clinical decision-making
- *Stage 7*: Plan
- *Stage 8*: Do
- *Stage 9*: Review progress.

Stage 1: Explain the Rationale and Gain Patient 'Buy-in'

In the session it is important to explain the LICBT CR intervention to enable patients to appreciate the underpinning theory. If adopting an intervention combining CR with BE (Farrand et al., 2015) it is important to give an overview of the rationale behind both techniques and the protocol informing the transition to BE. However, if the LICBT cognitive intervention solely focuses on CR (Richards and Whyte, 2010), the rationale need only address Stages 1 to 5.

Clinical Example

Presenting Rationale of the LICBT Cognitive Intervention Combining CR Progressing to BE

Based on the problem statement we constructed together it appears you're struggling with depression. We discussed behavioural activation that we'd commonly recommend in cases like yours but given that your thoughts currently cause you a lot of distress and you find yourself ruminating a lot on them, you'd like to try a cognitive intervention. The intervention I will explain combines two techniques that aim to give you the skills to evaluate your thoughts in a more objective way and if needed test them out. The first technique, called cognitive restructuring, teaches you to examine evidence that supports and contradicts the hot thought linked to your low mood causing you most distress and then re-evaluate it in light of the evidence. Some people find that by challenging their hot thought in the light of the evidence the belief they had in the hot thought reduces, helping them overcome their emotional problem. If you're happy with progress at this point you can choose to end the intervention. However, although at this point the amount of belief some patients hold in their hot thought has gone down and they logically know the thought is not accurate, they still find it impacts on their emotion. If this is the case it can be helpful to move onto behavioural experiments that support you to construct a real-life experiment to directly test the thought out to create further evidence that allows you to re-evaluate your hot thought. You will be supported by me to work through the cognitive intervention at a pace that suits you. Learning to evaluate your thoughts can help you manage the low mood you're experiencing. Being able to recognise unhelpful thoughts and manage these will improve your emotional difficulties and allow you to return to the things that are important to you. How does this sound?

It is important to ensure the patient appreciates that they have the opportunity to ask questions. You may like to have some printed information that explains the intervention in more detail ready to be handed, or if working over the telephone, sent to the patient.

Stage 2: Identify Unhelpful NATs

After explaining the cognitive intervention, the next step within the assessment session is to support the patient identify some of their NATs. Encourage the patient to write them down in the Thought diary as they are being identified (Worksheet 12.1).

Worksheet 12.1   Thought diary

Time/date	Situation (What? Where? With whom? etc.)	What emotion did you notice? What rating would you give this out of 100 (where 0 is minimal or no emotion and 100 is the worst you have ever felt)	What thoughts did you notice? What went through your mind?	Any other observations about this situation?

Within the constraints of the session time available, the patient should be supported to work through the Thought diary within the session. Depending on the time available and the level of understanding expressed by the patient, initially support them with one or two NATs to subsequently facilitate between-session homework.

Clinical Practice

Supporting the Thought Diary within the Session

1. Support the patient to identify NATs related to specific situations that lead to an emotional shift likely to be associated with the probable diagnosis.
2. Record the emotion(s) linked to the situation and rate using the 0–100 scale.
3. Identify the NAT(s) that arise as a result of the situation/emotion and rate the belief in the NAT(s).
4. Select the NAT with the highest belief rating causing the most distress as a *hot thought* to initially work on.

It is important to make NATs capable of being tested by ensuring they are thoughts and not questions, emotions or physical sensations. Sometimes the patient may write questions or 'What if' statements in the Thought diary that will be unspecific (Kennerley et al., 2016). The Thought diary, to be completed between sessions, should therefore be reviewed within the session to ensure that identified thoughts are amenable to testing. In the event that thoughts are not able to be tested the patient could be asked to reframe them as a statement. 'What ifs' can be reframed by asking the patient what the statement would mean if it was true.

Clinical Example

Reframing a 'What if' Statement

Practitioner: Thanks for completing the Thought diary. How did you find it?
Patient: I found myself often getting caught up in my thoughts. However, once it became more of a habit it was easier.
Practitioner: It's great to see you've made progress. I can see you've written down a number of thoughts related to the situation 'Phoning a friend to arrange a coffee'. It's good to put as many of the thoughts down as you can. I see one of them is a 'What if?' thought and I'm not sure how

easy it'll be to work with. It's not very specific and you may struggle to challenge it. I wonder if it may be a good use of time within this session to have a go at turning it into more of a testable thought?

Patient: OK, but I'm not sure how.

Practitioner: Sometimes with 'What if' thoughts it's easier to think about what the thought might mean to you if it were true. For example, you've written down, 'What if she is too busy to go for coffee with me?' If your friend was too busy, what would that mean to you?

Patient: Well that would mean she doesn't like me very much.

Practitioner: I can see that's an upsetting thought, but it'll now give us a thought you can apply the technique to. Do you think that's a true reflection of the 'What if' thought?

Generally, the NAT with the highest belief rating and causing the most distress will be chosen to work with as the hot thought (Beck et al., 1987). To enable the patient recognise progress, it is recommended that the belief rating should be at least 60 per cent or over (Richards and Whyte, 2011). Additionally, the hot thought chosen to work on should have been identified by the patient as the most amenable to change or modification (Kennerley et al., 2016). Consequently, whilst the patient may have identified several NATs during the assessment, it may not be these that are worked on if between sessions the patient begins to recognise that another NAT would be better to work on initially. Mentioning this at the end of the support session can be helpful.

Stage 3: Examine Thoughts and Search for Evidence

Using the Evidence recording and revised thought worksheet (Worksheet 12.2) the patient should write down the hot thought, rating the percentage belief (Beck et al., 1987).

Evidence should then be collected and assigned to either the Evidence for or Evidence against columns. To ensure the hot thought is evaluated as objectively as possible it is important that the patient gathers evidence for and against. Patients may struggle to identify objective evidence against the thought and write down opinions rather than facts. This should be checked within support sessions and, if needed, helpful questions can be asked to support the patient gather suitable objective evidence (Kennerley et al., 2016).

Worksheet 12.2 Evidence recording and revised thought

My hot thought		Belief in the thought (0–100)

Evidence for the thought	Evidence against the thought

My revised thought		Belief in the revised Thought (0–100)

The original emotion I felt	Strength of this emotion in light of my revised thought (0–100%)

Clinical Practice

Helpful Questions to Separate Fact from Opinion

- What evidence would I use for and against the thought?
- Take the thought to court and present your evidence to the judge. The evidence you present has to be based on facts, not your opinions.
- What would a trusted friend say?
- If your belief rating is, for example, 80 per cent, what makes up the other 20 per cent?

To help the patient with the LICBT cognitive intervention it may also be helpful to illustrate generalised thinking errors that are sometimes evident to reflect a style of thinking rather than a specific thought (Table 12.1).

Depending on the time available within the session, once the patient has begun to understand the process, ask them to complete the Evidence recording and revised thought worksheet, recognising any generalised thinking errors as between-session homework may be required in preparation for the next support session.

Stage 4: Using Gathered Evidence to Reconsider Thoughts

At this point, your patient should have gathered evidence for and against their hot thought that may have been supported by recognising generalised thinking errors. The patient should now consider the hot thought recorded on the Evidence recording

Table 12.1 Types of generalised thinking errors

Thinking Error	Examples
Mental Filter	Focusing on a random or isolated detail of an event. E.g. A person yawning is interpreted as meaning that the whole dinner party is a disaster, ignoring the positives or focusing on negatives.
Mind Reading	Making assumptions about what others think in the absence of evidence.
Prediction	Predicting a negative outcome whereby one previous negative experience is used to predict similar outcomes in ALL future situations.
Compare and Despair	"Everybody else is doing OK and I'm not!" "They're coping, why can't I?" "Nobody else is struggling with these problems."
Catastrophising	Thinking the worst possible thing will happen, while ignoring more likely alternatives.
Labelling/Mislabelling	Judging self or others on the basis of one mistake or event.
Emotional Reasoning	"It feels bad, therefore it IS bad!"
Black and White Thinking	All or nothing; either something works out perfectly or it is a disaster.
Critical Self	Total blaming of self for events where a negative outcome is a shared responsibility; "It's all my fault, I'm not good enough."

and revised thought worksheet in light of evidence gathered. Regardless of whether the hot thought has changed or not, it is important that the patient re-rates their belief in the thought and emotion rating. In the next support session, the Evidence recording and revised thought worksheet should be reviewed and the impact of any changes on emotion explored.

Stage 5: Review Progress Using CR

Following the use of CR, it is important to review progress *within-session* to inform clinical decision-making with appropriate actions taken (Chapter 6). If the patient has failed to reach recovery, clinical decisions to be made depend upon the cognitive approach taken. In all cases, decisions reached should be presented at case management supervision (Chapter 9).

Clinical Practice

Decision-Making Following the Use of CR

- *Reached recovery*: Discharge
- *No progress*: Present options to the case management supervisor
- *Some progress but patient has not reached recovery*: Consider the benefits of moving to BE when:
  - New evidence is considered helpful to test the revised thought
  - Belief in the NAT has fallen but there is little improvement in the emotion rating.

During clinical decision-making, maintain awareness that a limited number of sessions is a key characteristic of LICBT. This will likely be a consideration of the case management supervisor (Chapter 9).

Stage 6: Plan

Help the patient identify a hot thought or revised, more balanced thought identified during CR to serve as the basis of the BE and rate the level of belief (0–100%) they have in this thought (Worksheet 12.3).

It is then important to work collaboratively with the patient to identify how they are going to test the thought out bearing in mind session length.

Worksheet 12.3 Behavioural experiments plan

Thoughts to be put into action	
The thought I want to put into action is:	I believe this thought (0–100%) [%]
Designing the experiment	
I am going to test this thought by:	
What?	
Where?	
When?	
Who?	
Predicting the worst	
I predict the worst that will happen is:	I think this will happen (0–100%) [%]
Predicting an alternative:	I think this will happen (0–100%) [%]
Possible barriers	
The following things may get in the way:	
Overcoming barriers	
I might overcome these barriers by:	

Clinical Practice

Supporting the BE within the Session

- Identify the What? Where? When? and With whom? (the four Ws) for undertaking the BE
- Design the BE
- Support the patient to make predictions about the worst and alternative outcomes, rating how likely they believe these will arise
- Support the patient to consider any barriers that might stop them from conducting the BE.

COM-B (Michie et al., 2011) is a useful tool to consider potential barriers (Chapter 8). These barriers then need to be addressed to minimise any difficulties with conducting the BE. This enables the patient to anticipate possible barriers, making the BE more likely to be completed.

Stage 7: Do

The four Ws (Chapter 2) and COM-B should have enhanced the likelihood that the patient will carry out the BE. However, it is helpful to use common factor skills to normalise potential difficulties that may be encountered or empathise when the patient has struggled to engage with or complete the BE (Chapter 5). Ultimately, this stage is down to the patient to complete between sessions, unlike HICBT where in-vivo work may be carried out within sessions and on occasions and when needed outside of the office.

Many patients will struggle to remember the details of the BE if they do not record it. Therefore, using a Behavioural Experiments Review worksheet (Worksheet 12.4) is helpful to ensure that the LICBT practitioner and patient have something to review within the next support session.

It may be that the patient has struggled to complete all worksheet sections between sessions. If so, *within-session* the patient should be made aware that they should try to complete up to What happened? This can then be used as the focus of the next support session for further problem-solving (Chapter 6).

Stage 8: Review

The final stage is to review the Behavioural experiments review worksheet, working with the patient to elicit any areas of the worksheet not completed (Worksheet 12.4).

Worksheet 12.4 Behavioural experiments review

Thought to be put into action	
The thought I want to put into action is:	I believe this thought (0–100%) [%]
My original prediction	
I predicted the following would happen:	I believe this thought (0–100%) [%]
What happened?	
My learning	
From this behavioural experiment I have learned:	
Revising my original thought	
I would now change my original thought to:	
I believe this new thought (0–100%) [%]	I believe my original thought [%]
Changing behaviour	
Based on my new thought I'm going to do the following differently:	
Next steps	
Other behavioural experiments I may want to try:	

Supporting the patient to complete the worksheet should comprise a discussion around what the patient has learnt conducting the BE and whether there has been any change to the NAT being tested. It is important to re-rate the belief in the NAT regardless of whether it has been revised or any belief remains.

A discussion with the patient surrounding the impact the BE may have had on their emotion and what they might do in the future if faced with similar NATs helps to draw this intervention to a close. It might be that the patient wishes to apply BEs to another thought, in which case the LICBT practitioner can support this. However, if further sessions are agreed during case management supervision (Chapter 9), it is important to reduce the intensity of support to ensure that the patient is engaging fully with BE and adopting guided self-help principles.

Reflection Point

Reflect on how you might apply a cognitive intervention with patients whose first language is not English or have an intellectual disability.

Challenges with LICBT Cognitive Intervention

The LICBT cognitive intervention can present several challenges to patients with respect to engaging with the specific factors associated with the intervention. The LICBT practitioner should address challenges within support sessions and it may be helpful to consider the utility of the COM-B model (Michie et al., 2011) to overcome barriers (Chapter 8).

Key Point

Common Challenges

- Difficulty challenging thoughts with high initial belief ratings
- Small and limited improvement
- Difficulty supporting the BE between sessions.

Difficulties Challenging Thoughts with High Initial Belief Ratings

Rather than representing unhelpful thoughts that arise in the here and now, thoughts having high initial belief ratings have the potential to represent intermediate or core beliefs. Initially, try to support the patient to identify other situations to enable them to elicit NATs that can be worked on. If the patient is unable to identify any NATs, at case management supervision (Chapter 9) consider the appropriateness of referral to Step 3 HICBT for a longitudinal formulation with multi-strand interventions better able to address enduring cognitive distortions (Chapter 1).

Small and Limited Improvement

It is important for the patient to understand that cognitive change can take time and most importantly practice. This should be made clear when providing the theoretical rationale during the assessment session. Additionally, use common factor skills to ensure that the patient is made aware of progress that has been made during the review of intervention progress within support sessions. This could involve emphasising improvement in the severity of the mental health difficulty being treated as demonstrated by changes in the routine outcome measures (Chapter 6).

Difficulty Supporting the BE between sessions

An HICBT therapist has greater flexibility to support a patient undertake a planned in-vivo BE, potentially being able to support the patient outside of the treatment room (Bennett-Levy et al., 2004). Given shorter sessions and limits placed on LICBT practice, the LICBT practitioner is unlikely to be able to provide such support. On these occasions, the practitioner could adopt the COM-B model (Michie et al., 2011) within treatment sessions to help the patient overcome barriers to completing the BEs. This could involve the patient identifying someone they know and trust who is able to provide support to undertake their BE and potentially be involved in reviewing how it went when completing the worksheet.

Summary

Cognitive interventions have been widely and successfully used in HICBT with a growing LICBT evidence base (Beck et al., 1987; McMillan and Lee, 2010). LICBT cognitive interventions vary from the use of CR alone to reduce belief in NATs (Richards and Whyte, 2011) to approaches incorporating BE to directly test a NAT and create further evidence to reduce belief (Farrand et al., 2019a). This chapter has focused on applying LICBT cognitive interventions to reduce distress, presenting a five-stage CR protocol with an additional four stages adopted when CR progresses to the use of BEs. Whilst cognitive interventions are an important tool in the LICBT toolkit, cognitive change takes time. When evidence based for the mental health problem being treated therefore, a behavioural intervention may represent a better approach to accommodate briefer session times associated with LICBT.

Assessing Your Understanding

Declarative

Multiple Choice Questions

1. Behavioural experiments are different from cognitive restructuring as they…
   [Select all that apply]
   (a) …do not need a thought to be utilised as an intervention
   (b) …generate further evidence to help challenge a thought
   (c) …conduct a thorough review of the available evidence to challenge a thought
   (d) …are used to reduce belief in a NAT
   (e) …are the first stage of exposure

2. Cognitive change is generally a slow process. This is because... [Select all that apply]

    (a) ...cognitive interventions often take longer to become familiar with

    (b) ...a robust understanding of what constitutes a thought available for change is required

    (c) ...many patients do not have the intellectual capacity for a cognitive approach

    (d) ...a behavioural approach should always be engaged with first

    (e) ...an LICBT practitioner always needs to deliver both CR and BEs consistent with a single-strand approach

Procedural

Self-Practice/Self-Reflection

- Keep a Thought diary over the next week, recording thoughts around situations that have an emotional (but manageable) impact.
- Rate the emotion and belief linked to the situations.
- Apply CR-specific factors to one of your thoughts that have a belief rating of over 60 per cent.
- Design, plan and carry out a BE to help generate new evidence for your revised thought following CR. Reflect on difficulties you faced with the above and how you would go about addressing these when working with a patient.

  Answers to Assessing Your Understanding questions can be found in the appendix on p. 336.

Further Reading and Resources

Clark, D.A. (2013) Cognitive restructuring. In S.G. Hoffman (ed.), *The Wiley Handbook of Cognitive Behavioral Therapy*. London: Wiley & Sons. (pp. 23–44)

McMillan, D. and Lee, R. (2010) A systematic review of behavioral experiments vs exposure alone in the treatment of anxiety disorders: a case of exposure while wearing the emperor's new clothes? *Clinical Psychology Review*, 30, 467–78.

To access the online resources accompanying this chapter, please visit: https://study.sagepub.com/farrand

13

Graded Exposure Therapy
Climbing Ladders to Health

Mark Papworth

Learning Objectives

By the end of this chapter you should be able to:

- Critically appraise the theoretical rationale associated with the exposure therapy model used in low-intensity CBT
- Demonstrate an understanding of the principles associated with the low-intensity model of graded exposure
- Apply principles associated with supporting a patient to engage with low-intensity graded exposure for the treatment of specific phobias
- Recognise and overcome common difficulties experienced by patients when engaging with graded exposure

---

Intervention Description

A specific phobia is a disorder consisting of a marked and persistent anxiety or fear, caused by at least one object or situation that results in significant impairment or distress. Phobias have been categorised as being linked to animals (e.g. snakes), situations (such as driving) and the natural environment (for instance, heights); although not all phobias fit into these categories (such as a fear of clowns). Names for individual phobias are generally constructed by suffixing 'phobia' (*phobos* means 'fear' in Greek) to the Greek word for the feared object or situation. For example, arachnephobia (or arachnophobia) refers to a fear of spiders where the Greek word for spider is *arachne*. Lists of these names are available online, for example phobialist.com or en.wikipedia.org/wiki/List_of_phobias.

This chapter does not cover blood-injury and injection phobias where an adapted approach involving the use of applied tension is required (Ost and Sterner, 1989). Furthermore, social phobia (social anxiety disorder), where an individual is anxious about the possible scrutiny of others, is not recommended for treatment with low-intensity CBT (NICE, 2013).

Exposure Approaches

Exposure therapy consists of a number of approaches and formats, all of which involve a reduction in anxiety through controlled exposure to the feared object or situation (the stimulus). Covering several different approaches, exposure therapy has been used as a single-strand treatment (Chapter 1) for several anxiety problems since the 1960s (Barlow and Durrand, 1999; Rosqvist, 2005). It is used as a component intervention within several protocols informing high-intensity cognitive behavioural therapy (HICBT; Leahy et al., 2012).

Key Point

Modalities of Exposure Therapy

- *Graded or hierarchical*: Exposure conducted in stages
- *Single session*: Stages occur over the course of a single morning or afternoon (Ost, 1989)
- *Flooding*: Patient exposed to a stimulus in a single, longer session with a view to making them become initially as anxious as possible (Stampfl and Levis, 1967).

Only graded exposure therapy (GET) is addressed in this chapter given that it is the only approach that is consistent with the LICBT method.

Key Point

Characteristics of GET That Make It Consistent with LICBT

- Most manageable approach to adopt on a guided self-help basis
- LICBT sessions are commonly restricted to no more than 30 minutes duration
- Approach most commonly adopted within supporting LICBT self-help texts (e.g. Bourne, 2015; Farrand and Sheppard, 2018; Williams, 2012).

Exposure Format

The format of the exposure refers to the manner in which the stimulus is presented to patients. It consists of in-vivo and in-imagination, the latter of which can include the use of virtual reality (VR). Within the in-vivo format, the patient is presented with the feared stimuli live, in real life and in real time. With in-imagination exposure, these stimuli are focused upon purely internally through use of the person's imagination or through the use of VR. The in-imagination format has been considered to be a helpful approach when used to build up to in-vivo exposure or where it is not practicable to use real stimuli, for example with a fear of thunderstorms.

Evidence Base

A recent meta-analytic review (Wolitzky-Taylor et al., 2008) confirms that amongst all psychological interventions, exposure is potentially one of the most potent. In comparison to both waiting-list and placebo control groups, a large effect size was found for exposure therapy at follow-up. This was larger than found in similar comparisons using other psychological interventions for the treatment of depression, panic disorder and generalised anxiety disorder (Westen and Morrison, 2001). Within the review, exposure treatments were also found to be significantly more effective than non-exposure treatments (e.g. applied relaxation). More tentative findings have also highlighted that the in-vivo approach is more effective, with the multiple (graded) session modality being advantageous over single-session alternatives (Wolitzky-Taylor et al., 2008). Subsequent reviews have had a narrower focus, for example in the effectiveness of the use of VR. Many patients are reported to prefer this approach (Garcia-Palacios et al., 2007) with a meta-analysis reporting no significant differences between VR and in-vivo exposure (Carl et al., 2019).

Theoretical Rationale

Exposure is conceptualised as a behavioural approach. This assumes that phobias are developed primarily through and maintained by two stages of conditioning (Mowrer, 1947). In the first stage (Pavlov, 1903), a classical conditioning process occurs where a neutral stimulus (e.g. a dog) is paired with an unconditioned stimulus that produces an anxiety or fear response (such as a dog bite). This results in a conditioned response whereby a fear response becomes triggered by exposure to dogs.

The second stage (Skinner, 1938), is an operant conditioning process where the avoidance of dogs is negatively reinforced through the reduction of fear, for example crossing a road to avoid a dog. Where an individual is repeatedly exposed to a dog

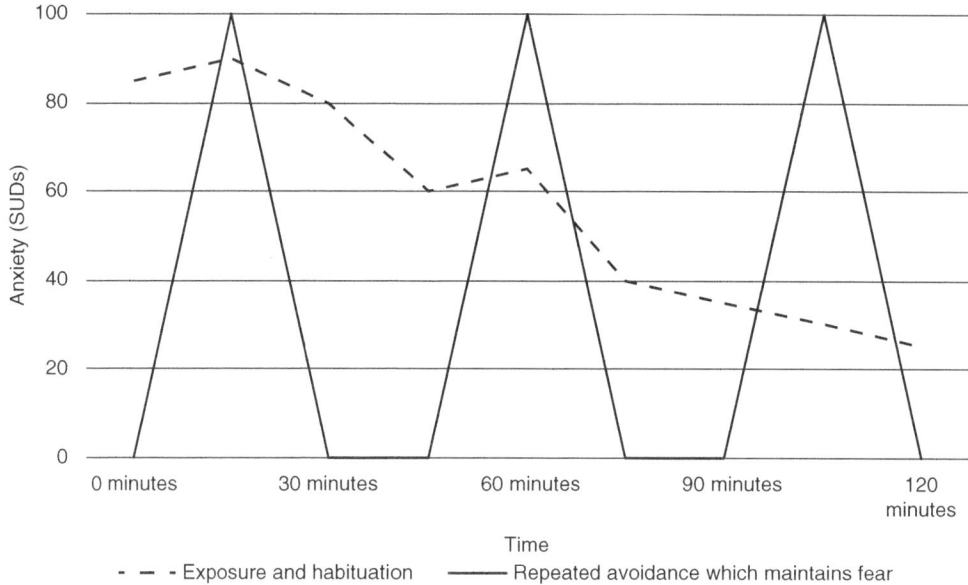

Figure 13.1   Anxiety levels associated with coping strategies of avoidance (escape) and exposure (with habituation)

(conditioned stimulus) and crosses the road to avoid it (avoidance), the individual has repeated experiences of negative reinforcement (Figure 13.1).

Although the individual's level of fear drops rapidly with avoidance, it is quickly raised again at subsequent exposure to dogs and so fear is maintained (solid line). A problem statement and maintenance cycle for this process is described (Figure 13.2).

Problem statement: I feel terrified when close to dogs; I avoid parks and countryside footpaths, and certain people who have them as pets. Near to dogs my heart races and I breathe heavily; I try desperately to escape as I think that they will bite me. I can't socialise with some people with dogs or relax in green spaces.

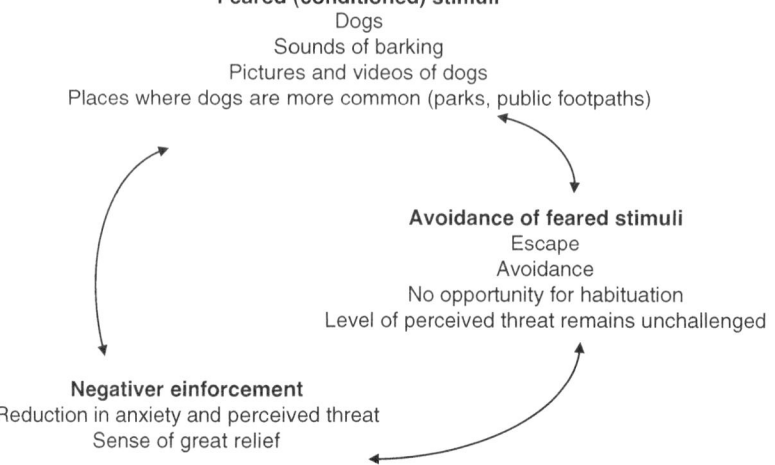

Figure 13.2   Azid's problem statement and maintenance cycle

Key Point

Additional Factors Considered Relevant to the Development of Phobias

- *Preparedness (Seligman, 1971)*: 'Pre-programmed' to fear 'natural' stimuli providing an evolutionary advantage (e.g. fear of spiders or snakes minimises the possibility of the receipt of a venomous bite).
- *Observation (Bandura, 1973; Rachman, 1977)*: Acquisition of fear through the observation of others (e.g. a parent modelling a fear response associated with clowns to a child).
- *Verbal information (Wilson, 1968)*: For example, being told by a parent that dogs will bite.

Exposure operates by deconditioning the individual's response to the conditioned stimulus, enabling the individual to overcome their avoidance by experiencing the stimulus (during practice sessions) whilst preventing avoidance. When avoidance is prevented, the level of fear reduces over time – a process called habituation (broken line; Figure 13.1).

Application of Graded Exposure

GET is an important approach adopted for all common anxiety disorders treated at Steps 2 and 3 of a stepped care mental health service delivery model (Chapter 1). Within LICBT specifically, GET is adopted as a single-strand treatment for mild to moderate presentations of specific phobia, agoraphobia and panic disorder (Chapter 3). Within multi-strand HICBT treatment protocols (Leahy et al., 2012), graded exposure is adopted alongside other CBT techniques (Part II) in the treatment of panic disorder, agoraphobia, generalised anxiety disorder, social anxiety disorder, post-traumatic stress disorder, specific phobia and obsessive-compulsive disorder (Chapter 3). It has also been conceptualised as being an active component in other treatment interventions and therapies, for example within eye movement desensitisation and reprocessing (Rosqvist, 2005; Wolitzky-Taylor et al., 2008).

Specific Factors: Supporting Graded Exposure

Graded exposure was first described within an LI context in the IAPT clinical support materials (Richards and Whyte, 2011), although it had been previously described in a similar form (e.g. Lovell, 1999). It is expanded upon below to consist of a six-stage protocol.

Clinical Practice

Intervention Stages

- *Stage 1*: Explain exposure principles and obtain informed consent
- *Stage 2*: Identify feared/anxiety provoking stimuli
- *Stage 3*: Grade stimuli creating an exposure hierarchy
- *Stage 4*: Set-up conditions for habituation
- *Stage 5*: Patient follows exposure hierarchy
- *Stage 6*: Review progress.

Worksheets included in a range of LICBT self-help interventions can be used both to help structure GET and as a record during exposure sessions (e.g. Bourne, 2015; Farrand and Sheppard, 2018; Papworth, 2020). Consistent with a LICBT approach, worksheet exercises should be supported within sessions. The patient should then be encouraged to fully engage with the self-help intervention as between-session 'homework' to consolidate learning (Chapter 6).

Stage 1: Explain Exposure Principles and Obtain Consent

As with all LICBT interventions, within sessions it is important to explain exposure to patients in an interactive manner that enables them to appreciate the underpinning theory supporting the LICBT model. This is essential as they will have received advice to confront their fears many times previously from well-meaning others, but in a way that may have been perceived to be unachievable.

Key Point

Content of Exposure Psychoeducation (Bourne, 1998; Rosqvist, 2005)

- *Evolutionary value of the fight or flight response and preparedness*. If the patient asks, describe the factors involved in the development of phobias (conditioning, modelling and verbal communication).
- *Role of avoidance in maintaining fear*: Emphasising that, whilst a natural response, avoidance negates the opportunity for extinction.
- *Habituation and its evolutionary value*: Deconditioning (or 'unlearning') occurs after experiencing the feared stimulus in the absence of negative consequences, enabling the conservation of valuable bodily resources that fuel the fight or flight response.
- *Graded*: How grading allows control over the level of anxiety/fear experienced.

Common examples/analogies can be helpful to illustrate the process (e.g. the use of incremental steps when learning to swim – grading; getting used to being in a cold swimming pool over time – habituation) and how this is applicable to GET. Whilst it is always important to obtain verbal consent before implementing an intervention, it is a particular consideration with GET as it involves the patient taking significant perceived risks, enduring higher levels of discomfort and it requires a great deal of persistence.

Stage 2: Identify Fear/Anxiety Provoking Stimuli

Fear/anxiety-provoking stimuli are objects or situations that are avoided or, at times, experienced with discomfort. They will be relevant to the patient's goals for therapy and should cluster around a theme that informs the nature of the phobia, which is identified through questioning. Questions asked during assessment (Chapter 2) will help to elicit this information and begin to inform the next stage of GET. The use of the IAPT Phobia Scales can also facilitate this. To establish the full range of stimuli, consideration should be given to the most feared circumstances, situations that may cause the mildest of discomfort and those lying between these two ends of the hierarchy.

Clinical Example

Questions to Elicit Feared/Anxiety-Provoking Stimuli

- What situations or objects are you fearful of?
- Are there any situations or objects that you would like to stop avoiding?
- What sorts of things do you do that you find help you to reduce the level of fear?
- Is there anything about [the situation/object] that would make it more or less intense for you?

If there is more than one feared/anxiety-provoking stimulus identified during assessment, usually the stimulus representing the priority for the patient is selected for treatment.

Stage 3: Grade Stimuli and Create an Exposure Hierarchy

Situations identified in Stage 2 should be rated out of 100 for fear/anxiety or in terms of the challenge the stimuli present. The situation causing the most distress is usually included at, or near, the maximum rating. Once rated, these can then be ordered into a hierarchy or ladder with the most feared situation at the top and least feared towards the bottom, with no large gaps between the steps or rungs. Generally, 8 to 12 steps on the ladder are sufficient (Bourne, 1998). Fewer steps may present the patient with too much challenge within the therapy or mean that aspects of the exposure hierarchy are not sufficiently represented. Once started within the session, the patient can be encouraged to complete the hierarchy between sessions, prior to the next support session (Table 13.1).

Once the hierarchy has been completed, it can be helpful to ask the patient a number of questions to ensure exposure tasks are well planned prior to being attempted.

Table 13.1 Exposure hierarchies for phobias relating to a) phobia of dogs (Azid) and b) phobia of driving over bridges (June)

Step of hierarchy	a) Situation	a) Azid's fear level	b) Situation[1]	b) June's fear level
12	Play 'fetch' with large dog, give them treats	100	Drive over Redheugh Bridge (very high, low sides, road close to edge), outer lane, with child on back seat	100
11	Local park at busy time of day, sit on bench near people with dogs	95	Drive over Redheugh Bridge (very high, low sides, road close to edge), outer lane, solo	95
10	Stroking large dog on lead	95	Drive over Redheugh Bridge (very high, low sides, road close to edge), inner lane, solo	85
9	Large, excited dog playing games at far side of room on lead	90	Drive over Tyne Bridge (high, more enclosed), outer lane, solo	85
8	Large, calm dog sitting at far side of room on lead	80	Drive over Tyne Bridge (high, more enclosed), inner lane, solo	80
7	Play 'fetch' with small dog, give them treats	80	Drive over Scotswood Bridge (medium high), outer lane, solo	75
6	Stroking small dog on lead	75	Drive over Scotswood Bridge (medium high), inner lane, solo	70
5	Small, excited dog playing games on lead at far side of room	60	Passenger in car driving over Redheugh Bridge (very high, low sides, road close to edge), outer lane	60
4	Small, calm dog sitting at far side of room on short lead	50	Passenger in car driving over Tyne Bridge (high, more enclosed), outer lane	50
3	Local park at a quiet time of day, sit on bench	40	Drive over Swing Bridge (very low, small), solo	50
2	Video of dogs	20	Drive over Swing Bridge (very low, small) with friend in passenger seat	45
1	Pictures of dogs	10	Video of driving over bridges, driver viewpoint	15

[1]Information regarding bridges available from www.bridgesonthetyne.co.uk

---

Reflection Point

With respect to phobias associated with wasps, driving around roundabouts and flying in an aircraft, reflect upon possible exposure hierarchies for these.

Clinical Example

Questions to Help Prepare for an Exposure Task Relating to a Dog Phobia

- When are you going to do the first exposure task?
- Who will bring the dog to the house?
- What type of dog would you consider to be small and what type large?
- How big should the room be for when you are in the room with the dog?
- What does the dog owner need to know to ensure they can support the exposure task?

Stage 4: Set-up Conditions for Habituation

Four necessary conditions should be followed to maximise the effectiveness of GET (Richards and Whyte, 2011).

Clinical Practice

Necessary Conditions for Exposure in GET

- Graded
- Prolonged
- Repeated
- Without distraction.

Graded

Discuss with the patient where they can start on their hierarchy. Whilst this decision should be patient led, the patient is likely to be able to choose a task they have identified as causing up to 50 per cent fear/anxiety, just before or at the start of exposure (Zayfert and Becker, 2007). Instructions for the practice session should be overviewed using suitable self-help materials and discussed as appropriate. When understood, patients should progress through their hierarchy in the graded fashion described in Stage 3.

Prolonged

Exposure to each task in the hierarchy should be prolonged in order to allow habituation to occur. In some instances, this may take as long as two hours; more usually 30 to 90 minutes is sufficient. However, it is important that time is *not used* to determine how long the patient should remain in the situation. Instead, it should be stressed that the patient remains in the situation until their level of fear/anxiety, sometimes termed subjective units of distress (SUDs), has reduced by at least 50 per cent from the rating noted just before or when they started the exposure task (e.g. from 80 to 40). For some tasks, consideration may be required to ensure exposure can be undertaken until SUDs have reduced by 50 per cent. For example, a person with a phobia associated with driving across bridges was instructed to repeatedly drive over a bridge, turn the car around and drive over the same bridge again until their SUDs had reduced to the appropriate level (Table 13.1, June, her clinical example is also below).

Repeated

Exposure should be repeated once per day on at least three to five days a week, but ideally daily (Bourne, 1998; Zayfert and Becker, 2007). The success of GET can be strengthened by varying the context of the exposure task (Craske et al., 2008). For instance, in GET for dog phobia, a wide variety of dogs and parks might be used (i.e. in steps 3–12 of Azid's hierarchy, Table 13.1).

Without Distraction

To maximise the potential for habituation, it is important that patients allow themselves to fully experience their fear/anxiety. This entails instructing them not to distract themselves as this is likely to serve as a safety behaviour to reduce their discomfort. Whilst specific to the individual, common types of safety behaviours include playing on a smartphone, listening to music, seeking reassurance, closing eyes or only engaging in activities with another person present. It can be helpful to support the patient to recognise any specific safety behaviours that they have. On occasion, tasks involving safety behaviours can be included within an exposure hierarchy if a task that involves dropping the behaviour is included at a higher step (Table 13.1, steps 2 and 3 of June's hierarchy).

Clinical Example

Case Study and Problem Statement: June

June was excited to have moved area with her new family, but she was immediately presented with a difficulty. To get to her new job in a solicitor's office she was required to drive across a bridge (the Redheugh Bridge). This presented significant challenges. For as long as she could remember, her father had avoided driving over bridges saying they made him feel scared. June had managed previously to drive across some small bridges (with significant difficulty) but had more recently not been able to do so following her maternity leave. After many months of having to leave 40 minutes earlier to drive to work to avoid the bridge, she decided to seek treatment. During the first session, the mental health practitioner (Alex) discussed graded exposure therapy with her and highlighted the '4 rules' that make the approach most likely to be effective. Within the session, they started to create an exposure task (Table 13.1, step 3 of June's hierarchy). Whilst three of the rules seemed fairly straightforward, June struggled to understand how 'prolonged' could be achieved, given that it would take less than a minute to drive over the bridge. The prolonged condition meant that she should drive over the bridge for as long as it took her anxiety to drop to 50 per cent of the baseline rating. Problem-solving the issue with Alex, they identified a way to achieve 'prolonged' by driving over the bridge, turning the car around and driving back again for as many times as needed for habituation to occur. This seemed overwhelming, but June felt that if she did this initially with a friend, it would be more achievable (Table 13.1, step 2 of June's hierarchy).

> *Problem statement*: I feel scared of driving over bridges; I drive long distances to avoid them. The thought of facing a bridge makes me come out in a hot sweat; I think that I will lose control of the car and drive over the edge. I spend much more time driving than I need to and I avoid travelling south of the river.

Stage 5: Patient Follows Exposure Hierarchy

Once the patient has completed their exposure hierarchy outside of the session, they should be encouraged to begin exposure task practice sessions as soon as possible after each support session. This helps to avoid dangers associated with procrastination that can add further credibility to the patient's fear and worsen it (Rosqvist, 2005). Patients should record their SUDs at the start of the practice session, at peak distress and at the end of the task. Noting down ratings at regular intervals (e.g. every five or ten minutes) can help with this task. Ratings can be recorded on worksheets included within self-help materials or by using other recording tools such as those included in smartphone applications.

Stage 6: Review Progress

Patient progress regarding the between-session practice sessions and movement up the exposure hierarchy should be reviewed during support sessions (Chapter 6). Whilst moving to the next task in the hierarchy should always be negotiated with the patient, typically by a point when the peak rating for a task is around 20 per cent, they should be encouraged to move onto the next step of the hierarchy (Zayfert and Becker, 2007). The process is then repeated, progressing up the hierarchy until the patient's symptoms fall within an acceptable range (Figure 13.3 illustrates the pattern of progression).

With continued progress, patients should be encouraged to take increasing responsibility for making decisions to move to the next step of the hierarchy and troubleshoot independently. To support troubleshooting, between-session homework tasks should be reviewed using the capability, opportunity, motivation – behaviour change model (COM-B; Michie et al., 2011) prior to the end of each support session (Chapter 8). In regard to homework agreed, it may be helpful to check if the patient is adequately motivated to complete it – for example, checking if the patient is sufficiently confident in their ability to do so. It can also be determined if the patient has sufficient opportunity – for example, adequate time in the day or ability to

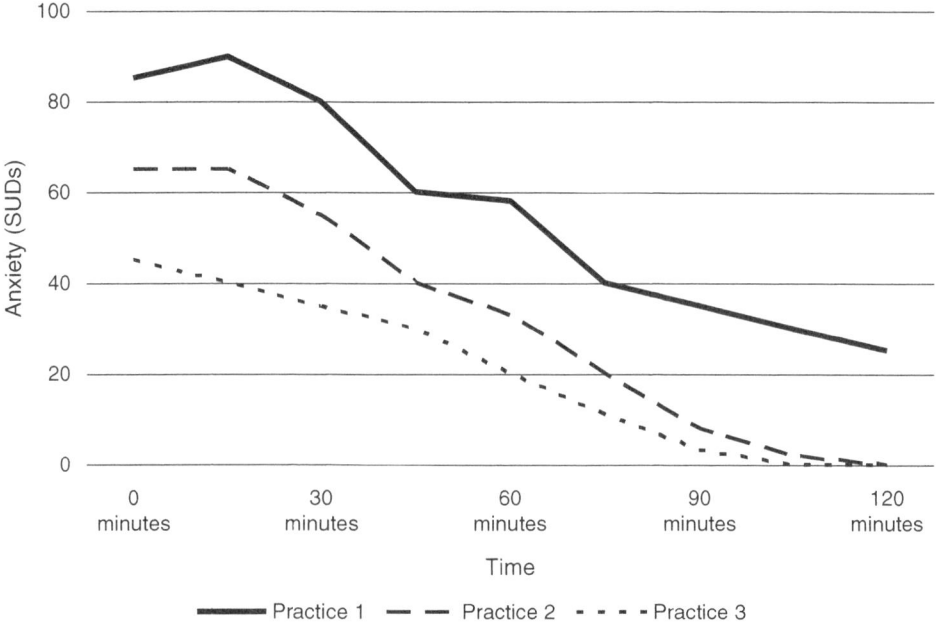

Figure 13.3 Reduction in anxiety levels with repeated exposure and habituation

enlist the necessary help of others. Many of Azid's tasks involve other people's dogs (Table 13.1); steps 2, 4 and 5 of June's hierarchy involve others as well. Finally, are they capable of completing the tasks – for example, has the patient fully understood the principles behind the approach?

Challenges Implementing Exposure Therapy

Challenges that arise with GET can often be resolved through the application of the COM-B model (see Papworth, 2019). Where possible, setbacks should be positively framed as learning opportunities rather than failures. However, some issues are commonly encountered (Bourne, 1998; Bourne, 2015; Rosqvist, 2005).

Key Point

Common Challenges

- Medication and alcohol
- Lack of success
- Motivation
- Co-morbid depression.

Medication and Alcohol

Psychotropic and some other medications may interfere with exposure by inhibiting anxiety and impeding habituation, and are therefore not usually recommended for the treatment of phobias (NHS, 2018). Consideration should also be given to the influence of alcohol or non-prescribed drugs. If possible, explore with the patient and/or their primary care physician whether use can be reduced or stopped.

Lack of Success

Sometimes patients underestimate the distress that they will experience or overestimate their ability to cope. This can result in the early termination of a practice session. A number of solutions can be applied on these occasions.

Clinical Practice

Solutions to Lack of Success

- Production of an intermediate step on the exposure hierarchy between the step successfully achieved and the one that the patient is struggling with. Consider facilitating the use of a safety behaviour at this step that is to be dropped at the next rung of the hierarchy.
- Use of an in-imagination exposure task to precede a step in the hierarchy. However, evidence suggests in-imagination is less effective than in-vivo exposure (Wolitzky-Taylor et al., 2008). Therefore, this should only be adopted when another suitable step cannot be identified.

Motivation

Due to high levels of anxiety that patients may foresee when engaging with GET, they may lack the motivation to engage. On these occasions, describe the specific factors (Chapter 5) associated with GET, highlighting that in Stage 3, situations that they feel are within reach will be identified which will allow them to start the process in a manageable fashion. Alternatively, some individuals may lack the motivation to follow through with the treatment more generally and in such instances motivational interviewing strategies may be helpful (Chapter 8; Miller and Rollnick, 2012; Papworth, 2019).

Co-morbid Depression

Up to 90 per cent of individuals with an anxiety disorder also experience depression (Gorman, 1997). Moderate to severe levels of depression may inhibit the processing of the exposure experience; it is therefore advisable to treat the depression first. Milder levels of depression may not interfere with GET and, with these patients, Rosqvist (2005) recommends adopting a data-driven approach. If habituation occurs within practice sessions but an expected reduction of SUDs does not occur between practice sessions, it is likely that symptoms of depression are impeding anxiety treatment. In such an instance, the depression should be treated before continuing with GET.

Summary

This chapter has overviewed the LICBT exposure model and its role in treating phobias, with research evidence highlighting it as an effective intervention. Exposure works through a process of deconditioning where the patient remains in the presence of the conditioned feared stimulus until habituation occurs. This is undertaken in a graded, prolonged and repeated basis, without distraction. LICBT exposure is accomplished by supporting the patient to follow a guided self-help process that follows a six-stage protocol.

Assessing Your Understanding

Declarative

Multiple Choice Questions

1. Which are among the four conditions necessary for effective exposure treatment? [Select all that apply]
    (a) Graded
    (b) Timely
    (c) Prolonged
    (d) Repeated
    (e) With distraction
2. Whilst decisions relating to exposure treatment should always be made in collaboration with the patient, which of the following guidelines are recommended? [Select all that apply]
    (a) A hierarchy should consist of 15 to 20 steps
    (b) Exposure should start at the bottom of the hierarchy and progress to the top
    (c) Exposure sessions should ideally be undertaken daily
    (d) The patient should remain in the exposure session until their SUDs have reduced by 50 per cent
    (e) When the patient's peak SUDs rating is less than 50 per cent they are usually able to move onto the next step of the hierarchy

Procedural

Self-Practice/Self-Reflection

Do something you find challenging over the next week. Plot your SUDs over the duration of this experience.

Reflect upon the pattern of your SUDs and influences upon it.

Adopt therapeutic principles to reduce the level of anxiety or fear linked to this experience. Reflect upon any challenges you experienced.

Answers to **Assessing Your Understanding** questions can be found in the appendix on p. 337.

Further Reading and Resources

Papworth, M.A. (2020) *How to Beat Fears and Phobias One Step at a Time*. London: Little Brown Books.

Wolitzky-Taylor, K.B., Horowitz, J.D., Powers, M.B. and Telch, M.J. (2008) Psychological approaches in the treatment of specific phobias: a meta-analysis. *Clinical Psychology Review*, 28, 1021–37.

To access the online resources accompanying this chapter, please visit: https://study.sagepub.com/farrand

14

Exposure Therapy and Response Prevention for Obsessive-Compulsive Disorder

Taking on the Challenge

Judith Gellatly, Rebecca Pedley, Penny Bee and Karina Lovell

Learning Objectives

By the end of this chapter you should be able to:

- Analyse obsessive-compulsive disorder and how it can present in patients assessed for low-intensity cognitive behaviour therapy
- Critically appreciate the theoretical rationale for the use of cognitive behaviour therapy using exposure and response-prevention for patients with obsessive-compulsive disorder
- Apply exposure and response-prevention in supporting patients with obsessive-compulsive disorder
- Appreciate potential barriers and facilitators faced when implementing exposure and response-prevention for obsessive-compulsive disorder

---

What is OCD?

Obsessive-compulsive disorder (OCD) is a debilitating condition (e.g. Markarian et al., 2010) characterised by the presence of obsessions and/or compulsions.

Key Point

Characteristics of Obsessions and Compulsions

- *Obsessions*: Persistent and repetitive unwanted intrusive thoughts, images, ideas or doubts that provoke marked anxiety and distress.
- *Compulsions*: Repetitive rituals or behaviours carried out in response to the obsessive symptoms with the aim of alleviating or avoiding anxiety/distress. Compulsions can be overt (observable behaviours) or covert (mental acts).

Patients most commonly present with a range of common obsessions and compulsions (Table 14.1) but can present with either obsessions or compulsions in isolation (American Psychiatric Association, 2013).

OCD, alongside other anxiety disorders, is ranked by the World Health Organization (WHO, 2017) as the sixth largest contributor to non-fatal health loss globally, with a lifetime presence of approximately 2 per cent (Ruscio et al., 2010). It negatively impacts upon functional impairment and quality of life of individuals and their families (Jacoby et al., 2014; Macy et al., 2013; Subramaniam et al., 2013). The exact cause of OCD is not clear. Some believe it is hereditary, while others

Table 14.1 Common obsessions and compulsions

Obsession	Examples	Compulsion
Aggressive	Fear of harming others or self, violent or horrific images, responsibility for something terrible happening	Reassurance seeking, excessive checking to ensure feared act not conducted
Contamination	Fear of or disgust at self or others being contaminated - e.g. by environmental contaminants, infections, animals	Washing or cleaning rituals
Magical thoughts, superstition	Lucky/unlucky numbers, colours/words - e.g. number 13; superstitious fears	Avoidance - e.g. not taking a bus if it contains an unlucky number; performance of repetitive rituals, touching, tapping, rubbing
Religious	Concerns about being immoral, sacrilege and blasphemy	Reassurance-seeking, praying, seeking forgiveness
Sexual	Forbidden or perverse sexual thoughts, images or impulses - e.g. of being a paedophile, acting sexually inappropriately towards others	Conducting rituals to counteract thoughts, avoidance of triggering situations/ environments
Somatic	Concern with illness or disease	Reassurance-seeking - e.g. attending multiple GP appointments
Symmetry, exactness	Thoughts that things need to be done in a specific way	Ordering, balancing and arranging
Miscellaneous	Need to know or remember insignificant things; fear of saying things or not saying the right thing	Mental rituals, involving others to reassure

propose that it develops following a traumatic life event or is the result of a chemical imbalance in the brain (Yaryura-Tobias and Neziroglu, 1997). Research evidence has identified a delay in treatment help-seeking of up to ten years following the onset of symptoms with an evidence-based intervention not being received until 17 years following onset (Hollander et al., 1997). This delay may be influenced by factors such as lack of knowledge about OCD, stigmatisation, fears of negative consequences or the normalisation of symptoms or seeing symptoms as a 'quirk' (Lovell and Bee, 2008; Marques et al., 2010; Pedley et al., 2019; Robinson et al., 2017; Vuong et al., 2016).

Consequently, given the length of time OCD may be experienced before help-seeking, it is likely to be ingrained and have a significant impact on daily functioning (Subramaniam et al., 2013). In developing treatment goals, patients may therefore place more importance on restoring their ability to engage with, or conduct, daily activities rather than reduce symptoms. Unlike other common mental health conditions, OCD rarely improves without treatment (Visser et al., 2014). Co-morbidity is commonly associated with an OCD diagnosis (Torres et al., 2006), with mood disorders being most frequently documented (Denys et al., 2004; LaSalle et al., 2004).

OCD is classified in the International Classification of Diseases (ICD-10; WHO, 1992) and the Diagnostic and Statistical Manual of Mental Disorders (DSM-5; American Psychiatric Association, 2013) (Table 14.2).

Whilst both classification systems are complementary, there are differences in the approaches adopted.

Table 14.2 Differences in classification of OCD between ICD-10 (WHO, 1992) and DSM-5 (APA, 2013)

ICD-10	DSM-5
A. Obsessions and/or compulsions must be present on most days over a two-week period	**A.** Presence of obsessions, compulsions, or both
B. Obsessions and compulsions share the following characteristics – all must be present: • Recognised as the patient's own thoughts or impulses, not imposed by any external influences • Repetitive and unpleasant, with at least one obsession or compulsion acknowledged as unreasonable or excessive • Unpleasant for the individual • Effort made to resist the obsessions/ compulsions where at least one is unsuccessfully resisted	**B.** The obsessions or compulsions are time-consuming (e.g. take more than one hour per day) or cause clinically significant distress or impairment in social, occupational or other important areas of functioning
C. Obsessions and compulsions cause distress or interfere with patient activity	**C.** The obsessive-compulsive symptoms are not attributable to the physiological effects of a substance (e.g. a drug of abuse, a medication) or another medical condition
D. Not diagnosed in the presence of schizophrenia or Tourette syndrome	**D.** The disturbance is not better explained by the symptoms of another mental disorder

Intervention Description

Guidance for the management of OCD is provided by the UK National Institute for Health and Clinical Excellence (NICE; NICE, 2005) who recommend using a stepped care model (Chapter 1; Bower and Gilbody, 2005). Stratified decision-making to inform treatment decisions for OCD within the stepped care model focuses on the severity of symptoms and functional impairment with management using high-intensity CBT (HICBT) recommended for treatment at Step 3 or above. Exposure and response prevention (ERP) of up to ten hours of therapist time delivered individually or in a group for patients is recommended as the gold-standard high-intensity treatment at Step 3.

Key Point

Exposure and Response Prevention

- *Exposure*: Therapeutic confrontation to a feared stimulus in imagination or in vivo until fear subsides through a process known as habituation.
- *Response prevention*: Making a choice to resist performing the compulsive behaviour.

Evidence Base

ERP is one of the most researched interventions for OCD and represents the most favoured and successful HICBT intervention. Comprehensive meta-analyses have reported large effect sizes for CBT in comparison to controls (Ost et al., 2015), with reduced but moderate effects persisting at follow-up (Olatunji et al., 2013). Recent systematic reviews comparing LICBT interventions for OCD with HICBT control conditions have also supported effectiveness with larger effect sizes associated with increased therapeutic contact (e.g. Pearcy et al., 2016; Wootton, 2016). Findings are broadly supportive of NICE pharmacological and psychological management approach recommendations; however, there remains a paucity of evidence for the management of OCD using a stepped care approach (Skapinakis et al., 2016; Lovell and Bee, 2008).

Unlike many other LICBT interventions that have derived their evidence base from HICBT, the Obsessive Compulsive Treatment Efficacy Trial (OCTET) was a multi-site RCT conducted within IAPT settings (Lovell et al., 2017). This study tested the effectiveness of LICBT with ERP delivered using guided self-help (GSH) and computerised CBT (cCBT) interventions, compared with waiting list for HICBT serving as a control. Although cCBT did not produce significant benefits, modest statistically significant effects of GSH were found. However, the effect did not reach clinical significance and effectiveness of GSH was not sustained at 12 months. However, over 12 months early access to treatment did result in significant reductions in the uptake of HICBT, which did not appear to compromise patient outcomes. Following involvement in the OCTET trial, patients receiving support from psychological wellbeing practitioners (PWPs) for both LICBT interventions were interviewed about their experiences of treatment. Perspectives were variable and largely dependent on individual factors such as preference for personalisation and value of interpersonal face-to-face relationships (Knopp-Hoffer et al., 2016). The support provided by PWPs was valued, as was the ease of access and increased privacy when delivered over the phone. PWPs recognised the benefits of both approaches in terms of increasing patient access and choice; however, they remained concerned about supporting OCD with LICBT. Lack of confidence highlights the need for training to address anxieties in the PWP workforce (Gellatly et al., 2017).

Theoretical Rationale

Work conducted in the 1930s, exploring the aetiology and treatment of OCD, focused on the theory of fear and avoidance (Mowrer, 1939). Influenced by this work, ERP was first described by Meyer (1966) and considered to be the first behavioural intervention for OCD. It has subsequently been refined by notable behaviour therapists such as Isaac Marks (Marks, 1973).

Key Point

ERP Implementation Criteria for OCD (Abramowitz, 2006; Foa and Kozak, 1986)

- Exposure to fear must be conducted to provoke the obsessional fear causing heightened anxiety or distress.
- Exposure should be conducted without the patient engaging in associated compulsion(s).
- Repeatedly confronting the fear will result in habituation resulting in reduced levels of anxiety/distress.
- With habituation, patients will be able to face increasingly fearful situations or stimuli.

Meeting these criteria, however, does not always ensure success. Some patients may be unable to refrain completely from performing their rituals and approximately 50 per cent are still likely to meet clinical levels of severity following treatment (Abramowitz, 2006). During the final scheduled support session (Chapter 6), the

LICBT practitioner should work collaboratively with the patient to review progress and a decision be made as to whether additional support is required. For patients who have been unable to engage in LICBT or where progress has not been adequate, this may involve *stepping up* to HICBT and/or being offered a pharmacological intervention (SSRI).

Application of Exposure and Response Prevention

Guidance from NICE (2011b) and *The Improving Access to Psychological Therapies Manual* (National Collaborating Centre for Mental Health, 2018) propose that mild to moderate symptoms of OCD with mild functional impairment can be treated at Step 2 using LICBT (Chapter 1). However, given that many patients delay help-seeking for up to ten years following symptom onset (Hollander et al., 1997), restricting LICBT to patients with milder functional impairment is likely to result in many cases being stepped up (Chapter 4). At Step 3, patients should be offered HICBT including ERP, at times alongside a selective serotonin reuptake inhibitor, SSRI (Chapter 10; NICE, 2005).

Specific Factors: Supporting Exposure and Response Prevention

Specific factors associated with the ERP intervention inform the basis of the written LICBT intervention addressed in this chapter (*Obsessive Compulsive Disorder: A Self-Help Book*, modified from Lovell and Gega, 2011). When supporting the four stages of the intervention, the LICBT practitioner should enable the patient to understand the purpose and specific factors associated with each stage of the intervention. As with other LICBT interventions addressed in Part II, relapse prevention should also be completed at Stage 5.

Key Point

Intervention Stages

- *Stage 1*: Assessment
- *Stage 2*: Explaining the ERP process
- *Stage 3*: Conducting ERP
- *Stage 4*: Continuing to conduct ERP.

Stage 1: Assessment

During assessment it is important to collaborate with the patient to explore their understanding of OCD and the way it can impact on multiple areas – home, work, relationships, social life – of their daily life. As they may have been experiencing OCD for some time before seeking help, impact on day-to-day life may be significant (Torres et al., 2006). This can be distressing for some patients but addressing impact is an extremely important part of the process. The case study about Laura outlines the difficulties faced by an individual with OCD and the goals identified (Chapter 2) with the support of an LICBT psychological practitioner.

Clinical Example

Case Study: Laura

Laura is a 43-year-old married woman with a child aged two. She has fears about contamination and dirt, in particular germs in food picked up from the environment, other people and animals. She is petrified about contaminating others, particularly her child, and causing them to become sick and potentially die. Due to these thoughts, Laura's rituals involve extensive washing routines. Leaving the house has become difficult as she believes it will increase the risk of contamination and if she is able to leave, when returning she removes all outer clothing, shoes and disinfects anything brought into the house, making her child and husband do the same. Each night she disinfects all surfaces in the house, focusing specifically on her child's bedroom, the kitchen and bathroom, cleaning out the fridge every three days and throwing out any food that has not been used. Shopping is a challenge too, with Laura wearing gloves to reduce the chance of infection. Laura cannot trust her own judgement and seeks reassurance from her husband. Laura has little face-to-face contact with friends and family as she does not want them visiting the house and finds it extremely difficult to meet them elsewhere. She continues to work where she finds a fear of contaminating her family is reduced but also finds it difficult, fearing colleagues may expose her to germs. Rituals to overcome anxiety are performed daily in the working environment and impact her ability to get tasks done on time. She avoids invitations from colleagues to go out for lunch or after-work drinks. Her child is due to attend playgroup soon but she does not think it will be possible as it will involve contact with other parents and children who may pass on germs. Laura estimates that her cleaning rituals occupy approximately six hours of her day and frequently more at weekends. She indicates that the time she spends on rituals is lost time with her child.

To fully identify what is being experienced it is also important to ensure the patient appreciates both obsessions and compulsions associated with their lived experience. In order to normalise their experience, it can be helpful to highlight that OCD is a common problem, affecting individuals regardless of gender, age or ethnicity.

Stage 2: Explaining Exposure and Response Prevention

Using the LICBT ABC cognitive behavioural model (Richards and Whyte, 2011), work collaboratively with the patient to help them understand their lived experience of OCD in the here and now.

Key Point

Using the Patient ABC Model to Help Patient to Understand OCD

- *What we feel (autonomic; physical sensations)*: This includes increased heart rate, difficulties breathing, experiencing 'butterflies' in the stomach and sweating. Some sensations may be experienced mentally, such as 'feeling out of control' or 'detached from reality'.
- *What we do (behaviours)*: There may be excessive ritualistic behaviours such as checking, counting or washing. There may also be things that are avoided due to the anxiety that they cause. Some people may avoid particular things or situations entirely or engage only if safeguards are put into place. Reassurance from others is often sought to ensure that any fears held are untrue or that rituals have been conducted correctly.
- *What we think (cognitions)*: Obsessive thoughts or intrusive images are experienced. Thoughts about the impact that OCD is having on their lives and others' may also be experienced.

Reflection Point

Reflect upon ways you could adapt your explanation of ERP for patients experiencing different OCD presentations to aid understanding.

The way in which these three parts of OCD are experienced can be thought of as a vicious circle of OCD (Figure 14.1).

Explain that for the symptoms to improve, a CBT approach is a recommended treatment. Discuss what CBT is, highlighting that the term refers to a variety of different types of interventions delivered by different practitioners working in different

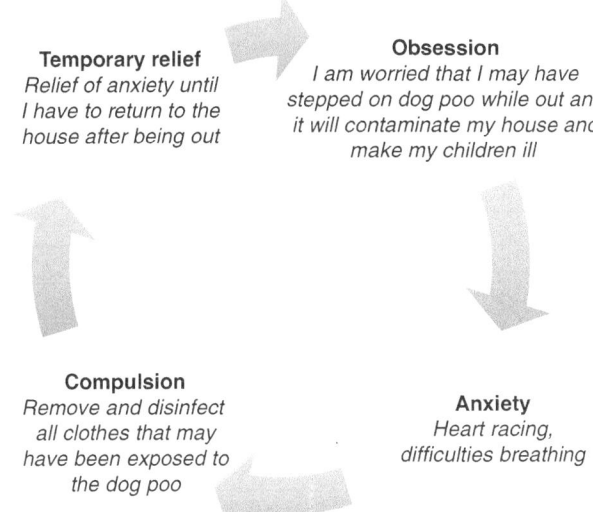

Figure 14.1 Vicious circle of OCD

settings and includes individual or group LICBT (including ERP) using structured self-help materials delivered face-to-face or by telephone. Highlight that the intervention recommended by the Department of Health for OCD is ERP and provide further information to enable patients to appreciate the technique.

Clinical Practice

Useful Information to Patients when Adopting ERP

- Rituals are carried out to avoid situations when faced with high levels of anxiety or distress (give specific examples provided by the patient). Explain that whilst the rituals bring relief it will only be in the short-term and when faced with the trigger again, the anxiety/distress will return.
  - Exposure involves gradually being faced with the obsessive thoughts, images, objects or situations that cause anxiety
  - Response prevention refers to stopping the rituals conducted to alleviate the anxiety or distress caused by obsessive symptoms.
- Therefore, ERP provokes short-term anxiety but provides lasting relief. This contrasts with the short-term relief and long-term anxiety arising if rituals continue to be engaged in.
  - The risks that patients will be asked to take do not differ from the kinds of 'risks' that people who do not experience OCD would take.

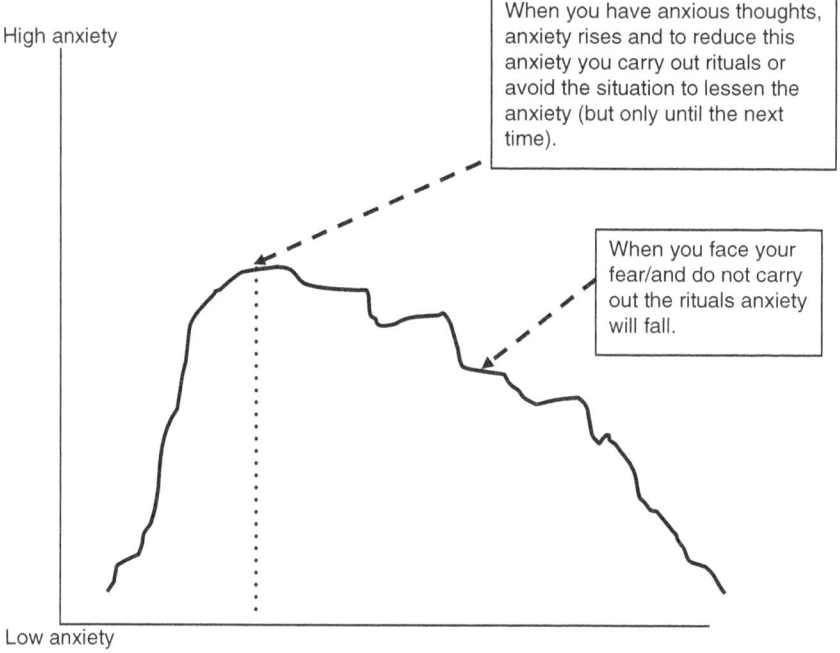

Figure 14.2 Pattern of anxiety during exposure and response prevention (Lovell and Gega, 2011. Reproduced with permission)

To ensure that the patient has understood ERP and the mechanism of action, ask them to explain how it works and to identify what they believe would happen if they were stopped from carrying out the rituals. It may be helpful to supplement patient discussion with the use of a diagram (Figure 14.2).

If the patient continues to struggle and time within the session permits, it may be useful to elicit the rationale with the patient using their own vicious circle to identify where it can be broken and how.

Stage 3: Conducting ERP

When conducting ERP there are four rules that should be followed to maximise a successful outcome. Rules 1 to 3 are the same as those adopted with exposure for simple phobia (Chapter 13).

Key Point

- *Graded*: Gradually facing fears, starting with something that causes little or minimal anxiety/distress, rated at about 30 per cent, gradually building up to more difficult and challenging situations or stimuli.
- *Repeated*: Repeating the exposure is important. Being exposed to the feared situation over and over again will gradually reduce anxiety/distress and the situation will feel more comfortable.
- *Prolonged*: It is important to face the feared situation for long enough to reduce anxiety/distress by approximately 50 per cent.
- *Prevent*: The ultimate aim is to stop the conduct of rituals.

Reflecting upon goals set during the assessment process, work collaboratively with the patient to identify manageable and achievable small steps (Chapter 6). This will involve devising weekly targets and each week identifying daily targets to meet. Create a hierarchy of an identified feared situation, listing the easiest to hardest derived from Laura's case study (Figure 14.3).

Consistent with LICBT working, ensure that between-session 'homework' is well defined and make the patient aware that if they meet the prolonged rule during exposure they may wish to move to the next hierarchical step. Within the session, it can also be beneficial to work collaboratively with the patient to complete a goals sheet to identify one or two steps as homework (Worksheet 14.1).

Explain how to use the *Exposure* goal diary, which involves noting the goal completed and rating the anxiety experienced before and after exposure.

Hardest

↑ Avoid wearing gloves when shopping

↑ Avoid disinfecting floors every evening

↑ Leave shoes and clothes by the front door after being out of the house without disinfecting

↑ Put shopping away without disinfecting

↑ Have friends and family visit

↑ Have friends and family visit without disinfecting the house afterwards

↑ Socialise with friends and family outside of the home environment

Easiest

Figure 14.3 Graded hierarchy ranging from easiest to hardest exposure situations

Worksheet 14.1   Exposure goal diary

GOALS				
Goal 1			Goal 2	
Anxiety: rate how anxious you felt before and after you did the task using the rating scale below				

0 no anxiety	2 little anxiety	4 moderate anxiety	6 much anxiety	8 extreme anxiety
Goals I completed			**Anxiety before**	**Anxiety after**

Step 4: Continuing to Conduct ERP

Over the remaining sessions it is important to be mindful that progression will be different for each patient.

Clinical Practice

Specific Support for Patients to Engage with ERP

- Continue to repeat the step until the rules of exposure have been met.
- Use specific factors to support the patient to break the steps down into further, more manageable but still anxiety provoking, steps (Chapter 6).
- Explain that whilst behaviour may change, unhelpful thoughts can remain (cognitive lag).
- If practical barriers to complete goals as homework are identified, consider applying COM-B (Chapter 8; Michie et al., 2011).
- Use common factors (Chapter 5) to demonstrate empathy to help the patient recognise that difficulties engaging with ERP can be common.
- Reiterate the theoretical rationale supporting ERP.

Consistent with the aim of LICBT support sessions (Chapter 6), patients struggling to implement ERP should be supported to revisit their goals and hierarchy to continue engagement.

Summary

This chapter has focused on the LICBT treatment of OCD using ERP as the recommended and effective approach for people experiencing mild levels of functional impairment (NICE, 2005). ERP involves patients confronting their fears without conducting the associated compulsive behaviours. Success is reliant on exposure being graded, repeated and prolonged, and specific factors similar to those adopted for the LICBT treatment for simple phobia (Chapter 13). LICBT including ERP has been tested in the largest trial of psychological therapies for OCD worldwide (Lovell et al., 2017). In the short-term, guided self-help delivered at LI using ERP is beneficial and significantly reduces stepping up to HICBT in the longer term. The experiences of individuals with OCD and their engagement with ERP will vary. Therefore, adopting common factors (Chapter 5) to work in a collaborative manner and aid understanding of ERP and support exposure activities is a vital aspect of implementation.

Assessing Your Understanding

Declarative

Multiple Choice Questions

1. Which of the following are possible symptoms of OCD?
   (a) Fear of pushing someone onto a railway line
   (b) Keeping excessive amounts of carrier bags and junk mail
   (c) The need to think of a pleasant image to counteract a bad thought
   (d) Avoiding going on holiday abroad due to fear of flying
   (e) Avoiding children due to fear of causing harm
2. Which of the following is important when conducting ERP?
   (a) Always keep exposure activity under 15 minutes
   (b) Repeat exposure over time
   (c) Start with the least anxiety provoking activity/situation
   (d) Monitor change in distress before and after exposure
   (e) Ensure exposure is always undertaken with someone trusted by the patient

3.   Which of the following are possible ways to assist patients receiving ERP?
    (a) To ensure engagement do not discuss the possibility of relapse
    (b) Draw a vicious circle diagram based on the patient's OCD experience
    (c) Let patients know to stop ERP if they experience uncomfortable levels of anxiety
    (d) Revisit and evaluate progress with patient goals set at the start of treatment
    (e) Ask the patient to explain their understanding of how ERP works

Procedural

Self-Practice/Self-Reflection

•   Think about something you find difficult or challenging and develop an exposure hierarchy. Reflect upon any barriers you would face if asked to work through it.
•   Using the case study in the chapter, identify what barriers and facilitators you think Laura may face when implementing ERP. How could you help Laura overcome these?

    Answers to **Assessing Your Understanding** questions can be found in the appendix on p. 337.

Further Reading and Resources

Locked short film (www.ocduk.org/features/locked)

Lovell, K. and Gega, L. (2011) *Obsessive Compulsive Disorder: A Self-Help Book*. Manchester: University of Manchester.

OCD UK (ocduk.org)

Veale, D. (2007) Cognitive-behavioural therapy for obsessive-compulsive disorder. *Advances in Psychiatric Treatment*, 13, 438–46.

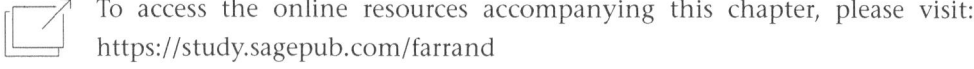 To access the online resources accompanying this chapter, please visit: https://study.sagepub.com/farrand

15

Worry Management

A Practical Solution to a Problem of Hypotheticals

Faye Small and Katie Lockwood

Learning Objectives

By the end of this chapter you should be able to:

- Critically appraise the theoretical rationale for the low-intensity cognitive behavioural therapy worry management intervention
- Demonstrate an understanding of specific factors associated with the worry management intervention
- Apply specific factors associated with the worry management intervention for a patient experiencing generalised anxiety disorder
- Appreciate and address some of the common problems a patient may experience when working with worry management

---

Intervention Description

National Institute for Health and Clinical Excellence (NICE) guidance recommends high- and low-intensity cognitive behavioural therapy (HICBT and LICBT) for the treatment of generalised anxiety disorder (GAD; NICE, 2011a). Recommendations for LICBT extend beyond guided self-help and include self-administered CBT self-help and guided psychoeducational groups (NICE, 2011a). Guidance for the LICBT treatment of GAD does not, however, specify any particular protocol, although a number of specific techniques have been adopted within a guided self-help format such as recognition of physical symptoms, cognitive restructuring and relaxation (Lucock et al., 2008; Van Boeijen et al., 2005). Adopting all techniques within an intervention represents a multi-strand approach and is therefore not consistent with the focus on single-strand interventions that characterise the LICBT clinical method (Chapter 1). On this basis, the low-intensity model for the treatment of GAD has adopted a behavioural approach to treatment in line with many other low-intensity interventions. The low-intensity worry management protocol described is based on the models of Borkovec et al. (1983) and Dugas and Ladouceur (2000).

Key Point

Adopted techniques from HICBT Interventions

- Worry awareness
- Stimulus control
- Problem-solving, where considered necessary.

Lack of confidence in problem-solving ability is a common feature of GAD. However, patients with GAD have largely been shown to be proficient in their ability to problem-solve (Dugas et al., 1997). As such the option of moving to problem-solving is only considered following discussions in case management supervision (Chapter 9) regarding the necessity to continue treatment. This approach is comparable to that adopted within the cognitive restructuring and behavioural experiments (Chapter 12) LICBT intervention, with progression to behavioural experiments only undertaken when required.

Evidence Base

Although mainly consisting of multi-strand approaches, NICE (2011a) recognises a strong CBT evidence base for the treatment of GAD (Leichsenring et al., 2009; Linden et al., 2005; Wetherell et al., 2003). The development of a single-strand approach for the treatment of GAD has primarily arisen from the stimulus control protocol (Borkovec et al., 1983) of which component parts are also highlighted in the Roth and Pilling CBT competency framework (Roth and Pilling, 2007a). Whilst a specific evidence base for the adoption of stimulus control as a singe-strand intervention is currently lacking, professional consensus for its efficacy exists.

Theoretical Rationale

The theoretical rationale informing the worry management intervention is based on the premise that patients engage in worry behaviours in an attempt to avoid potential future threats, problem-solve potentially arising problems or manage anticipatory anxiety (Borkovec and Inz, 1990; Borkovec and Roemer, 1995). As the threat is future focused and therefore hypothetical, a standard behavioural avoidance associated with the fight or flight response is not possible (Borkovec and Newman, 1998). Cognitive avoidance is employed as an alternative coping strategy, where worrying is used in an attempt to problem-solve potential threats and avoid thinking about the feared outcome. Cognitive avoidance therefore seeks to reduce discomfort associated with uncertainty (Borkovec et al., 1983; Dugas and Ladouceur, 2000).

Worry management requires the patient to interrupt the worry process and identify their unhelpful worries about hypothetical situations. Stimulus control is then practised as an alternative to worrying. Central to stimulus control is the practice of postponement of worry. The patient learns to disengage from hypothetical worries and instead refocus on the here and now. This replacement behaviour enables the focus on potential threat to be minimised and helps to reduce the associated anxiety-related cognitions (Borkovec, 2002). In order to support the patient to disengage from their worries, a predetermined time is allocated in which hypothetical worries will be revisited. Through utilising this process of stimulus control the patient learns that they are able to intentionally reduce or increase worrying at will (Newman and Borkovec, 2002).

Application of Worry Management

Worry management represents a single-strand intervention for GAD to be adopted where there has been no significant improvement after education and active monitoring (NICE, 2011a). Whilst worry is transdiagnostic, the application of worry management for common mental health problems is restricted to the treatment of GAD.

Specific Factors: Supporting Worry Management

Specific factors associated with worry management, worry awareness, stimulus control and problem-solving inform the basis of the Managing Your Worries written LICBT intervention (Farrand et al., 2019b) addressed in this chapter. To fully engage with the intervention the patient should be supported to understand the purpose (Why?) and specific factors (How?) associated with each stage of the intervention.

Clinical Practice

Intervention Stages

- *Stage 1*: Explain GAD and the LICBT intervention
  - Stage 1a: Collaboratively discuss the vicious cycle
  - Stage 1b: Present the LICBT treatment rationale
  - Stage 1c: Review important life areas
- *Stage 2*: Identify and record worries (worry awareness)
- *Stage 3*: Classify worries (worry awareness)
- *Stage 4*: Worry time (stimulus control)
  - Stage 4a: Schedule
  - Stage 4b: Record worries
  - Stage 4c: Refocus on the present moment
  - Stage 4d: Engage with worry time
  - Stage 4e: Review.

When supporting the intervention, it is essential that the patient appreciates the importance of between-session home practice (Kazantzis et al., 2000) that informs the basis of the support sessions (Chapter 6).

Stage 1: Explain Worry Management

Stage 1a: Collaboratively Discuss the 'Vicious Cycle'

The LICBT practitioner should work collaboratively to enable the patient to appreciate the LICBT model of GAD (Westbrook et al., 2007).

Clinical Example

Explaining GAD

Worrying is a behaviour most people do from time to time and, in some ways, it can be helpful, making us feel more alert, prepared and in control. However, if we start to believe worrying is helpful across all situations, it can become problematic and a vicious cycle of worry can be created. We might find ourselves worrying about a lot of things a lot of the time; it can start to feel out of control and get in the way of our lives. Extensive worry about uncertain situations is key to generalised anxiety disorder. You told me you often worry that your partner might have a traffic accident on his way home from work. Understandably this makes you feel really anxious and distressed. When worries such as this pop into your head you will start to think of all the possible negative outcomes that might happen and what you might be able to do to prevent them. Often people with generalised anxiety disorder will try to cope with uncertain situations by continuing to worry to make the situation feel more certain and relieve the discomfort associated with uncertainty. You indicated that when you come up with a solution to one of the possible negative outcomes, whilst providing some momentary relief, you will then have another worry about why the solution might not work or about a different outcome. This will make you feel anxious again and so the cycle continues.

Rather than presenting a generic model, the practitioner should encourage the patient to consider how *their* experience is consistent with the model. Depending on patient preferences, using a diagram to represent the presenting problem in the here and now as the foundation of the explanation may enhance collaborative working (Figure 15.1).

Problem statement: My main problem is feeling on edge and anxious most of the time but it can be worse at night. I feel very tense and get frequent headaches. I worry a lot, struggle to relax and seek a lot of reassurance from my partner. I think things like, 'What if my partner has an accident on the way home?', 'What if he leaves me?', 'What if I lose my job and we go bankrupt?'. As a consequence, my relationships have been put under strain and I'm not as productive in work.

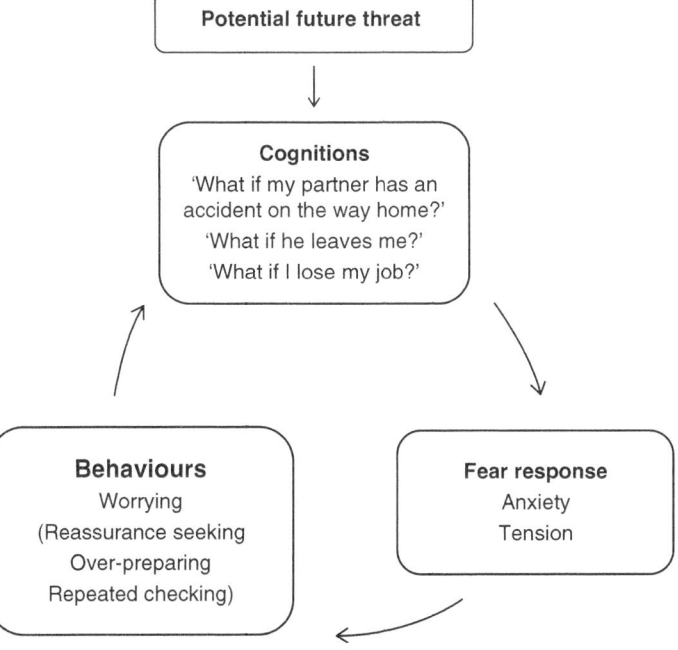

Figure 15.1 Jordan's problem statement and vicious cycle of worry

Stage 1b: Present the LICBT Treatment Rationale

The LICBT practitioner should highlight the theoretical rationale underlying the Managing Your Worries intervention (Farrand et al., 2019). It is good practice for the practitioner to highlight how the intervention disrupts the vicious cycle (Figure 15.1). This will highlight how it will enable the patient to develop helpful coping strategies and help to motivate them to engage with the intervention between sessions.

Clinical Example

Worry Management

There is research to suggest that techniques used as part of a worry management intervention can be really effective to break the vicious cycle we have just discussed. This intervention supports you to notice when you are worrying and helps you interrupt this behaviour so you are able to get on with your day without worry and anxiety impacting so significantly on you. When you become skilled at identifying your worries we can look at more helpful ways to manage them. Some of the worries might be ones that can be solved but many of them may be what we call hypothetical worries and so we need a different way to address them. Together we can also look at techniques called worry postponement and worry time. This allows you to manage your worries in a more helpful way by scheduling a dedicated time of the day to worry about them, rather than allowing them to disrupt your life whenever they occur. Where there may be practical solutions to any worries you are having that you may be struggling to think about, it may be possible to consider ways to support you problem-solve these.

Stage 1c: Important Life Areas

Support the patient to identify their important life areas, with identification of around five areas often sufficient. This will enable the patient to prioritise any practical problems identified in the next stage and help normalise distress associated with worries centred on these important life areas. This information can be helpfully recorded on the Areas of my life that are really important to me worksheet (Worksheet 15.1).

Completing and referring to this worksheet will be helpful during subsequent support sessions and enhance treatment engagement.

Worksheet 15.1   Jordan's areas of my life that are really important to me

	List here the five most important things in your life right now:
1	Relationship with my partner
2	Family's wellbeing
3	Doing well in work
4	Relaxing at the weekends and during holidays
5	Making time for my friends

Stage 2: Identify and Record Worries

Work collaboratively within the session to support the patient to begin routinely noticing, identifying and recording their worries to enhance worry awareness. In order to practise stimulus control, the patient must first learn to identify the range of triggers for their worry (Borkovec et al. 1983). The patient should be supported to practise intervening in the worry process as early as possible, given that a higher occurrence and longer duration of engagement with worry will continue to reinforce worry as a coping strategy and maintain GAD (Borkovec and Newman, 1998). At this early stage in treatment the patient will not have alternative coping strategies in place. However, enhancing worry awareness by pausing to identify and record individual worries each time worrying is noticed should be considered a form of intervention that disrupts the worry cycle itself. After being supported to recognise one or two worries within the session, the patient should also be supported to begin using a Worry Record to capture worries identified between sessions. The patient should be encouraged to record individual worries as close to the time they occur as possible. To provide useful information about potential triggers, the patient should be encouraged to record the date and time when the worry occurred (Worksheet 15.2).

When capturing worries, the patient should also record wider information associated with their worries.

Clinical Practice

Information to Collect Associated with Worry

- Date and time
- Situation
- Thought associated with the worry
- Anticipated outcome
- Emotions.

Worksheet 15.2   Jordan's worry worksheet

Date and time	The situation	What are you thinking?	What do you fear might happen?	What emotions are you feeling?
Tuesday, 10 am (I had this worry over and over again on this day!)	Charlie driving to Manchester for work today	The roads are really busy around there and it's a long way – what if she has an accident?	Somebody might crash into her and she might be seriously hurt or might die	Frightened, on edge
Tuesday, 8 pm	Charlie still isn't back home	She should have been home by 8 pm. Where is she? What if something really bad has happened?	She might be in hospital, she might be paralysed and never walk again or she could be dead	Really stressed out Really scared
Wednesday 7.30 am	Getting ready for work, there's a team meeting this morning at 9.30 am	What if there's nowhere to park? What if I walk in late to the team meeting?	I'll miss something important and then I won't know what's going on and I won't be able to do my job properly. I'll get put on performance management!	Anxious Stressed
Wednesday, 1 pm	I received an email from the gas company with a final reminder to submit a meter reading	What if I don't submit it on time?	They may cut off the gas and we'll have no hot water, won't be able to shower and then how will I be able to go to work?	Overwhelmed Really anxious
Wednesday, 11 pm	Lying in bed thinking about how many worries I had today, I gave up trying to record them	I think I'm getting worse. What if I never get better?	I'll be like this forever and Charlie will leave me and I'll lose my job	Sad Hopeless

Capturing the precise thought associated with the worry is important given that patients will sometimes record negative thoughts that do not represent a worry but are more closely associated other common mental health difficulties. On these occasions, within the following support session the practitioner should collaboratively work with the patient to determine if worry management or another intervention would be the best focus.

Reflection Point

Reflect upon ways you would support a patient who is unable to read or write to complete a worry record?

Stage 3: Classify Worries

Once the patient is successfully and routinely identifying and recording worries as they occur, they should be supported to classify the worry as practical or hypothetical.

Key Point

Worry Classification

- *Practical*: Based in reality in the here and now and can be practically addressed and solved.
- *Hypothetical*: Do not have tangible evidence to support their existence or problems that cannot be solved given that the feared outcome is currently beyond control.

Depending on how quickly the patient is able to appreciate Stage 2 and the time available, Stage 3 may also be supported in the same session. At this point the patient should be supported within the session to use a worry classification tool to classify each worry as they arise between sessions (Figure 15.2).

Through the process of classification, the patient may identify that they have a mixture of both practical and hypothetical worries, which require very different interventions. Both interventions involve substantial time and effort to practice and master. Whilst practical worries can be addressed using a low-intensity problem-solving intervention (Chapter 16), hypothetical worries are addressed by continuing onto Stage 4 of worry management. When deciding which intervention would be most beneficial, the patient should be supported to identify whether it is their practical or hypothetical worries that are most problematic. Classifying worries should be recorded on the My types of worry worksheet, where they will also be grouped according to worry type (Worksheet 15.3).

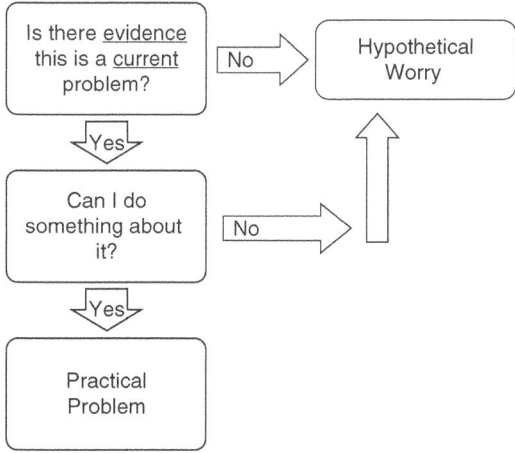

Figure 15.2 Worry classification tool

Worksheet 15.3   Jordan's my types of worry

Not important	Important and can be solved	Important and cannot be solved
What if the coffee shop is closed when I get to the station? I could really do with a coffee on the train.	What if I don't submit the gas meter reading on time and they overcharge us or cut off the gas?	What if Charlie has an accident on the way home and is hurt or dies?
What if they don't have our favourite bread in the supermarket and I have to get an alternative? They always run out.	What if I miss something important in the meeting and can't do my job properly?	What if there is nowhere to park and I'm late for the meeting (I've already got up two and a half hours before the meeting, there's nothing else I can do!)
		What if Charlie leaves me?
		What if I lose my job?

At this point it is helpful for the patient to identify if each worry is important or whether it can be easily dismissed with no negative consequences. This will enable the patient to focus on the worries having most impact.

Stage 4: Worry Time

Where the patient has identified hypothetical worries as the most relevant focus, Worry Time should be introduced. Following the categorisation of worries in Stage 2, the patient is encouraged to postpone their worries and revisit them at an agreed time set aside for worry. Having a set time to return to their worries helps the patient let go of worries and gain more control of their anxiety during the rest of their day. Patients may report that they find letting go of worries difficult, but this can be supported through the use of refocusing (Stage 4c) and knowing that the worries will be revisited again during worry time.

Clinical Example

Worry Time

Now we have recognised you have two different types of worry, hypothetical and practical, and you feel the hypothetical ones are more problematic, the next stage of the intervention is introducing worry time. We use worry time to help you postpone your worries throughout the day, knowing that you will return to them later. This should be easier than trying to let them go altogether. Scheduling worry time will enable you to focus on your worries during a set time period rather than worrying all day as you currently do. Whilst this can initially be difficult, through practice and the use of refocusing you will get better at postponing your worries and taking back control.

Step 4a: Schedule Worry Time

Working collaboratively, worry time should be scheduled in advance and where possible scheduled at the same time and location every day and follow a few rules (Borkovec et al., 1983).

Clinical Example

Rules of Scheduling Worry Time

- Ideally the patient should not schedule close to bedtime as once in bed it can be harder to switch the worries back off.
- Schedule at a suitable time and place where the patient will not be interrupted. The same time and place should be used every day.
  - If the daily routine varies or is unpredictable, the patient should try to schedule worry time as close to the same time as possible. If a different time must be chosen, the patient should try at least to engage with worry time in the same location.
- Learning from the experience of setting too much or too little time, the patient should schedule the amount of worry time that feels appropriate.
  - If a time in excess of 60 minutes is chosen, support the patient to consider if this period can be regularly accommodated within their day
  - Worry time should be scheduled as a task in its own right, rather than at a time the patient already worries.

Step 4b: Continue to Record Your Worries

Initially scheduling time for worry will not stop the patient worrying. Consequently, the patient should be encouraged to continue writing their worries down as soon as they notice them. Worries should be postponed and written on the Worry Time worksheet (Worksheet 15.4) and revisited during the scheduled worry time.

This step, in combination with Step 4c, may help reduce the impact of the worries at that particular time. If the same worry recurs, it does not mean that the intervention is being used incorrectly and this experience should be normalised. The recurrent worry can be recorded each time it is noticed, or the patient may prefer to keep a tally of how many times it recurs. Encourage the patient to remind themselves that the worry has been recorded and will be given adequate attention during worry time. Recurrent worries can be distressing and use of common factor skills (Chapter 5) is important in supporting the patient through this experience. This difficulty is likely to improve as the patient adopts this new routine of managing worries, but it can require considerable persistence in the early stages.

Worksheet 15.4   Jordan's my worry time

	Worry time
My scheduled worry time is: Every day, 6 pm	
	My hypothetical worries
1	What if Charlie has an accident on the way home and is hurt or dies?
2	What if there is nowhere to park and I'm late for the meeting?
3	What if I miss something important in the meeting and can't do my job properly?
4	What if Charlie leaves me?
5	What if I lose my job?
6	
7	
8	
9	
10	

Step 4c: Refocus on the Present

Once worries have been written down and sent for worry time, the patient refocuses on the present. This is a key stage in the intervention as refocusing on the present moment reduces engagement with the worry process and enables the patient to start to take control of their worries and associated anxiety (Borkovec et al., 1983; Borkovec and Newman, 1998). Refocusing and letting go of the worries can be difficult for the patient to engage with and in this instance several specific factors can be adopted.

Clinical Practice

Specific Factors Supporting the Patient to Refocus and Let Go

- Encourage the patient to re-engage with the activity they were doing when they started worrying.
- Encourage focusing on the task in the present using all the senses (Borkovec and Sharpless, 2004).
- Change tasks or move to a different room.

The main purpose of refocusing is to encourage the patient to be present in the here and now, enabling them to let go of the future focus that comes with worrying. Rather than continue with the problematic worrying behaviour, this new response to individual worries encourages the patient to re-engage with daily life, including their important life areas. The patient should be supported to recognise that whilst they are encouraged not to worry in the present, scheduled worry time has been established to enable them to revisit the worries they have experienced during the day.

Step 4d: Engage with Worry Time

Between sessions, the patient should be encouraged to revisit their My Worry Time worksheet during their allocated time to worry and use this time solely to worry about the worries listed. Whilst revisiting the worksheet, patients should be encouraged to follow a few simple rules.

Clinical Practice

Simple Rules

- The patient may choose to worry mentally or they may find it easier to write things down whilst worrying.
- Put a cross through any worry that had been written down that is now no longer considered to be a worry.
- Worries identified as having a practical solution can be problem-solved. If the patient needs help with this, it can be supported using the problem-solving intervention (Chapter 16) following discussion in supervision. Problem-solving should be undertaken outside of worry time.
- Patients should be encouraged to try and worry for the full duration of the scheduled worry time.
- Worry time should be solely used to worry.

If the patient is unsure how to worry voluntarily during worry time, encourage them to give it their best shot, informing them that different people will experience the time they have set aside for worry time in different ways and you will review this with them during your next session. It is important that the patient does not give up on worrying during worry time too early and use this time for another activity. The practitioner should remind the patient that worry time can be a difficult technique to engage with and will take practice.

Step 4e: Review

After the patient has completed their scheduled time to worry, they should move on to the Worry Time Review worksheet (Worksheet 15.5). The review gives the

Worksheet 15.5   My worry time review

What have I learnt during worry time?
Try to think about what you've learnt during worry time. For example, what have you noticed using worry time? Are some of your worries practical worries? Were you having lots of worries about the same thing? Are some of the worries no longer bothering you?
I wasn't late for the meeting so that turned out fine. There was lots of parking.   Charlie was fine but I just find this worry keeps coming back.   I told Carol I was worried about being late and she said that Mike keeps notes anyway and emails them around after the meeting so I wouldn't have missed anything.

patient an opportunity to take an objective look at their worries when they are not in a heightened state of anxiety. The patient should be supported within the session to begin to complete the worksheet and continue this as part of their home practice plan. Using the prompt questions on the worksheet, the patient may become aware of a number of outcomes.

Clinical Practice

Common Learning from Worry Time

- Some worries are no longer relevant or the issue that led to the worry has passed.
- As the worries are future based, despite worrying there is still nothing that can be done.
- Some worries have a practical component that can be actioned through problem- solving.
- Some worries now seem trivial.
- It is hard to worry about your worries at a later stage.
- Not as much time is needed in worry time as first believed.
- It is hard to worry about worries in one go.

Patients may find that over time the amount of time spent worrying outside of worry time reduces and the amount of time needed within worry time also reduces. Worry management takes practice and can be very difficult for someone who is used to focusing on their worries all of the time. In subsequent sessions, it is also helpful to review the patient's understanding of the rationale for worry management. This helps to consolidate understanding of the intervention and component parts during support sessions (Chapter 6).

Challenges with Worry Management

Encouragement to persevere with the intervention and, where necessary, problem-solve any difficulties is important (Table 15.1). Specific and common factors should be utilised to enable the patient to make progress and overcome any difficulties that arise. Revisiting the rationale and component parts of the intervention may help the patient recognise and resolve common difficulties associated with the intervention. The use of common factor skills such as empathy and funnelling are important here to support the patient. At all times it is important to maintain a collaborative approach to support the patient's learning (Beck et al., 1979).

Solutions intended to overcome difficulties experienced by the patient should respect the key principles of the intervention rationale and not encourage drift into a multi-strand approach (Waller, 2009). Be sure to let the patient give the intervention a good try before considering moving on, making sure all key steps are included in order to give the patient the best opportunity to apply the intervention in full.

Summary

This chapter has focused on the Managing Your Worries (Farrand et al., 2019) LICBT intervention for the treatment of GAD. Although the rationale and process of worry management have been drawn from established models of GAD (Borkovec et al., 1983; Dugas and Ladouceur, 2000) employed within HICBT, the protocol adopted within LICBT represents a single-strand intervention informed by specific factors associated with worry awareness (Dugas and Ladouceur, 2000) and stimulus control (Borkovec et al., 1983). This focus is achieved by supporting the patient to engage with four intervention stages – explain, record, categorise, worry time. It is recommended that future research specifically focus on examining the evidence base for LICBT worry management.

Table 15.1 Common difficulties experienced by patients engaging with worry management

Difficulty	Specific or common factor to address difficulty
It is too difficult or distressing to identify and record specific worries	• Provide verbal empathy and normalise this experience early on in treatment. • Encourage the patient to start by writing down the main theme of the worry. • Support the patient to practise writing down more specific worries within the session. • As a practice exercise write down worries retrospectively, when the associated emotional intensity has reduced. Ultimately, worries need to be recorded as and when they occur. • Use of various apps can be helpful but ensure you are familiar with how they work and that they meet the conditions of the intervention.
Use of worry behaviours to try to solve hypothetical worries	• Support the patient to consider whether the behaviour actually solves a problem or whether it functions purely to reduce the uncertainty around a situation, e.g. repeatedly texting your partner every time they travel on a motorway. • Consider whether this behaviour is helpful in managing anxiety or whether the relief is temporary. Further worries are likely to develop around the uncertainty which remains. • Consider whether the 'worry behaviour' disadvantages the patient in any way and whether it is a functional long-term solution.
Unable to refocus after recording worries at night	• Make sure that the worry record can be easily accessed during the night and that any worries are properly recorded and classified. • The patient should remind themselves that they will return to any hypothetical worries in their worry time the next day. The worries are not discarded but it is not helpful to engage with them at this point. • Practical problems should also be written down and can be problem-solved at a more reasonable time. • Refocusing can be more difficult at night when there is less going on but encourage the patient to refocus on their present-moment experience, such as the touch of the pillow or duvet, or physical sensations associated with breathing.
Reluctance to revisit worries which have been forgotten or are no longer impacting during worry time	• Normalise this concern and provide verbal empathy – worry time can be a daunting prospect for many patients struggling with worry. • Remind the patient that the intervention takes practice and that they will have your support in the next session. • Revisit the rationale for worry postponement and worry time. • Discuss the alternative, which would be to continue to worry frequently and for significant periods of time with no reduction in impact on valued life areas.

Assessing Your Understanding

Declarative

Multiple Choice Questions

1. Which is the main target of change within the Managing Your Worries intervention? [Select all that apply]
    (a) Physical tension
    (b) Reassurance seeking
    (c) Cognitions concerning uncertain situations
    (d) Worry process
    (e) Behavioural activation

2. Worry is a form of ____ avoidance. [Select all that apply]
   (a) Behavioural
   (b) Cognitive
   (c) Emotional
   (d) Autonomic
   (e) Adaptive
3. Which of the following techniques should be used to support worry postponement immediately after a worry has been identified and recorded? [Select all that apply]
   (a) Refocus on the present moment
   (b) Distraction
   (c) Re-engage with the task at hand
   (d) Worry suppression
   (e) Seek reassurance from a supportive friend or family member

Procedural

Self-Practice/Self-Reflection

- During the next week, keep a worry record for yourself and at the end of the week categorise worries as 'Not important', 'Important and can be solved' or 'Important and cannot be solved'. Reflect upon any challenges you experienced.
- Schedule yourself a regular time each day during the next week for worry time. Practise worry postponement and refocus on the present moment whenever you notice a worry which is 'important and cannot be solved'. Practise worry time as scheduled and reflect upon this experience using the Worry Time Review worksheet. Reflect upon any challenges you experienced.

> Answers to **Assessing Your Understanding** questions can be found in the appendix on p. 337.

Further Reading and Resources

Borkovec, T.D., Wilkinson, L., Folensbee, R. and Lerman, C. (1983) Stimulus control applications to the treatment of worry. *Behaviour Research and Therapy*, 21, 247–51.

Dugas, M. J. and Ladouceur, R. (2000) Treatment of GAD: targeting intolerance of uncertainty in two types of worry. *Behavior Modification*, 24, 635–57.

 To access the online resources accompanying this chapter, please visit: https://study.sagepub.com/farrand

16

Problem-Solving

Doing What It Says on the Tin

Georgina Miles

Learning Objectives

By the end of this chapter you should be able to:

- Critically appraise the theoretical rationale underpinning problem-solving therapy
- Demonstrate an understanding of specific factors associated with a low-intensity problem-solving intervention
- Apply specific factors associated with supporting a patient engage with a low-intensity model of problem-solving
- Formulate common difficulties experienced by patients when engaging with a low-intensity problem-solving intervention and support the patient's continued engagement

---

Intervention Description

Problem-solving (PS), or problem-solving therapy as it is often referred to, is an intervention that 'does what it says on the tin', supporting the patient to solve problems and difficulties they face in everyday life effectively. PS therapy was first outlined by D'Zurilla and Goldfried (1971) and involved teaching the patient a step-by-step protocol to approach problems head-on to find and apply potential solutions. It has been adopted for the treatment of depression and anxiety across a variety of health-care settings and adapted for different patient populations (Cuijpers et al., 2018) – for example, older adults (Kirkham et al., 2016), middle-aged and older armed forces veterans (Kasckow, et al., 2014), ethnic minorities (Unlu Ince et al., 2013; van't Hof et al., 2011) and patients with long-term physical health conditions such as chronic-obstructive pulmonary disease (Lee et al., 2015) and cancer (Hopko et al., 2011). Additionally, PS therapy has been delivered using a variety of formats, including supported self-help groups (Lee et al., 2015), psychoeducational groups (Dowrick et al., 2000) and online CBT based programmes (Warmerdam et al., 2010). As well as being used as a treatment, PS therapy has also been reported to be effective as a preventative measure for long-term sickness absence (Lexis, et al., 2011). Given an emphasis on supporting patients with common mental health difficulties returning to work, such application is of particular relevance to LICBT practitioners working within the IAPT programme (Chapters 1 and 20).

Evidence Base

Randomised control trials (RCTs) have demonstrated the effectiveness of PS therapy compared to psychological interventions such as behavioural activation (Hopko et al., 2011) and pharmacological interventions (Bell and D'Zurilla, 2009; Malouff et al., 2007; Mynors-Wallis et al., 1995). A meta-analysis has reported PS therapy to be an effective treatment for depression with small effect sizes comparable to those reported for other psychological treatments for depression (Cuijpers et al., 2018). Significant heterogeneity was highlighted in this meta-analysis, however, which was partly explained by three different types of PS intervention included in the analysis (Cuijpers et al., 2018).

Key Point

Main Types of Problem-Solving Therapy

- *Extended (E-PS)*: Often conducted in a group format of 10–12 sessions focusing on enhancing PS skills alongside changing cognitions that may interfere with PS (D'Zurilla and Nezu, 1982).
- *Brief (B-PST)*: Core features of PS originally developed to be delivered individually within primary care to patients in nine sessions or less (Mynors-Wallis et al., 1995).
- *Self-examination therapy (SET)*: PS skills central to an intervention adopted within an individual guided self-help or group format enabling patients to identify major goals in their life, focus on problems of personal value and accept situations that cannot be changed (Bowman et al., 1995).

No significant differences were found between the three types of PS treatment, although E-PS treatments with ten or more sessions had a larger, but non-significant, effect size. However, with E-PS therapy representing a multi-strand intervention combining problem-solving with cognitive restructuring techniques (Chapter 12) delivered over a larger number of treatment sessions, it would not meet criteria for a LICBT intervention (Chapter 1). With some potential adaptations, however, both B-PST and SET could be seen as representing an LICBT intervention.

The LICBT PS intervention implemented within the Improving Access to Psychological Therapies (IAPT) programme (Richards and Whyte, 2011) is informed by B-PST (Laurence Mynors-Wallis, 2010) and represents the basis of this chapter. That SET was originally developed as a guided self-help PS intervention to be supported in up to six sessions makes it a particularly appropriate addition to the LICBT PS portfolio. However, it is worth noting that little research has examined the effectiveness of either of these PS interventions as an LICBT intervention delivered by a mental health practitioner workforce for the treatment of mild to moderate common mental health problems.

Theoretical Rationale

Problem-solving is recognised as a mediator between challenging life events and wellbeing (D'Zurilla and Nezu, 2007). Effective and adaptive problem-solving ability is proposed as a mechanism maintaining positive wellbeing, reducing impact from stressful life events on emotional wellbeing and enhancing recovery from emotional difficulties (Nezu et al., 1986). Conversely, challenges with problem-solving are associated with increased likelihood of experiencing a range of common mental health difficulties such as depression (Nezu et al., 1986) and anxiety (Pawluk et al., 2017). The impact of these mental health difficulties can be heightened through poor problem-solving ability (Nezu et al., 1986) which enhances and maintains the main symptoms (Figure 16.1).

Whilst most adults have good enough problem-solving ability when faced by one or two coexisting problems, when faced with multiple problems, especially in the presence of a mental health difficulty, problem-solving ability may be impaired.

Application of Problem-Solving

As practical problems can impact symptoms associated with both depression and anxiety, the LICBT PS intervention can be applied across all common mental health difficulties recognised for treatment at Step 2 of a stepped care service delivery model (Chapter 1). To determine suitability for this intervention it is helpful to work collaboratively with the patient to identify any practical problems that may be exacerbating their presenting difficulty and symptoms.

Problem statement: Over the last few months I have been feeling stressed and overwhelmed due to lots of pressures in everyday life. I have been working long hours to try to help this, but this has meant that I am constantly tired and irritable and I have been seeing much less of my family and spending less quality time with my children. I have also been avoiding addressing problems elsewhere. As a result, I have thoughts of 'I can't cope' and 'I'm a bad parent'. This is impacting on my relationships with others.

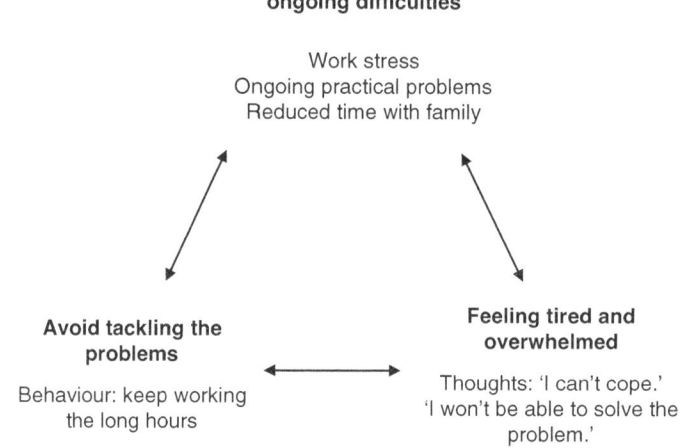

Stress and pressure from ongoing difficulties

Work stress
Ongoing practical problems
Reduced time with family

Avoid tackling the problems

Behaviour: keep working the long hours

Feeling tired and overwhelmed

Thoughts: 'I can't cope.'
'I won't be able to solve the problem.'

Figure 16.1 Jamie's Problem statement and maintenance of symptoms

Clinical Practice

Clinical Decision-Making Informing Problem-Solving

- Recognise the extent to which practical problems may be associated with, and having an impact on, the presenting problem
- Assess problem-solving ability
- Determine if poor problem-solving ability may affect the patient's ability to break their vicious cycle and make changes elsewhere
- Provide patient choice.

It is important to remember that LICBT PS is an intervention in its own right and should only be used as a single-strand intervention (Chapter 1). On occasions where assessment suggests the patient may benefit from using an LICBT PS intervention alongside other CBT interventions, clinical decision-making should consider the advantages of stepping the patient up to Step 3 (Chapter 4). However, the large evidence base for PS interventions as a single-strand intervention should not be overlooked (Cuijpers et al., 2018). Where clinical decisions have been reached, they should be presented at case management supervision for further discussion (Chapter 9).

Specific Factors: Supporting Problem-Solving

The Brief-PS LICBT intervention addressed in this chapter (Mynors-Wallis and Lau, 2010) provides an eight-stage framework to address a range of practical problems whilst drawing on pre-existing abilities to reduce symptoms associated with common mental health problems. Specific factors are informed by those reported within the LICBT clinical support materials (Richards and Whyte, 2011) that formed the basis of the PS intervention implemented within the IAPT programme (Richards and Whyte, 2011).

Clinical Practice

Intervention Stages

Stage 1: Explain LICBT problem-solving
Stage 2: Identify the problem to be worked on
Stage 3: Generate a variety of potential solutions to the problem
Stage 4: Complete a pros and cons analysis of the generated ideas
Stage 5: Select the most appropriate solution to put into action
Stage 6: Plan implementation
Stage 7: Carry out the plan
Stage 8: Review
- If the solution worked, complete the cycle for the next problem
- If the solution did not work, repeat steps 5–7.

Consistent with LICBT, the patient should be supported within the session to engage with the LICBT PS intervention (Farrand et al., 2019; Mynors-Wallis and Lau, 2010).

Stage 1: Explain Problem-Solving

In a manner consistent with the patient's level of comprehension, the rationale for the LICBT PS intervention, detailing the theoretical basis and highlighting why the intervention may be helpful to address their presenting difficulties, should be presented. The LICBT PS intervention or worksheet adopted should be introduced at this point and specific factors overviewed (Worksheet 16.1).

Once specific factors regarding the PS intervention have been explained, the use of common factor skills to elicit patient understanding is important (Chapter 5). If the patient understands the approach and is willing to continue, Stage 2 should

Worksheet 16.1 Example of an LICBT problem-solving worksheet

Problem-solving worksheet

Identify the problem

Potential solutions (Generate as many as possible)

Advantages and disadvantages (Continue on a separate sheet if necessary)			
Solution:		Solution:	
Advantages	Disadvantages	Advantages	Disadvantages
Solution:		Solution:	
Advantages	Disadvantages	Advantages	Disadvantages
Solution:		Solution:	
Advantages	Disadvantages	Advantages	Disadvantages

Chosen solution

Implementation plan What are you going to do? When are you going to do it?

Review How did it go?

be introduced. If the patient struggles to appreciate how the approach will benefit them or chooses another evidence-based LICBT intervention, signposting options to address the practical problems identified is a consideration. However, signposting may also be proposed by the patient as a potential solution during Stage 3. To promote engagement with the PS intervention it is important the patient is not led to consider signposting or other solutions within the session.

Stage 2: Identify Problem to Be Worked on

The next stage of LICBT PS intervention (Richards and Whyte, 2011) is to support the patient get started with the intervention to identify a problem they want to tackle first within the session. Depending on the patient's presenting difficulties and the types of practical difficulties that may be faced, the nature of support will vary. For example, symptoms that arise with depression – such as lack of volition, lethargy and poor motivation (Chapter 3) – may serve as initial barriers to PS. In this case, considering an LICBT intervention such as behavioural activation to target these symptoms directly may be preferable (Chapter 11).

Clinical Practice

Support to Get the Patient Started

- Identify a suitable practical problem to work on.
- Given the difficulty identifying a solution to a vague or wide-ranging problem, ensure that each problem identified is stated as specifically as possible – for example, if the patient identifies 'financial problems' to work on, support should help break the problem down into more specific examples, such as overdue electricity bill, car MOT, mortgage.
- If the patient struggles to identify a practical problem to work on, provide support to create a problem list (Worksheet 16.2) to write down as many practical problems faced as possible.
  - Problems *graded* in terms of difficulty can be helpful
  - The patient is supported to select the problem considered most acceptable to approach first
  - It is important to consider the consequences of not completing any identified practical problems within deadlines. If any problem presents with substantial consequences but is considered overwhelming, potential sources of community support or advice should be identified for contact.

Worksheet 16.2 Jamie's problem list

Problem list	
Main problem area	Main problem area
Work	*Financial*
Specific problems *Not getting on with colleagues* *Having to cover for two colleagues who are off on* *long-term sick leave* *Current project is behind* *Getting to work*	Specific problems *Credit card payment is overdue* *Always running out of money towards the end of the* *month* *Car MOT*
Most difficult to solve	Most difficult to solve
Current project is behind *Not getting on with colleagues*	*Always running out of money towards the end of the* *month*
Medium difficulty solving	Medium difficulty solving
	Credit card payment is overdue *Car MOT*
Least difficult to solve	Least difficult to solve
Getting to work *Having to cover for two colleagues who are off on* *long-term sick leave*	
Selected problem *Having to cover for two colleagues who are off on long-term sick leave*	

Given limited time available it is likely that the problem list will be started within session but completed between sessions.

Stage 3: Generate a Variety of Potential Solutions to the Problem

Without considering viability, difficulties or practicality, generate as many potential solutions to the selected problem as needed. The focus in this stage should be on quantity not quality with the following tips followed.

── **Key Point** ──────────────────────────

Useful Tips to Generate Potential Solutions

- 'Quantity breeds quality' (D'Zurilla and Goldfried, 1971, p. 115): Creativity and thinking of potential solutions not previously considered sensible should be encouraged.
- Reject nothing no matter how ridiculous (Richards and Whyte, 2011): No matter how seemingly unreasonable a solution sounds, do not reject it at this stage.

Worksheet 16.3   Jamie's problem selection and potential solutions

Problem-solving worksheet
Identify the problem
Having to cover for two colleagues who are off with long-term sickness
Potential solutions (Generate as many as possible)
Quit my job *Continue as I am currently - do nothing* *Speak to manager and discuss difficulties managing workload* *Refuse to do the extra work* *Delegate more responsibilities* *Ask colleagues for help* *Organise a team night out to boost morale* *Book some annual leave*

Stage 4: Complete a Pros and Cons Analysis of the Generated Ideas

A detailed consideration regarding the advantages and disadvantages of the identified solutions and judgement about their suitability should be completed. Areas such as access to resources needed, acceptability to self or others, feasibility, likelihood of success should be considered.

Worksheet 16.4   Advantages and disadvantages analysis

Advantages and disadvantages (Continue on a separate sheet if necessary)			
Solution: *Quit my job*		Solution: *Continue as I am currently - do nothing*	
Advantages	Disadvantages	Advantages	Disadvantages
Would no longer have the stress *Would have lots of spare time*	*Don't have another job to go to* *Would be more stressed due to financial issues* *Could lose house if we can't pay the mortgage* *Would miss my job as it's something I am good at*	*Easy to do as I'm already doing it*	*It's not working*

(continued)

Worksheet 16.4   Advantages and disadvantages analysis (Continued)

Solution: *Speak to manager and discuss difficulties managing workload*		Solution: *Refuse to do the extra work*	
Advantages	Disadvantages	Advantages	Disadvantages
They may not know how much work I currently have to do They may be able to take some of the responsibilities from me They could help with some of the tasks themselves	They may just expect me to continue working as I am I may be seen as less capable than colleagues	I would finish work on time and get to spend more time with my family	I would still be stressed due to not meeting the demands of the job I may be seen as a troublemaker at work I would be letting my colleagues down

Solution: *Delegate more responsibilities*		Solution: *Ask colleagues for help*	
Advantages	Disadvantages	Advantages	Disadvantages
It would help to manage some of the tasks I am working on I am probably taking on too much myself and should already have delegated some tasks to others It will give others more opportunity to get different types of experience	It would put extra pressure on the team They may not be up to standard to complete the tasks as they need to be done	It's a supportive team so there would be lots of people who are prepared to help me out	I may be seen as a failure or not coping by colleagues

Solution: *Organise a team night out to boost morale*		Solution: *Book some annual leave*	
Advantages	Disadvantages	Advantages	Disadvantages
We haven't had a team night out in ages It would be a good way to support working relationships	I don't have time It wouldn't solve the problem of reducing my workload	I really could do with some time off It would give me time to catch up on things around the home and do things I enjoy I would have more time to spend with my family	I don't have time for annual leave The problems will still be waiting for me when I go back I wouldn't want to go back

Stage 5: Select the Most Appropriate Solution to Put into Action

Select a solution that appears to have the best chance of success, is achievable and can be completed with the resources available.

Stage 6: Plan Implementation

Plan how the solution will be undertaken by using the four Ws (Richards and Whyte, 2011) to make the plan explicit.

Key Point

The four Ws:

- *What*: The solution to put into action selected from Stage 5.
- *Where*: The place or location where the solution will be carried out.
- *When*: Select an appropriate time to apply the solution.
- *With whom*: Consider anybody else who may be needed to implement the solution.

Using an LICBT PS worksheet (Richards and Whyte, 2011), intervention (Farrand et al., 2019) or something readily accessible (e.g. mobile phone, diary), it is important to ensure a plan is written down. If practical barriers are identified within the session or experienced between sessions, the Capability, Opportunity, Motivation - Behaviour (COM-B) framework (Chapter 8; Michie et al., 2011) can be applied to amend or make the implementation plan more explicit.

Stage 7: Carry out the Plan

The plan should be undertaken as practice between sessions, with progress and outcomes recorded as the basis of the next support session. It is important that both successful and unsuccessful solutions are recorded to inform the review of progress within a session.

Stage 8: Review

Within the support session, information-gathering and common factor skills should be used to elicit how the solution went and any learning acquired. If the solution was carried out as planned and was successful in solving the problem, the intervention can be applied to the next problem. If unsuccessful, another solution identified within Stage 5 should be selected and the subsequent stages repeated.

Reflection Point

Consider the process of going through the problem-solving steps and reflect on any challenges you may have experienced.

Problem-Solving Challenges

An advantage of problem-solving as an LICBT intervention is that alternative solutions are nearly always available where an applied solution has been unsuccessful. When unsuccessful, the LICBT practitioner should apply the COM-B framework or use specific factors to address practical challenges engaging with the intervention within the session (Chapter 8; Michie et al., 2011).

Clinical Practice

Common Challenges

- Plan considered too overwhelming to complete
- Solution has not worked
- Patient cannot think of any new solutions
  - Patient selects a solution thought not to work.

Plan Considered Too Overwhelming to Complete

If the patient has been struggling to problem-solve for a long time or is experiencing a mental health difficulty that impacts on their problem-solving ability, it is understandable that they may initially consider themselves to be overwhelmed. There are several ways the patient can be supported on these occasions.

Clinical Practice

Supporting the 'Overwhelmed' Patient

- Break an identified solution into smaller steps
- Consider alternative solutions that the patient initially considered less overwhelming
- Adopt the COM-B framework to potentially identify more acceptable ways to implement.

Solution Has Not Worked

- Support the patient to consider other solutions
- Whilst the solution may have failed, consider helping the patient adapt the learning to another solution
- Encourage the patient to go back to previous solutions.

LICBT Practitioner Does Not Believe Patient Solution Will Work

- Maintain an approach based on 'collaborative empiricism' (Tee and Kazantzis, 2011)
- The patient should generate solutions and only be guided through the LICBT-specific factors by the LICBT practitioner; it is not the practitioner's role to predict outcomes.

Summary

This chapter has looked at PS therapy as an intervention that is as effective as others available (Cuijpers et al., 2018). The LICBT PS intervention adopted can be used across a range of common mental health difficulties recognised as suitable for treatment at Step 2 (Chapter 1). The LICBT PS intervention implemented within the IAPT programme is informed by the brief-PST model (Mynors-Wallis et al., 2000) and follows an eight-stage protocol – define the problem, consider potential solutions, weigh up the advantages and disadvantages, select, plan, carry out the solution, review. Providing a structure to support patients to address overwhelming practical problems, the intervention teaches patients a structured technique they can then apply for any subsequent difficulties, thereby overcoming avoidance and addressing symptoms of common mental health problems.

Assessing Your Understanding

Declarative

Multiple Choice Questions

1. What are the main types of problem-solving therapy? [Select all that apply]
    (a) Problem reduction therapy (PRT)
    (b) Brief PS (B-PS)
    (c) Crisis management
    (d) Self-examination therapy (SET)
    (e) Extended PS (E-PS)
2. What factors are important in assessing suitability for PST? [Select all that apply]
    (a) Determining if poor problem-solving ability may affect the patient's ability to break their vicious cycle and make changes elsewhere
    (b) Identifying if there are any practical problems exacerbating the current symptoms
    (c) Determining whether the patient wishes to focus on depression or anxiety symptoms
    (d) Considering whether the patient is avoiding tackling practical problems
    (e) Providing the patient with choice of treatment and collaborative decision-making
3. How might the patient be supported to tackle a problem when they are feeling overwhelmed? [Select all that apply]
    (a) Encourage the patient to break the problem down into smaller steps
    (b) Grade problems into a hierarchy
    (c) Begin with the easiest quick win to boost patient confidence
    (d) Adopt the COM-B framework to potentially identify more acceptable ways to implement
    (e) Encourage the patient to tackle the most overwhelming problem first to get it out of the way

Procedural

Self-Practice/Self-Reflection

Over the next week, set aside some time to consider any *practical* problems you are currently experiencing

*   Apply the problem-solving steps
*   Carry out the plan you have set for yourself
*   Review the extent to which it was successful.

Answers to **Assessing Your Understanding** questions can be found in the appendix on p. 337.

Further Reading and Resources

Cuijpers, P., De Wit, L., Kleiboer, A., Karyotaki, E. and Ebert, D. (2018) Problem-solving therapy for adult depression: An updated meta-analysis. *European Psychiatry*, 48, 27–37.

Marrinan, T. (2019) Treatment strategies. In M. Papworth and T. Marrinan (eds), *Low Intensity Cognitive Behaviour Therapy: A Practitioner's Guide*. London: Sage. pp. 221–79

Mynors-Wallis, L. and Lau, M.A. (2010) Problem solving as a low-intensity intervention. In J. Bennett-Levy, D.A. Richards, P. Farrand, H. Christensen, K.M. Griffiths, D.J. Kavanagh, et al. (eds), *Oxford Guide to Low Intensity CBT Interventions*. Oxford: Oxford University Press. pp.151–8

 To access the online resources accompanying this chapter, please visit: https://study.sagepub.com/farrand

17

Sleep Management

Steps to a Good Night's Sleep

Sophie Brooks

Learning Objectives

By the end of this chapter you should be able to:

- Critically appraise the theoretical rationale informing a low-intensity cognitive behavioural therapy sleep management intervention
- Apply declarative knowledge concerning how the sleep management intervention can be used to support a patient with poor sleep
- Apply specific factors associated with the low-intensity cognitive behavioural therapy sleep management intervention
- Recognise common difficulties experienced when engaging with sleep management and demonstrate appropriate decision-making to support the patient overcome them

What Is Insomnia?

The DSM-V (APA, 2013) classifies insomnia as a predominant feeling of dissatisfaction with sleep quantity or quality, for at least three months, accompanied by one (or more) of the following symptoms:

1. Difficulty falling asleep
2. Difficulty staying asleep (characterised by waking up frequently and difficulty getting back to sleep after waking)
3. Waking up early in the morning and unable to get back to sleep.

To meet the diagnostic criteria the sleep difficulties must:

- Cause significant distress or significantly impair important areas of functioning (e.g. social, occupational)
- Occur three or more nights per week
- Occur despite adequate opportunity for sleep
- Not be better explained by another sleep–wake disorder or co-existing physical or mental health condition
- Not be better explained by substance use (e.g. medication, recreational drugs).

It is important to be aware of other health issues or sleep disorders, such as sleep apnoea (NICE, 2015a) and restless leg syndrome (NICE, 2016), for which low-intensity CBT (LICBT) sleep management is not the recommended treatment. To increase awareness of these presentations, refer to the DSM-V (APA, 2013) and NICE guidelines (NICE, 2015b) and consider referral to the GP for further exploration if necessary.

Intervention Description

Within Great Britain approximately 30 per cent of people have disrupted sleep most nights (Sleep Council, 2017) with sleep difficulties identified as both a symptom and risk factor for a range of mental health disorders (Dolan-Sewell et al., 2005). It is likely therefore that people experiencing common mental health problems may also be experiencing some form of sleep difficulty. Sleep management as an LICBT intervention is informed by a multi-component treatment, cognitive behavioural therapy for insomnia (CBT-I; van Straten et al., 2018). Variations are used across the literature base but CBT-I is likely to include a combination of techniques (Table 17.1).

Further research is needed if superiority of a singular component of CBT-I is to be established, although attempts have been made to compare and evaluate techniques. Briefer behavioural versions of CBT-I without formal cognitive components have

Table 17.1 Components of CBT-I

Technique	Overview
Sleep hygiene	General advice on how someone may improve sleep (e.g. reduce caffeine, ensure bed is comfortable)
Stimulus control	Behavioural technique intended to strengthen the association between bed and sleep and reduce cues for behaviours not conducive to sleep
Sleep restriction	Behavioural technique in which time spent in bed is initially restricted to an individualised amount of time. Improves sleep efficiency, quality of sleep and time taken to fall asleep
Cognitive therapy	Cognitive techniques to challenge unhelpful beliefs about sleep that may be maintaining difficulties
Relaxation therapy	Formally taught relaxation techniques to reduce anxiety or tension that prohibit sleep – e.g. progressive muscle relaxation, diaphragmatic breathing
Paradoxical intention	Patients instructed not to make any effort (intention) to fall asleep and remain passively awake. Intended to eliminate anxiety and pressure experienced around the need to fall asleep

been effective in primary care: brief behavioural treatment for insomnia (BBTI; Troxel et al., 2012) and abbreviated cognitive behavioural insomnia therapy (ACBT; Edinger and Sampson, 2003). Furthermore, research comparing full CBT-I to standalone stimulus control therapy (SCT) and to sleep restriction therapy (SRT) has demonstrated equally positive outcomes across each treatment (Epstein et al., 2012). This suggests that these behavioural techniques are individually sufficient for therapeutic change. It should be noted that whilst this evaluation of behavioural techniques contained no structured cognitive components, cognitive elements did at times accompany sleep hygiene (Epstein et al., 2012). Additionally, it has been argued that the importance of cognitive elements within CBT-I should not be overlooked (Lancee et al., 2019). However, no controlled studies evaluating standalone cognitive therapy have been identified (NICE, 2015b) and there is insufficient evidence to recommend cognitive therapy as a standalone intervention (Morgenthaler et al., 2006).

Based on these considerations and the single-strand nature of LICBT work, LICBT sleep management focuses on supporting patients make behavioural changes using principles of SCT or SRT, with the addition of sleep hygiene information. If necessary and relevant, high-intensity CBT can be offered to target negative automatic thoughts or worries if the behavioural routes are contraindicated or declined by the patient.

Evidence Base

A meta-analysis has concluded that CBT-I, delivered either in full or as component parts, is an effective treatment for insomnia (van Straten et al., 2018). CBT-I has been shown to be effective for patients experiencing psychiatric and physical health co-morbidities (Geiger-Brown et al., 2015), older adults and chronic users of hypnot-ics (Morgenthaler et al., 2006). Furthermore, research has demonstrated CBT-I to be more effective than hypnotic medication in the long-term (Mitchell et al., 2012), and is therefore recommended for the long-term management of insomnia in prefer-ence to medication (NICE, 2015b). Wider research highlights how CBT-I represents a particularly suitable intervention to be delivered within an LICBT framework.

Key Point

Characteristics of CBT-I consistent with LICBT:

- Effective via a number of delivery methods:
  - Self-help (Ho et al., 2015; van Straten and Cuijpers, 2009)
  - In an online format (Seyffert et al., 2016)
  - With telephone support (Arnedt et al., 2013)
  - Via a group (Koffel et al., 2015) and within a primary-care group setting (Espie et al., 2007)
  - Face-to-face (van Straten et al., 2018).
- Can be delivered effectively by primary care counsellors (Morgan et al., 2004), primary care nurses (Espie et al., 2007) and nurse practitioners with no previous training in sleep medicine (Buysse et al., 2011).
- Four to eight sessions are considered to be the optimal dose (van Straten et al., 2018; Anderson, 2018b).

Similarly, Espie (2009) has highlighted that delivering CBT-I within a stepped-care model (Chapter 1) is likely to be a cost-effective way of improving access to treat-ment for the high proportion of people requiring psychological help for their sleep difficulties.

Whilst CBT-I is well supported, it remains necessary to consider NICE guidelines (2015b) before adopting sleep management. Where sleep difficulties are identified during assessment as arising secondary to a common mental health difficulty, treat-ment should focus on the primary problem (NICE, 2015b), unless the patient makes an informed choice that addressing their sleep difficulties is their priority concern.

Theoretical Rationale

LICBT sleep management is based on a two-process model of sleep regulation that identifies two biological mechanisms working together to regulate sleep (Borbély, 1982; Espie, 2006).

Key Point

Mechanisms Regulating Sleep

- *Homeostatic drive (or sleep drive)*: Mechanism by which the need for sleep accumulates with time spent awake. This mechanism means that the longer we spend awake, the stronger our need for sleep becomes.
- *Circadian sleep-wake cycle*: Biological cycle working over roughly a 24-hour period. In someone that sleeps well, the area of the brain linked to circadian rhythms will begin to decrease melatonin (hormone associated with sleep) with increasing levels of light in the morning and secrete cortisol (hormone associated with wakefulness) to wake them up. The opposite occurs in response to decreasing levels of light as the sun goes down.

In good sleepers these mechanisms are aligned with the brain responding to morning sunlight, recognising wake time, and the sleep drive replenished following a sufficient amount of sleep. Disruption in these mechanisms – for example, through enforced changes to the sleep–wake cycle (e.g. jet-lag, night shifts, staying up late) or behaviours that can disrupt the sleep drive – can result in a vicious cycle of sleep with the potential to create bad sleepers (Worksheet 17.1).

Worksheet 17.1   Example CBT vicious cycle for sleep difficulties

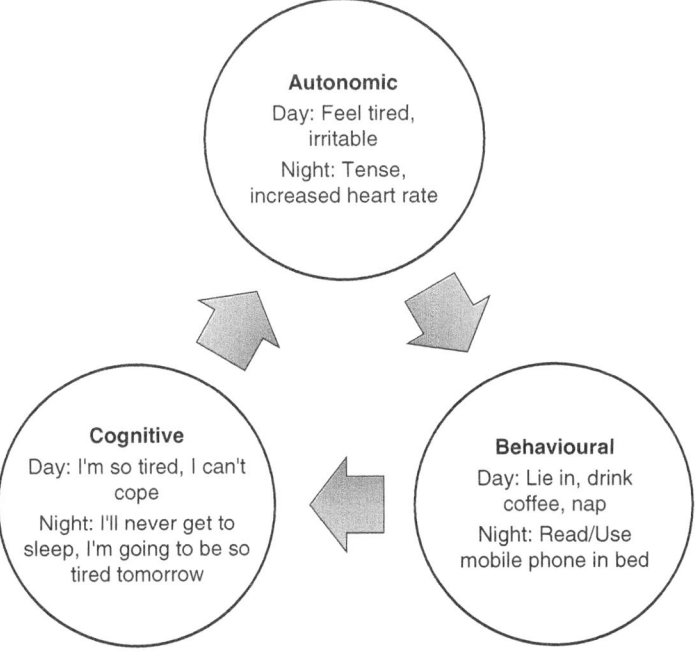

Autonomic
Day: Feel tired, irritable
Night: Tense, increased heart rate

Cognitive
Day: I'm so tired, I can't cope
Night: I'll never get to sleep, I'm going to be so tired tomorrow

Behavioural
Day: Lie in, drink coffee, nap
Night: Read/Use mobile phone in bed

Another factor perpetuating the vicious cycle of sleep difficulties is spending time awake in bed, becoming tense and frustrated whilst trying to get to sleep. This leads to a weakening of the association that bed = sleep and a strengthening of the association that bed = frustration, not getting to sleep and experiencing a sense of arousal. In this context, arousal refers to a state of heightened physiological and psychological activity. Arousal increases physical and mental alertness and is therefore incompatible with sleep. LICBT sleep management enables the realignment of the two drives through behaviour modification, which strengthens the association between being in bed and being asleep, leading to improved sleep.

Application of LICBT Sleep Management

Steps to a good night's sleep LICBT sleep management follows a 6-stage process over a number of sessions that can be collaboratively discussed in case management supervision (Chapter 9). CEDAR 'Steps to a Good Night's Sleep' workbook can be used to support the patient through the intervention.

Clinical Practice

Intervention Stages

- *Stage 1*: Provide psychoeducation
- *Stage 2*: Support the patient to begin a sleep diary
- *Stage 3*: Establish an appropriate behaviour modification route
- *Stage 4*: Implement behaviour modification
  - Stage 4a: Stimulus control therapy
  - Stage 4b: Sleep restriction therapy
- *Stage 5*: Review
- *Stage 6*: If necessary, consider alternatives – for example, LICBT cognitive restructuring or LICBT intervention for generalised anxiety disorder.

Stage 1: Psychoeducation

Whilst it is important for patients to understand the mechanisms that regulate sleep, the LICBT practitioner should consider the language used to explain these concepts.

Clinical Example

Explaining the Mechanisms Regulating Sleep

The need for sleep builds up during time spent awake (homeostatic drive). Our bodies follow a daily biological routine linked to daylight and darkness cycles and this controls when we feel tired, but this can become disrupted (circadian sleep-wake cycle).

To elicit the symptoms, collaboratively fill out an LICBT *Vicious Cycle* based on Worksheet 17.1. This can be used to highlight how behaviours adopted by the patient may be maintaining poor sleep and can additionally indicate whether unhelpful beliefs about sleep are also present. It can be a good opportunity to discuss and dispel common myths about sleep.

Clinical Example

Debunking Sleep Myths

- *'I should fall asleep straight away'*
  - Taking up to 30 minutes to fall asleep is considered appropriate and can be used as an indicator of good quality sleep, according to recommendations from the National Sleep Foundation (Ohayon et al., 2017).
- *'I should always get eight hours of sleep'*
  - The amount of sleep needed varies by age and individual, but the National Sleep Foundation (Hirshkowitz et al., 2015) guidelines suggest:
    - For adults aged 18 to 64 between seven and nine hours of sleep *is recommended*
    - For those aged 18 to 25 six to eleven hours *may be appropriate*
    - For those aged 26 to 64 six to ten hours *may be appropriate*
    - For adults aged 65+ between seven and eight hours *is recommended*; however, five to nine hours *may be appropriate*.
- *'I should be able to sleep through the night'*
    - It is normal to wake a number of times during the night. People without sleep difficulties may wake between two and eight times a night, depending on age (Anderson, 2018a).
- *'If I don't get a lot of sleep, I won't get what I need to function properly'*
  - Deep sleep (slow-wave, non-REM sleep) occurs early during sleep (Espie, 2010). Deep sleep is linked to the restorative and recovery functions of sleep (Dijk, 2010).

Sleep Hygiene

At this stage the LICBT practitioner should introduce sleep hygiene. Whilst there is insufficient evidence to support sleep hygiene as a standalone intervention (Morgenthaler et al., 2006), it is often included within the wider package of CBT-I and forms part of insomnia guidelines (NICE, 2015b).

Differentiating between tiredness (fatigue) and sleepiness (drowsiness) is an important part of psychoeducation.

Table 17.2   Sleep hygiene tips

Dietary factors	Caffeine, sugar, alcohol and nicotine can all have a negative impact on sleep. Where appropriate, support the patient to reduce safely or signpost to GP.
Comfortable bedroom	The optimum sleeping environment is approximately 16–18 °C and free from significant levels of light, noise and clutter. A comfortable bed and pillows are also recommended.
Daily activity	Increasing day-time activity levels can help build the sleep drive. High-intensity exercise can impact the ability to sleep so should be avoided one to two hours before bedtime (Stutz et al., 2019).
Reduce clock-watching	Watching the clock causes anxiety and frustration as we lay in bed, look at the clock and calculate, 'Only four hours left until my alarm. I'm going to feel awful!'
Reduce screen time	Screens on smartphones, TVs and tablets give off a blue light that can delay the release of the hormone melatonin and increase alertness. Limiting use of these devices in bed or before bedtime is preferable. Using a blue light filter can also help.
Night-time routine	Implementing a wind-down routine can put the brain and body in a state conducive to sleep – e.g. turning off phone notifications, lowering the light level, completing all chores by a set time before bed.
Shift attention to something neutral or enjoyable	Ruminating about lack of sleep or trying to command ourselves to get to sleep increases anxiety and tension, thereby reducing the likelihood of sleep.

Key Point

Differences between Tiredness and Sleepiness

- *Tiredness*: General lack of energy.
- *Sleepiness*: The state immediately before falling asleep when the body and mind struggle to stay awake, resulting in a range of symptoms which feel difficult to control, including:
  - Eyelids becoming heavy and hard to keep open
  - Difficulty holding the head up
  - Mind drifting and difficulty keeping focus.

Differentiation is key to improving sleep as patients should experience sleepiness before falling asleep, rather than going to bed to attempt to sleep when only experiencing tiredness. Supporting someone to recognise the difference between these states during the psychoeducation stage will lead to greater success with the behaviour modification techniques moving forward.

Stage 2: Support the Patient to Begin a Sleep Diary

Working collaboratively, the LICBT practitioner should support the patient within the session to begin gathering further information about their sleep using a sleep diary (Worksheet 17.2), beginning with the previous night.

Before the next support session the patient should complete the sleep diary every morning for the previous night. Consider allowing a two-week period between sessions to allow the patient to record adequate sleep information in the diary. To minimise clock-watching, it is important to highlight that timings do not need to be completely accurate. During the next support session, the sleep diary should be collaboratively reviewed and the patient should be supported to identify any unhelpful behaviours contributing to sleep difficulties.

Stage 3: Establish Appropriate Behaviour Modification Route

After reviewing the sleep diary the LICBT practitioner should use it to inform a collaborative discussion about which behavioural modification route, stimulus control therapy (SCT) or sleep restriction therapy (SRT), is indicated. The LICBT practitioner should discuss both options with the patient and use the information gathered, patient choice and clinical judgement to collaboratively agree on a treatment route. It is important that the patient has an understanding of the theoretical rationale of SCT and SRT.

Theoretical Rationale for SCT and SRT

Stimulus control therapy (SCT): Bed (and bedtime) can become associated with arousal/wakefulness when behaviours or activities leading to arousal (and therefore incompatible with sleep) repeatedly occur in bed. This might include watching TV, replying to emails, worrying or feeling frustrated. SCT intends to strengthen the association that bed = sleep and weaken the association that bed = arousal/wakefulness. This is done by reducing (controlling) activities (stimuli) that are incompatible with sleep so they are not done in bed (stimulus) or immediately before bedtime (stimulus).

Worksheet 17.2 Example sleep diary

	Monday	Tuesday	Wednesday	Thursday	Friday	Saturday	Sunday
Time woke up	8.20 am	8 am	8.30 am	8.20 am	8.15 am	7.30 am	8 am
Approx. duration of sleep (total sleep time/TST)	Unsure when fell asleep on Sunday	7 hours 5 mins (425 mins)	5 hours 55 mins (355 mins)	6 hours 50 mins (410 mins)	6 hours 25 mins (385 mins)	7 hours 10 mins (430 mins)	7 hours 30 mins (450 mins)
Time got out of bed	10 am	9.45 am	10.30 am	9.30 am	10 am	9 am	9.30 am
Amount of caffeine	4 coffees, 2 teas	4 coffees, 1 tea	6 coffees, 2 teas	4 coffees, 3 teas	4 coffees	3 coffees, 2 teas	3 coffees, 3 teas
Exercise	Walked dog, 30 mins	5k jog with friends	None	5k jog with friends	Walked dog, 90 mins	Countryside walk, 2 hours	None
Naps	None	1 x 50 mins	1 x 80 mins	1 x 40 mins	None	None	1 x 45 mins
What I did before bed	Ironing, watched TV. Used tablet in bed	Jog, pub, dinner at 9 pm, TV, read and used tablet in bed	Used tablet most of the evening and in bed	Jog, pub, dinner at 9 pm, cleaned bathroom, used tablet	Gave dog a bath, TV, played cards. Read in bed	Early dinner and theatre, read for a bit in bed	Cleaned kitchen, watched film, used tablet in bed
Time went to bed	10 pm	10 pm	10 pm	10.15 pm	11 pm	11 pm	10 pm
Time fell asleep	12 am	1.30 am	12.30 am	1 am	12 am	11.45 pm	12.15 am
Approx. no. times/ duration woke in night	1 x 15mins, 1 x 40 mins	2 x 5 mins, 1 x 1 hour	1 x 15 mins, 1 x 45 mins	1 x 30 mins, 1 x 20 mins	1 x 20 mins	1 x 15 mins, 1 x 30 mins	1 x 45 mins, 1 x 10 mins
Comments	Felt quite good today	Enjoy our jog and pub nights! Took ages to get to sleep but my book is really good so wasn't too bad!	Slept really badly and so tired today, couldn't be bothered to do much	Busy evening so slightly later to bed	Busy today as friend visiting and long walk with the dog. Later night as partner doesn't have to be up for work at the weekends	Another nice day, not too tired. Was nice to go out for dinner, shared a bottle of wine	Really tired after a big Sunday lunch so had a nap and a lazy afternoon

Sleep restriction therapy (SRT): People experiencing sleep difficulties often remain in bed, despite not sleeping, in a vain effort to get to sleep or catch up on sleep. This is rarely effective and can perpetuate sleep problems. People with sleep difficulties may also nap during the day, unhelpfully resetting the sleep drive. SRT reduces time in bed and daytime napping in order to temporarily create a minor sleep deprivation, thus increasing sleep drive and consolidating any sleep that may occur to the time spent in bed.

The theoretical rationales for SCT or SRT are not discrete, so deciding which option will be most beneficial may not always be clear-cut. A patient who uses their bed or bedroom for activities such as watching TV, reading or working or who reports high levels of arousal or anxiety whilst trying to fall asleep may benefit from SCT. A patient reporting spending a long time in bed at night but little time spent asleep and/or excessive daytime napping may find SRT helpful.

Stage 4: Implement Behaviour Modification

Stage 4a: Stimulus Control Therapy

If SCT is agreed upon, discuss which specific behavioural changes the patient would like to begin with (Table 17.3; Bootzin and Perlis, 2011).

Support the patient to think about how they might apply the specific behavioural change using the worksheet (Worksheet 17.3).

If appropriate, the patient may decide to make more than one behavioural change at once. Patients should be encouraged to maintain the changes made every week and add to these rather than replace them.

Stage 4b: Sleep Restriction Therapy

Where a collaborative decision to use SRT has been reached, discuss and implement the following set of instructions (Wohlgemuth and Edinger, 2000). The LICBT practitioner should support the patient to use the SRT worksheet (Worksheet 17.4).

Table 17.3   SCT behaviour changes

Behaviour change	Theoretical rationale	Considerations
Fixed wake-up time every day	Helps get the sleep drive back into sync. If the body learns what time to get up every day, it will start to become sleepy at the right time to ensure the right amount of sleep is experienced.	May seem unappealing as it includes getting up at the same time every day, including days off or when the patient has not slept very well!
Getting out of bed if lying awake for 15–20 minutes	Staying in bed when unable to sleep leads to physical feelings associated with anxiety and unhelpful thoughts. This strengthens the association that bed = awake. Getting up to do something enjoyable and relaxing can serve as a distraction to the inability to sleep. When sleepy, the patient can go back to bed, but may need to repeat.	Encourage the patient to consider what is likely to happen if they stay in bed. By getting out of bed, patients are accepting wakefulness but engaging in something worthwhile rather than becoming increasingly frustrated. Having a cosy space available can make getting out of bed seem less unappealing. Clock-watching is discouraged; therefore 15–20 minutes is an approximation.
Avoid lying in, going to bed before sleepy, and use bed for sleeping and sex only	Intention to establish association that bed = sleep. Spending time in bed whilst not asleep strengthens the unhelpful association that bed = awake.	The exception here is sex – this leads to a number of hormonal changes that can help us drop off more quickly and experience better quality sleep (Lastella et al., 2019).
No napping	Napping re-sets the sleep-drive, making it harder to get to sleep at bedtime.	Can be trickier for some people than others – for example, people with long-term health conditions. If people really need to nap, encourage them to nap in bed with a limit of around 15–20 minutes, setting an alarm to avoid unintentionally sleeping for hours. Napping earlier on during the day allows the sleep drive to build back up.

Clinical Practice

Steps Associated with SRT

- *Step 1*: Calculate total sleep time (TST)
- *Step 2*: Calculate initial time in bed prescription (TIB)
- *Step 3*: Support patient to apply TIB prescription
- *Step 4*: Calculate sleep efficiency
- *Step 5*: Use sleep efficiency to create new TIB prescription.

Step 1: Calculate Total Sleep Time

Support the patient to use their sleep diary to calculate how much time per night is spent asleep (total sleep time, TST). Converting this into minutes will be helpful when calculating sleep efficiency, it can then be converted back to hours when setting and implementing the time in bed prescription. Support the patient to acknowledge that their total sleep time is likely to be less than their time in bed (TIB).

Putting sleep changes into action: Stimulus control

Change:
1

Week commencing: *2/9/19*

Specific behavioural change to put into action: Fixed wake-up time everyday

How I can apply this: *Set an alarm for a reasonable time and then make sure I get up! Maybe I'll put the alarm clock at the other side of the room.*

What might get in the way: *If I'm still tired I won't want to get up!*

How might I overcome this: *Remind myself of why it is important, think about the long-term benefits (i.e. hopefully my sleep problems will get better).*

How did it go? (What went well? What didn't go well? What got in the way? How will I maintain this?)

Change:
2

Week commencing: *2/9/19*

Specific behavioural change to put into action: *Only use bed for sleep and sex.*

How I can apply this: *Watch box sets on sofa in spare room rather than in bed.*

What might get in the way: *I'm just in the habit of watching box sets in bed.*

How might I overcome this: *Keep my laptop in the spare room rather than bedroom, tell my partner to remind me if I go to watch box sets in bed, make the spare room cosier.*

How did it go? (What went well? What didn't go well? What got in the way? How will I maintain this?)

Change:
3

Week commencing:

Specific behavioural change to put into action:

How I can apply this:

What might get in the way:

How might I overcome this:

How did it go? (What went well? What didn't go well? What got in the way? How will I maintain this?)

Clinical Example

Calculating TST and TIB

Patient got into bed at 10 pm, fell asleep around 11.30 pm. Woke up at 1 am for 30 minutes. Fell back asleep at approximately 2 am, woke up at 6.30 am, got out of bed at 7.30 am.

- Slept 11.30 pm–1 am = 1 hour 30 minutes
- Slept 2 am–6.30 am = 4 hours 30 minutes
- TST = 6 hours (360 minutes)
- TIB = 9 hours 30 minutes (570 minutes).

Support the patient to use their completed sleep diary and calculate the TST for the last seven days. Add the TSTs together and divide by 7 to get the mean weekly TST. If the patient has kept the sleep diary for 14 nights between sessions, add up the TSTs and divide by 14 for the mean fortnightly TST. The mean TST (weekly or fortnightly) will be used moving forward.

Step 2: Calculate Initial TIB Prescription

To calculate the TIB prescription, add 30 minutes to the mean TST. The TIB prescription is the amount of time the patient should be spending in bed each night, regardless of whether they achieve sleep, with no napping during the day. The TIB prescription should never be less than five hours (Espie, 2010).

Clinical Example

Calculating TIB Prescription

- Mean TST = 6 hours + 30 minutes = 6 hours 30 minutes (390 minutes)
- TIB prescription = 6 hours 30 minutes (390 minutes).

Step 3: Support Patient Apply TIB Prescription

Maintaining fidelity to the intervention protocol, support the patient to adhere to the TIB prescription by collaboratively calculating new bed and wake times. Consider what time the patient needs to be awake in the morning and work backwards using the TIB prescription to identify a new bedtime.

Clinical Example

Calculating Bed and Wake Times

The patient's TIB prescription is 6 hours 30 minutes. They need to be up at 7 am. Subtracting their TIB prescription from their required wake time results in a prescribed bedtime of 12.30 am. If a 12.30 am bedtime feels too late, this could be shifted – for example, bedtime becomes 12 am and wake time becomes 6.30 am.

The patient should then implement the TIB prescription every night before the next support session and continue keeping their sleep diary, calculating the TST each night. The wake time should remain the same every day.

Step 4: Calculate Sleep Efficiency

Sleep efficiency (SE) refers to how much time in bed is actually spent sleeping. In the next support session look at the diary and the mean TST since the last session. Use the TIB prescription and mean TST to calculate sleep efficiency using the formula: **(Mean TST/TIB) x 100.**

Clinical Example

Calculating Sleep Efficiency

- Mean TST = 5 hours 30 minutes (330m), TIB prescription = 6 hours 30 minutes (390m)
- 330/390 = 0.85
- 0.85 x 100 = 85%.

In this example, SE is 85%, showing that 85 per cent of time in bed is spent asleep.

Step 5: Use Sleep Efficiency to Create New TIB Prescription

The TIB prescription is changed based on the patient's SE.

- If the SE is below 85 per cent, reduce the TIB prescription by 15 minutes.
- If the SE is between 85 and 89 per cent, the TIB prescription remains the same.
- If the SE is above 90 per cent, the TIB prescription can be increased by 15 minutes.

Putting sleep changes into action: Sleep restriction

Week commencing:

You will need to use your completed sleep diary to help you fill out this worksheet.

Calculate your mean weekly total sleep time (TST) by adding up how many hours you have spent *asleep* over the last seven days, converting this to minutes and dividing by seven. Put this in the box below. Then calculate your new time in bed prescription (TIB) by adding 30 minutes to your mean weekly TST, convert this back to hours. Write this in the box below.

Mean weekly TST (minutes)		TIB prescription	Minutes: Hours:

Your TIB prescription is the amount of time you will need to spend in bed over the next week. Record what time you want to wake up (keep this consistent) and then take away your TIB prescription from this to work out what time you need to go to bed.

Wake time		Bedtime	

Over the next week stick to your bedtime and wake time as recorded above. Keep filling out the sleep diary, making sure to track your TST. Use this worksheet to think about whether anything will get in the way of sticking to your bed and wake times. What might help you overcome these?

Potential barriers to my planned bed and wake times	What might help me to overcome these barriers?

After a week of going to bed and waking up at your new bed and wake times, calculate your sleep efficiency to see if you should adjust your TIB prescription. Firstly, you will need to re-calculate your mean weekly TST based on your most recent sleep diary, then calculate sleep efficiency using the following formula:

(Mean weekly TST ÷ TIB prescription) x 100.

Mean weekly TST (minutes)	÷	TIB prescription (minutes)	=	x 100
	÷			

This should give you a percentage. If this percentage is below 85%, reduce the initial TIB prescription by 15 minutes. If the percentage is between 85% and 89% keep the initial TIB prescription the same. If the percentage is 90% or over, add 15 minutes on to the initial TIB prescription.

Whether SCT or SRT is adopted, it is important to highlight that techniques will not instantly address sleep difficulties and that perseverance is required in the face of frustration. Difficulties with engagement and the potential for increased short-term tiredness when employing these techniques should also be acknowledged. The patient should continue to use the sleep diary while implementing behavioural changes to allow the impact on sleep to be tracked and reviewed during support sessions.

Stage 5: Review

During each support session the completed sleep diaries and worksheets should be collaboratively reviewed. Use this time to understand how the intervention is being applied and explore any challenges or non-concordance. If using SCT, support the patient to continue applying the original behavioural changes and come to a shared decision about any new changes (Table 17.3). If using SRT, support the patient to calculate their sleep efficiency and adjust TIB prescription accordingly, then plan how to implement the new TIB prescription.

When the patient is consistently feeling more satisfied with the quality and quantity of their sleep, they may consider ending SCT or SRT. It is important to discuss how sleep improvements can be maintained. Consider revisiting the vicious cycle and drawing attention to the unhelpful behaviours that may have been contributing to sleep problems initially. This can help the patient to identify if they are falling back into old habits and act to prevent this. Some patients may choose to continue using these strategies after treatment sessions have ended.

Stage 6: If Necessary, Consider Alternatives

At assessment, if sleep difficulties are caused mainly by excessive worrying or negative automatic thoughts, worry management (Chapter 15) or cognitive restructuring (Chapter 12) may be a more appropriate intervention. If the decision is made to commence LICBT sleep management but the patient reports their thoughts or worries being problematic (despite adhering to the behavioural changes), the LICBT practitioner may need to re-think. This should be discussed in case management supervision to consider stepping up for further assessment and treatment.

Challenges with Sleep Management

The COM-B model (Michie et al., 2011; Chapter 8) can be used to address challenges that may arise with the LICBT sleep management intervention. Maintaining common factor skills, giving clear information and framing setbacks as learning opportunities rather than failures are all important to maintain treatment engagement.

Reluctance to Engage

Behavioural changes associated with the LICBT sleep management intervention can be challenging, particularly in the short term where they may increase tiredness and feel counter-intuitive. As well as maintaining common factor skills (Chapter 5), several specific factors associated with the intervention should be implemented to address reluctance to engage.

Clinical Practice

Specific Factors Addressing Reluctance to Change

- Ensure the LICBT intervention rationale is understood. It facilitates informed and collaborative treatment decisions.
- Set the expectation at the start of treatment that it is going to be necessary to change behaviours to improve sleep. Stress that in the short term this has the potential to increase tiredness and may feel challenging.
- Reaffirm that many patients that continue to engage with the intervention between sessions experience improved sleep and reduced tiredness.

Contraindications

The LICBT practitioner should pay attention to a number of considerations before recommending SCT or SRT as these approaches are not suitable for everyone.

Key Point

Contraindications for Specific Populations

- *SCT*: People experiencing mania, epilepsy, parasomnias or those at risk of falls
- *SRT*: People with a history of bipolar disorder (or mania), obstructive sleep apnoea, seizure disorders, parasomnias or those at risk of falls.

SRT relies on the patient having the opportunity to sleep during their time in bed. This may not be possible for parents or carers with dependants who require attention during the night. SRT should not be offered if the patient will not have adequate opportunity to sleep during their allocated time in bed.

Potential to Increase Risk Undertaking Regular Activities

Given that SRT may initially cause increased tiredness or daytime sleepiness, the LICBT practitioner should ascertain whether this may increase levels of risk when undertaking regular activities, including caring or parenting responsibilities, driving or operating machinery. Where this is identified, the LICBT practitioner should advise the patient to stop making the behavioural changes and liaise with the GP, wider primary care team or employer to recognise potential actions that could be taken.

Summary

This chapter has considered the evidence supporting CBT-I, demonstrating that it is an effective way of improving sleep across a range of different populations and delivery modalities. LICBT sleep management (*Steps to a Good Night's Sleep*), which is closely informed by CBT-I, has been introduced with guidance around how an LICBT practitioner may use the intervention to support a patient experiencing sleep difficulties. The two key mechanisms behind sleep, the homeostatic sleep drive and circadian rhythms, are targeted by a six-stage intervention. After discussing these mechanisms with patients and gathering information using a sleep diary, behaviour modifications in line with either stimulus control therapy or sleep restriction therapy can be made. Modifying behaviours that maintain sleep difficulties acts to realign the homeostatic sleep drive and circadian rhythm resulting in improved sleep.

Assessing Your Understanding

Declarative

Multiple Choice Questions

1. Which of the following statements are incorrect? [Select all that apply]
   (a) It is normal to wake up a number of times throughout the night
   (b) Everyone needs to get eight hours of sleep a night
   (c) There are changes we can make that can help improve poor sleep
   (d) The amount of sleep we need changes with age
   (e) Not falling asleep instantly when going to bed is normal
2. Which of the following statements are *not* consistent with the theoretical rationale for LICBT sleep management? [Select all that apply]
   (a) Need for sleep accumulates over time
   (b) Napping makes it harder to sleep at night
   (c) Our levels of sleepiness are affected by light
   (d) It is unhelpful to associate bed with sleep
   (e) We have an internal rhythm that impacts when we feel sleepy

Procedural

Practise explaining the theoretical rationale behind LICBT sleep management to a friend or colleague.

Answers to **Assessing Your Understanding** questions can be found in the appendix on p. 337.

Reflection Point

Consider your attitude if someone suggested you needed to make the behavioural changes associated with SCT.

Further Reading and Resources

Bootzin, R.R. and Perlis, M.L. (2011) Stimulus control therapy. In M. Perlis, M. Aloia and B. Kuhn (eds), *Behavioral Treatments for Sleep Treatments: Practical Resources for the Mental Health Professional*. London: Academic Press. (pp. 21–30)

Espie, C.A. (2009) 'Stepped care': a health technology solution for delivering cognitive behavioural therapy as a first line insomnia treatment. *Sleep*, 32, 1549–58.

Morgenthaler, T., Kramer, M., Alessi, C., Friedman, L., Boehlecke, B., Brown, T., et al. (2006) Practice parameters for the psychological and behavioural treatment of insomnia: an update. An American Academy of Sleep Medicine report. *Sleep*, 29, 1415–19.

van Straten, A. and Cuijpers, P. (2009) Self-help therapy for insomnia: a meta-analysis. *Sleep Medicine Reviews*, 13, 61–71.

To access the online resources accompanying this chapter, please visit: https://study.sagepub.com/farrand

Part III
Adapting Low-Intensity CBT

18

Adapting Low-Intensity CBT to Accommodate Black, Asian and Minority Ethnic Patients

Supporting BAME!

Earlise C. Ward

Learning Objectives

By the end of this chapter you should be able to:

- Appreciate the ethnic and cultural context of patients during assessment, treatment planning and service delivery
- Achieve a level of knowledge of Black, Asian and Minority Ethnic populations necessary for a low-intensity CBT practitioner to provide culturally responsive mental health services
- Critically evaluate the application of a cultural adaptations framework to enhance the acceptability of psychological interventions for Black, Asian and Minority Ethnic populations
- Demonstrate a critical awareness of how a cultural adaptations framework has been applied to inform adaptations to a low-intensity CBT intervention for Black Americans

Background

Across England and Wales, the number of people with a White ethnic background made up 94 per cent of the population in 1991. Twenty years later this had reduced to 86 per cent with the number of people with Black, Asian and Minority Ethnic (BAME) backgrounds increasing from 6 per cent to 14 per cent (Figure 18.1).

With the exception of people with a White Irish background, there was an increase in the number of all other ethnic groups (Figure 18.2).

London represents the most ethnically diverse area in Britain, with an above average number of people from the African (7.0%), Indian (6.6%) and Caribbean (4.2%) BAME populations (Office for National Statistics, 2019).

Common Mental Health Problems Experienced by People from BAME Backgrounds

Little is known about the impact of mental health on people from BAME communities (Mental Health Foundation, 2016). However, compared to the White British

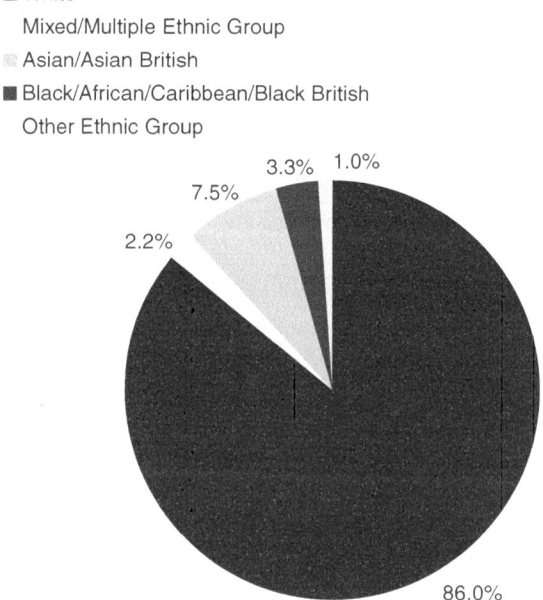

Figure 18.1   Percentages of ethnic groups in England and Wales, 2011 (Office for National Statistics, 2019)

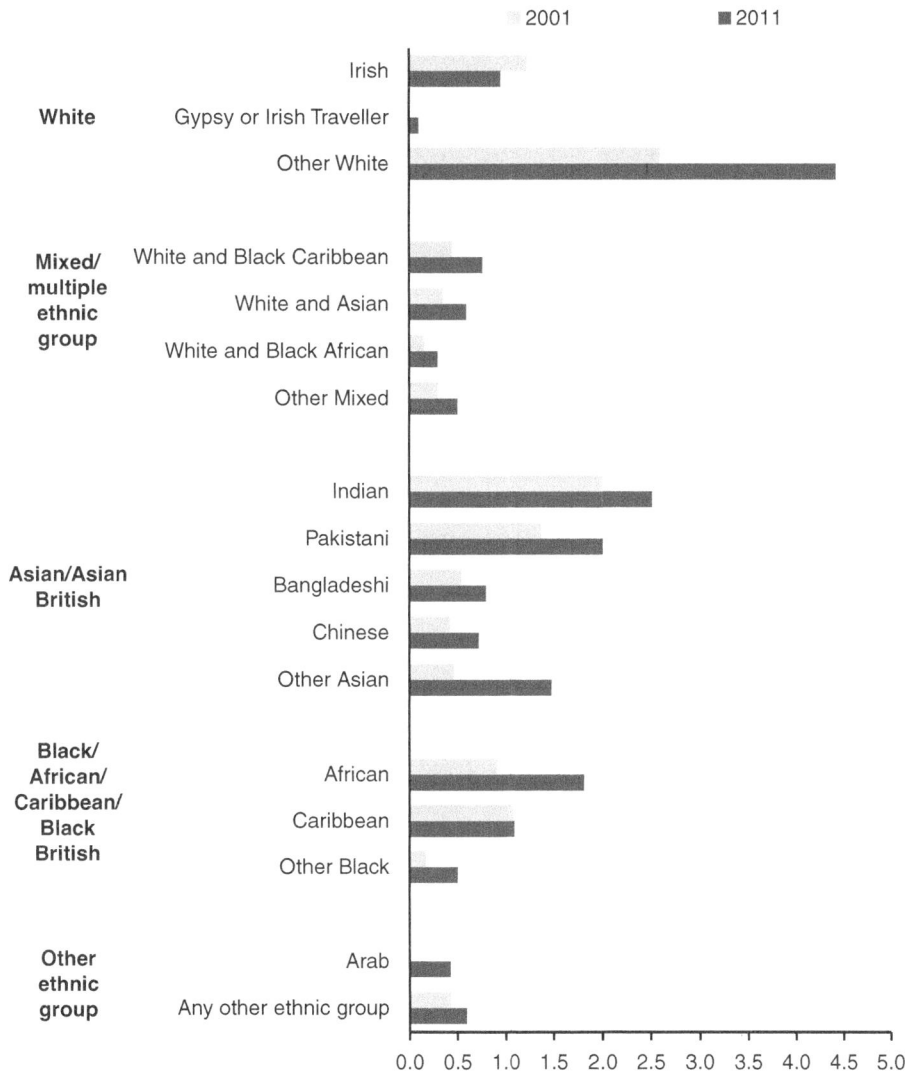

Figure 18.2 Percentage increases in specific ethnic groups in England and Wales, 2011 (Adapted from Office for National Statistics, 2019)

population, these communities have a higher prevalence of common mental health disorders reaching a rate of nearly one in four of the Black and Black British population reporting a problem in the last week (Figure 18.3).

Despite having the highest prevalence, however, Black and Black British adults also experience one of the lowest rates of referral for evidence-based psychological

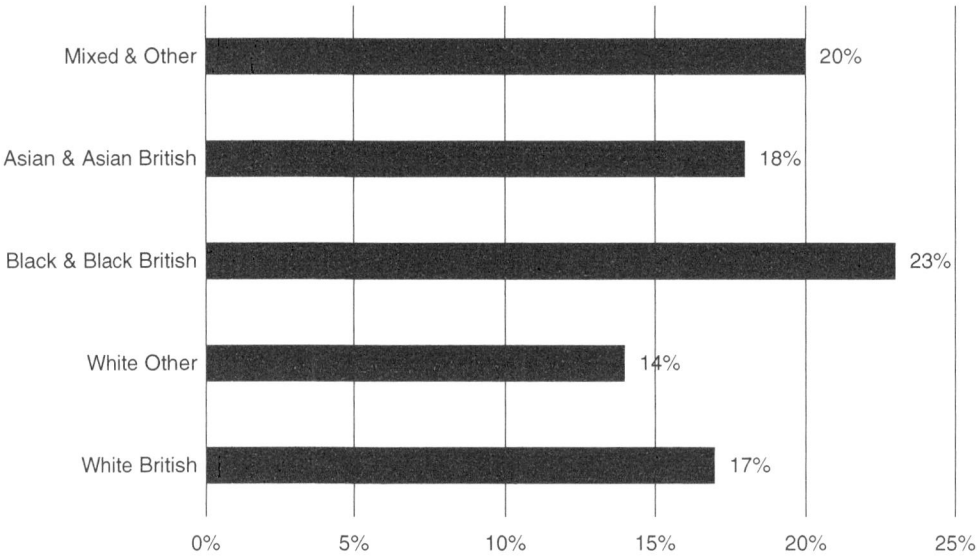

Figure 18.3 Reporting a common mental health problem in the last week by ethnicity, England 2014, age-standardised (McManus et al., 2016).

therapies and are under-represented within Improving Access to Psychological Therapies (IAPT) services (Table 18.1).

Adapting Psychological Therapy to Accommodate BAME Patients

Culturally adapted treatments/interventions (CAT/I) refer to any modification to evidence-based psychological treatments that involve changes in the approach to service delivery to accommodate the target population (Whaley and Davis, 2007).

Table 18.1 Referrals to the IAPT programme by ethnicity in 2016/17 (Baker, 2018)

Ethnic group	Referrals	Entering treatment (%)	Finishing treatment (%)
Asian or Asian British	60,578	78	40
Black or Black British	36,016	75	40
Mixed (Multiple)	29,150	73	39
White	1,016,523	76	46
Other	18,776	75	40

Key Point

Common Changes to Culturally Adapt Treatments and Interventions

- Nature of the therapeutic relationship
- Treatment components to accommodate specific characteristics of the BAME population related to:
  - Appearance and language
  - Cultural beliefs
  - Attitudes
  - Behaviours.

When adapting psychological therapy, it is important to understand the specific needs faced by each population separately and not assume that the same adaptation will equally accommodate all groups. Such an approach to adapt psychological therapies and inform a culturally sensitive mental health service was adopted within the Newham (London) IAPT demonstration site (Department of Health, 2009).

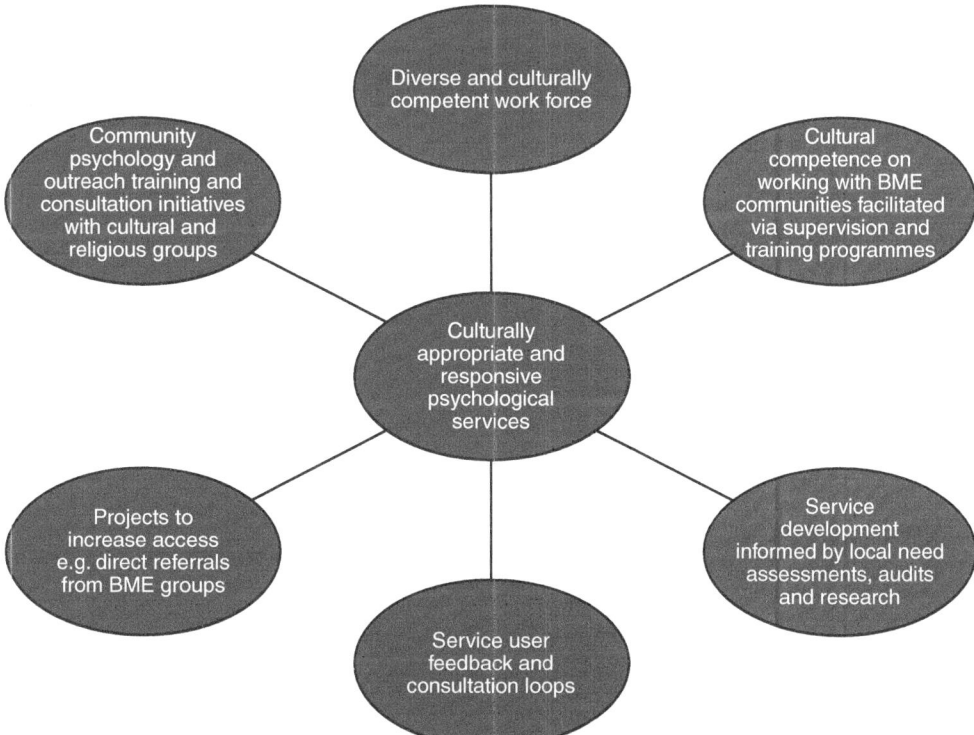

Figure 18.4 Developing a culturally sensitive IAPT service (Department of Health, 2009)

Best Practices

A number of recommendations have been reached to improve access and engagement with mental health services for people from BAME backgrounds (Department of Health, 2009).

Developing Local Care Pathways

Commissioners, managers, primary and secondary care clinicians should develop local care pathways in consultation with service users and community leaders. Collaboration is critical in enabling access to services for a range of under-represented groups. Working in partnership with service users is paramount in order to understand and overcome barriers that might hinder the effective shaping of local care pathways. Additionally, collaborating with voluntary community groups and faith sectors will improve access for BAME patients who may find it more difficult to access services via primary care, as will self-referral into services within the IAPT programme. In the IAPT Newham demonstration site (Department of Health, 2009), 49 per cent of self-referrals came from people from BAME communities, including 25 per cent with an Asian background and 17 per cent a Black background (Clark et al., 2009). The availability of self-referral for people with BAME backgrounds should therefore be actively promoted.

Workforce, Education and Training

Standardising educational curricula, content and training delivery represents a feature of the IAPT programme alongside a commitment for training providers to attract trainees who are representative of all parts of the community (Chapter 1).

Reflection Point

Reflect upon ways you could apply a cultural adaptations framework to improve access and enhance treatment acceptability for patients from a specific BAME community in the area covered by your service.

Key Point

Commissioners and Services

Commissioners and services should consider:

- Commissioning services that have bilingual practitioners who speak the language of local minority groups – practitioners fluent in British Sign Language (BSL) for deaf people, and independent translation services
- Ongoing professional development and training to build capability and cultural competence
- Ensuring people are given a choice in how evidence-based therapy is delivered
- Ensuring an appropriate skill mix and workforce representative of the local population to ensure people have a choice of clinician with respect to characteristics such as gender, physical differences and cultural background.

Adapting Treatments and Delivery for Specific BAME Populations

Ensuring LICBT interventions themselves are adapted to meet the specific needs and preferences of specific BAME populations can improve acceptability and enhance access.

Clinical Practice

Adaptations to Enhance Acceptability

- Provide the patient with the choice of gender and cultural background of the practitioner.
- Consider venues such as job and community centres.
- Adapt promotional materials to improve acceptability and engage with the community to promote the service to improve accessibility.
- Provide prompt and clear routes into the service, avoiding over-complicated referral processes or opt-in systems.
- Adapt session length to accommodate the use of interpreters.
- Include written communication and visual resources for people who do not speak English as their first language.
- Work in partnership with third-sector organisations and faith groups – they often have knowledge about the range of BAME communities within a local area and are often the first point of contact for individuals from BAME communities.

Culturally Adapting an Intervention for Black American Adults: Oh Happy Day Class

The *Oh Happy Day Class* (OHDC) is culturally adapted from the Coping with Depression (CwD) intervention (Ward and Brown, 2015). CwD has been validated within the White population based on research conducted across several countries (Cuijpers et al., 2009a; Lewinsohn et al., 1989). However, adaptations have not currently been made to accommodate a Black American community, which is important given significant disparities in mental healthcare recognised in Black Americans (U.S. Department of Health and Human Services, 2001; Williams et al., 2007).

Key Point

Disparities Affecting Black Americans

- Less access to, and availability of, mental healthcare, resulting in poorer quality mental health services being received (Anderson et al., 2001).
- Greater impact of major depressive disorder (MDD) – in comparison to White Americans, Black American adults (56.5%) report greater severity and disability associated with MDD (38.6%). Despite greater impact however, Black Americans have lower mental health service use.

In an effort to address unmet need regarding the treatment of depression in Black Americans, CwD was selected for adaptation because it is the most studied depression intervention. Adapting psychological therapies for a Black American population is of benefit, as when undertaken to enhance acceptability, positive outcomes are experienced (Griner and Smith, 2006).

Cultural Frameworks Guiding Adaptation of CwD to Create OHDC

Several frameworks exist to inform cultural adaptations of psychological interventions for people from BAME communities (Bernal and Domenech Rodríguez, 2017). These frameworks served to inform adaptation of the CwD programme (Cuijpers et al., 2009a; Lewinsohn et al., 1989) for the Black American community to create the OHDC intervention (Ward et al., 2009; Ward and Brown, 2015).

Framework to Adapt CwD for Black Americans

Afrocentric Paradigm

Nguzo Saba are seven humanistic principles originating in Africa to help facilitate a sense of direction, personal growth and meaning in one's life (Karenga, 1980, 1998).

Key Point

Nguzo Saba Principles

- Unity
- Self-determination
- Collective work
- Responsibility
- Cooperative economics
- Purpose
- Creativity
- Faith.

These principles were specifically created for Black families and have been effectively used with Black Americans in mental health and educational interventions (Bernal et al., 2009; Nicolas et al., 2009).

Ecological Validity and Culturally Sensitive Framework

Culturally sensitive elements can be used to inform the development and delivery of treatment interventions (Bernal et al., 1995; Bernal et al., 2009).

Key Point

Elements

- Language
- Metaphors
- Content
- Concepts
- Goals
- Methods
- Context.

This framework has been used to adapt depression interventions effectively for use with Puerto Rican Americans and Haitian-American youth in the US (Nicolas et al., 2009). Furthermore, it was especially helpful when developing LICBT interventions to target specific populations, such as armed forces veterans (Farrand et al., 2019a).

Cultural Adaptation Process

Several methods were used to culturally adapt the CwD (Cuijpers et al., 2009a; Lewinsohn et al., 1989) intervention to create OHDC for Black American adults. Similar approaches may be helpful when applied to adapt LICBT interventions to meet the needs of other populations.

Key Point

Method Adopted to Culturally Adapt OHDC (Ward et al., 2015)

- Examine attitudes and awareness of Black Americans regarding:
  - Experiences of mental health treatment and interventions (Ward et al., 2009)
  - Effective depression treatments (Beauchamp, et al., 2005)
  - Beliefs about mental illness, perceived stigma and preferred coping behaviours (Ward et al., 2009)
- Integrate study results into the OHDC LICBT intervention
- Review the Ecological Validity and Culturally Sensitive Framework and Nguzo Saba for integration into the OHDC LICBT intervention
- Conduct a series of pilot studies testing preliminary effectiveness, acceptability and feasibility of the OHDC LICBT intervention
- Use data from pilot studies to finalise the OHDC LICBT intervention to potentially examine effectiveness in a Phase III randomised controlled trial (Medical Research Council, 2019).

The cultural adaptation process included strategies identified by Black Americans as necessary for culturally sensitive care and thereby gave them a voice regarding their mental health needs. With respect to the OHDC LICBT intervention, the Black American voice highlighted the following adaptations as improving intervention acceptability (Ward et al., 2009).

Key Point

Recommended Cultural Adaptations

- Broaden reach of the OHDC intervention beyond older female members of the community – to address gross disparities in mental health treatment and outcomes experienced by middle-aged and younger Black American women and men.
- Change the name of the intervention from Oh Happy Day Depression Intervention to Oh Happy Day Class – it was felt that 'class' was less stigmatising than 'treatment sessions'.

Application of Cultural Frameworks

The Nguzo Saba principles and Ecological Validity and Culturally Sensitive Framework helped to inform adaptations to delivery of the OHDC to enhance engagement.

Key Point

Enhancing Engagement with the OHDC LICBT Intervention

- Provide the intervention within a group format with a strong psychoeducation focus
  - The first hour of class is the support group in which participants have the opportunity to share psychosocial issues with which they are struggling
  - The second hour of class consists of the psychoeducation component, which emphasises knowledge about depression, treatment options, healthy coping behaviours, and shifting perceptions of health and disability status.
- Facilitate intervention delivery through two mental health professionals drawn from the Black American community alongside a practitioner
  - Use of competent practitioners working closely with mental health professionals has been linked to positive health outcomes and cost effectiveness (Nicolas et al., 2009).
- Hold classes after work (5:30–7:30 pm).
- Provide food and music to help foster opportunities for social interaction, emotional comfort and group cohesiveness
  - Given the cultural salience of food and music in Black American culture, 30 minutes before intervention delivery, dinner is provided accompanied by jazz music and an instrumental version of 'Oh Happy Day' by the Edwin Hawkins Singers.

Summary

In the past 20 years there has been a large increase in people with Black, Asian and Minority Ethnic (BAME) backgrounds in the UK. Research highlights that whilst members of the BAME population experience higher rates of common mental health difficulties they have lower rates of service use. Given the growth of BAME and increased prevalence of common mental health difficulties it is important to ensure that members of communities representing diversity with respect to spiritual values, cultural norms and personal, family or social circumstances have equal access and benefit to mental health services.

As demonstrated by the development and adaptation of the OHDC (Ward and Brown, 2015), cultural adaptations frameworks have the potential to enhance acceptability of psychological interventions for BAME populations. This may serve to enhance the acceptability of LICBT interventions and improve access to mental health services. Practitioners supporting LICBT interventions with people from BAME communities should pursue professional development opportunities to increase their awareness, knowledge and ability to provide culturally responsive services.

Assessing Your Understanding

Declarative

Multiple Choice Questions

1. Which of the following elements are included in the Ecological Validity and Culturally Sensitive Framework? [Select all that apply]
   (a) Language
   (b) Persons
   (c) Metaphors
   (d) Mission
   (e) Content
2. Members of BAME communities are more likely to seek out which of the following as the first point of contact? [Select all that apply]
   (a) Third-sector organisations
   (b) Faith groups
   (c) Community leaders
   (d) Community nurses
   (e) General practitioners

Procedural

Self-Practice/Self-Reflection

- Contact third sector organisations or faith groups in your area that may be able to help improve access and reflect on factors that may explain any disparities between different BAME populations compared to the White population.

    Answers to **Assessing Your Understanding** questions can be found in the appendix on p. 338.

Further Reading and Resources

Beck, A., Naz, S., Brooks, M. and Jankowska, M. (2019) *Improving Access to Psychological Therapies: Black, Asian and Minority Ethnic Service User Positive Practice Guide.* British Association of Behavioural and Cognitive Psychotherapies. Available at www.babcp.com/files/About/BAME/IAPT-BAME-PPG-2019.pdf (last accessed 2 April 2020).

Bernal, G., Jiménez-Chafey, M. and Domenech Rodríguez, M. (2009) Cultural adaptation of treatments: a resource for considering culture in evidence-based practice. *Professional Psychology: Research and Practice, 40,* 361–8.

Department of Health (2009) *Black and Minority Ethnic (BME): Positive Practice Guide.* London: Department of Health.

Ward, E.C. and Brown, R. (2015) A Culturally Adapted Depression Intervention for African American Adults Experiencing Depression: Oh Happy Day. *American Journal of Orthopsychiatry,* 85, 11–22.

To access the online resources accompanying this chapter, please visit: https://study.sagepub.com/farrand

19

Adapting Low-Intensity CBT for Older People

Don't Let Misconceptions Get in the Way of Evidence-Based Treatment

Alessa Werson, Paul Farrand and Ken Laidlaw

Learning Objectives

By the end of this chapter you should be able to:

- Critically appreciate the evidence base for CBT when working with older adults
- Critically appreciate ageing and challenge common misconceptions associated with late life
- Demonstrate an awareness of the fundamentals associated with working with older adults in clinical settings
- Apply a range of adaptations to low-intensity CBT techniques to enhance assessment and support when working with older adults

---

Background

Cognitive behavioural therapy (CBT) for older adults is an effective mainstream treatment option for common mental health problems, such as depression and anxiety disorders. CBT is particularly appropriate as an intervention with older adults as a pragmatic, jargon-free approach that empowers people to manage their difficulties more effectively through the transmission of coping skills, while adopting a here and now problem-solving orientation (Chapter 1). However, much more has been written about the outcome of CBT with older adults than about the therapy process (Laidlaw, 2015; Laidlaw and Kishita, 2015). Therefore, a dearth of texts that talk about the *how to* of high- and low-intensity CBT (LICBT) with older adults remains.

Reflection Point

Reflect upon your personal attitude towards working with older adults and consider ways it may influence your practice.

Misconceptions of Ageing

Practitioners may be reluctant to adopt a CBT approach to work with older adults as a result of stigma or uncertainty over life experiences associated with later life and the potential to influence treatment (Laidlaw and McAlpine, 2008). Such misconceptions about CBT may have impact upon psychological treatment from access to treatment outcomes; however, many of these are unsupported.

Key Point

Common Misconceptions

- Older people are too set in their ways to change (Gowling et al., 2016)
- Older adults would not be amenable to modifying their thinking (cognitive restructuring) sufficiently for treatment to be effective (Gould et al., 2012; Wilson et al., 2008)
- Depression and anxiety in later life arises as a natural consequence of challenges and losses associated with ageing (Burroughs et al., 2006; Carstensen et al., 2011)
- Older adults are more reluctant to access psychological treatment compared to working age adults (Frost et al., 2019).

Gerontology Informing Clinical Practice

Given greater potential for complexity, co-morbidity and different values held by different age cohorts, it is unsurprising that practitioners who are untrained and lacking experience in geriatrics and gerontology may be less confident working with older adults. Research findings derived from gerontology (the science of ageing) may augment efficacious outcomes for CBT with older adults, and understanding normal aspects of ageing may serve to counterbalance negative age-stereotypical beliefs about working with older adults (Bryant and Koder, 2015). Data from large-scale longitudinal studies from gerontology testify that emotional change occurs across our entire lifespan, emotional regulation improving with better emotional stability (Carstensen et al., 2011). Evidence from gerontological research therefore debunks myths and negative stereotypes of older adults and may encourage practitioners to expect a good outcome from treatment (Karel et al., 2012).

Impact on Clinical Practice

As a consequence of these misconceptions, depression in older adults is often under-recognised, under-diagnosed and under-treated, with poorly treated depression associated with higher mortality rates and higher healthcare utilisation costs (Pocklington, 2017). Controversially, however, rather than depression in older adults being a natural outcome of challenges associated with ageing, it is less common when compared to the working age population (Fiske et al., 2009). Prevalence of depression appears to reach a peak in mid-life and declines subsequently (ONS, 2019), with older adults also reporting an increased sense of wellbeing and emotional stability (Carstensen et al., 2011).

Key Point

'Happiness is approximately U-shaped throughout the life-course; mental distress tends to reach a maximum in middle age' (Blanchflower and Oswald, 2008; p. 1746).

Evidence Base

Since the late 1970s and early 1980s there have been a number of published clinical trials of CBT for late-life depression. However, as a consequence of several methodological shortcomings, caution should be exercised before implementing the conclusions in clinical practice. Recent research employing more robust design has, however, identified CBT, behavioural activation and problem-solving as effective for the treatment of common mental health difficulties in older people (Cuijpers et al., 2013). CBT is one of the most systematically evaluated forms of psychological therapy with older adults (Laidlaw, 2015), with data indicating effectiveness for the treatment of depression in older adults regardless of age (Cuijpers et al., 2009, 2013; Frost et al., 2019; Laidlaw, 2015; Laidlaw and Kishita, 2015) and more generally for psychological therapy in later life (Huang et al., 2015). Indeed, in Improving Access to Psychological Therapy (IAPT) services, greater recovery rates are reported for older adults (Chaplin et al., 2015; Department of Health, 2009). Whilst CBT is efficacious with older adults, however, there remains an empirical question as to whether outcomes could be further enhanced with the development of an age-appropriate format for CBT. Older adults are at a different developmental stage from other adults and life challenges are often developmentally different.

NICE Depression Clinical Practice Guideline (90) and late life depression

In the updated NICE Clinical Practice Guideline (CG90) for depression (2019) there is a review of pharmacological management of depression in older adults and a limited review of structured psychological therapy for older adults despite there being a robust evidence for CBT beyond the papers cited. CG90 notes that depression diagnosis in later life can often be complicated by physical factors and physical comorbidity, as well as health beliefs of older adults. A number of randomised controlled trials (RCTs) examining CBT for older adults are included in the evidence base reviewed in CG90 and included in data making recommendation for treatment. Data from three RCTs generally support a cautious positive outcome for CBT in treating depression in older people. Additionally, data indicated that older adults may be less likely to drop out of treatment with CBT. In one of the RCT studies *not* included in the NICE review (Serfaty et al., 2009), participants were randomly allocated to three groups; CBT plus TAU, a talking control condition plus TAU, and TAU alone. Participants in the talking control group received support from a passive but empathetic practitioner. The participants in this group did less well than those receiving CBT. As such, these results discredit the myth that depressed older people are lonely and simply need a listening ear. The RCT study by Laidlaw et al. (2008) demonstrated that older people can benefit from CBT alone (i.e. older people receiving CBT but not also concurrently receiving antidepressants).

Group CBT

Group CBT has been evaluated in the prevention of depression recurrence (Wilkinson et al., 2009), but at present there is insufficient evidence from which to draw any clear conclusions regarding efficacy with older adults (NICE, 2019). Therefore, a need for large, high-quality randomised trials of CBT to assess the effectiveness and cost-effectiveness of CBT in people aged 75 and over, including in combination with antidepressant medication, remains.

Benefits of Psychological Therapies for Older Adults

Older adults often view psychological therapy as being as effective and acceptable as medication but with fewer unwanted side effects. Consequently, if given a choice, many would prefer to receive psychological therapy rather than psychotropic medications (Gum et al., 2006).

Key Point

Benefits of CBT for Older People

- Simple, but not simplistic, explanations of how to identify and challenge cognitions and strategies for behavioural change inform techniques that can be positively adopted.
- There is the potential to pass techniques and learning on to younger generations in older people's extended families.
- Living a life with ups and downs helps individuals appreciate their own and others' frailties and their own personal resources.
- CBT empowers older adults to believe that change is possible, at any age, and while not always easy, change can occur through cognitive and behavioural methods of problem solving.
- Where appropriate, LICBT may be especially appropriate given the greater focus on supported self-management (Chapter 1).

Adapting Practice

An interesting discussion arises from the evaluation of potential adaptations of CBT with older adults. Whilst there may be greater variability in life experience and presenting difficulties may be complex, adaptations or modifications may not necessarily be required to bring about beneficial change (Chand and Grossberg, 2013). That older adults seek support for similar reasons as younger adults, the intervention focus may remain the same overall.

Appreciating the Older Person's Perspective

To inform potential adaptations it can be helpful to appreciate whether a patient possesses a negative age stereotype where they expect old age to be characterised by frailty and degeneration. Negative attitudes on ageing affect perception of experiences in late life through mood-congruent bias, attributing depression to ageing rather than mood (Laidlaw, 2010). In some cases, therefore, it can be helpful for the

LICBT practitioner to gain an appreciation of the older person's perspective on the ageing process to help inform LICBT treatment planning in order to achieve the primary aim of reducing patient-centred rather than age-related symptoms (Laidlaw and McAlpine, 2008; Laidlaw, 2015).

The Five Cs

While symptom profiles for depression and anxiety disorders in older adults may not be different, presentation of concerns and problems may be qualitatively different from that of younger patients and can be captured as the Five Cs (Sadavoy, 2009).

Key Point

The Five Cs

- *Complexity* – the relationship and interaction of multiple factors including life events, stress, psychological development, and personality. When working with an older adult complexity could be presented in the form of multi-morbidity.
- *Chronicity* – having lived longer lives, diseases or illnesses may have been experienced for a longer time by older people which may affect older people by these being perceived as irreversible, and also impact on their presenting difficulties.
- *Co-morbidity* – older adults present a greater likelihood of experiencing more than one (interacting) physical or mental health condition.
- *Continuity* – lifelong development stemming from an older adult's environmental, psychological and physiological experiences.
- *Context* – wider factors impacting on the development of an illness or disease, including the older adult's physical, psychological, social and environmental circumstances.

The importance and relevance of the Five Cs for LICBT practitioners inexperienced in working with older adults is that LICBT interventions developed for working-age adults may present challenges when used with older adults. Additionally, it should not be forgotten that older people remain as much a heterogeneous group as working-age adults. The Five Cs will therefore require variable modifications in clinical settings (Laidlaw, 2010).

Problem Statements

Whilst it may not be necessary to adapt LICBT as a treatment for older adults, it seems logical to adapt LICBT techniques to suit the patient (Laidlaw, 2010). Emphasising

Table 19.1 Older person's presenting difficulty adapted into a problem statement

Presenting difficulty
Mrs Black is 86 years old and lives on her own. She experiences difficulties with panic disorder and depression, problems with her mobility and has long-term physical health conditions (atrial fibrillation, high blood pressure and osteoporosis).

Problem statement
My main problem is experiencing terrible physical feelings of panic. These are triggered by being on my own at night. I feel shaky and my heart is racing. I have tried medication to help with the panic attacks and my heart but nothing has helped. I think, 'Will I collapse and die?'. As a consequence, I think I am a burden to my family and I don't think the health professionals know what to do with me. I fear I will die alone.

patient-centred, symptom-focused treatment over age-centred treatment may benefit treatment outcome. Shifting focus to the patient's specific difficulties is facilitated by the problem statement (Chapter 3; Beckwith and Crichton, 2010) that captures the main presenting difficulties whilst illustrating the interaction between mental health and any co-morbid physical long-term conditions (Table 19.1).

Capability, Opportunity, Motivation – Behaviour (COM-B)

Implementing the COM-B model (Michie et al., 2011) as a tool in LICBT (Chapter 8) may be especially beneficial when setting treatment goals (Chapter 2), evaluating progress towards treatment goals during support sessions (Chapter 6) or at the end of a support session when the LICBT practitioner checks patient understanding of the homework and addresses any barriers to completion (Chapter 8). An example of the way the COM-B model can be applied to supporting LICBT with an older patient can be seen in Figure 19.1.

Selection, Optimisation with Compensation (SOC)

SOC fits well within a CBT treatment package as it complements the problem-focused orientation of this approach and can be seen as a form of problem solving when older people are faced with age-related challenges (Laidlaw, 2015). As a useful tool for CBT with older adults, SOC aids preserving function in later life where limits such as capacity are reached (Laidlaw et al., 2003). A strategy for actively coping with age-related changes, a patient allocates resources to a particular goal or role, promoting maximum gain and compensating (minimising) losses (Weiland et al., 2011). The stance of the SOC model is that successful development through life, and thus ageing, involves a process of selection, optimisation and compensation for preserving function (Baltes and Baltes, 1990).

Presenting difficulty

At 86 years of age Leonard lost his wife who had suffered from dementia and passed away shortly after a fall. Leonard was devastated and indicated that he thought, 'I am never going to get over this, we were married for 65 years'. Prior to accessing psychological services, Leonard had thoughts about taking his own life on two or three occasions but had never made a plan and no longer has thoughts about taking his own life. He is, however, anxious about living on his own.

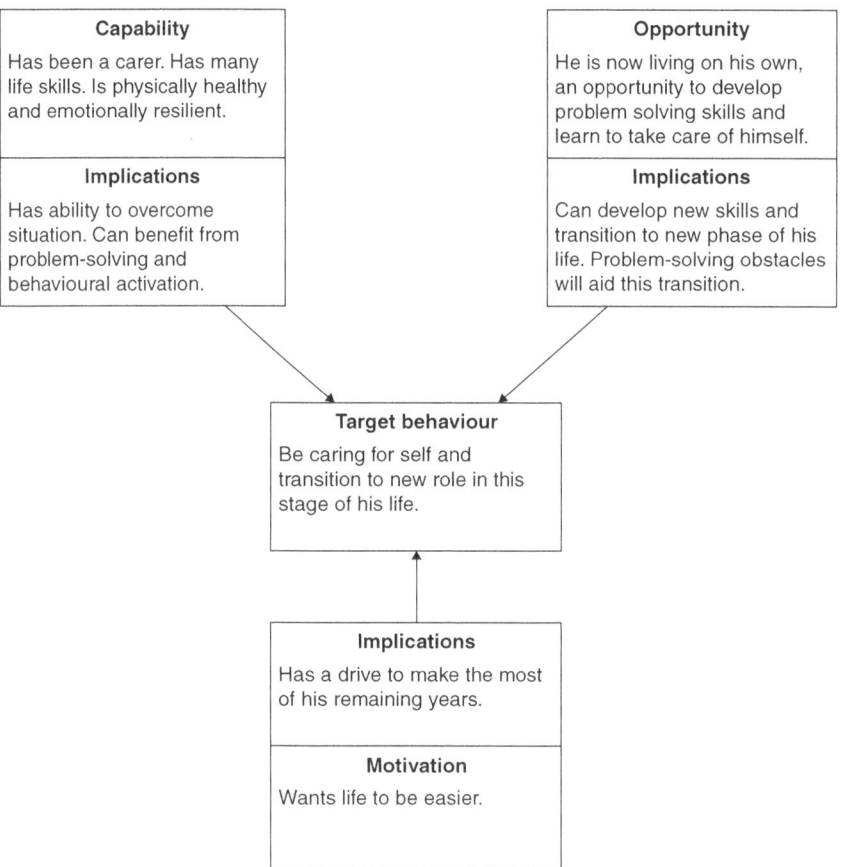

Figure 19.1   Example of the COM-B applied to the case of Leonard

Key Point

Components of the SOC Model

- *Selection*: Emphasis on particular outcomes, which may entail focusing on certain goals over others.
- *Optimisation*: A new strategy is practised prior to being put into place to increase the potential for goal achievement.
- *Compensation*: Involves reviewing the means by which a goal is achieved, assisting in the minimisation of losses.

Incorporating SOC may be particularly beneficial when an older adult faces challenges requiring adjustment and adaptation as it encourages resilience (Laidlaw, 2015). When used in CBT with older adults, these elements may be applied depending on the specific situation and within the capacity of the patient (Weiland et al., 2011).

Lifeskills: A Valuable Resource

Life experiences or lifeskills (Laidlaw, 2015) of older patients can be viewed as a positive and valuable resource to be drawn upon whilst supporting LICBT interventions. Lifeskills of older patients in CBT can be explored by the use of a simple technique called a timeline. A timeline allows patients to learn from, and profit from, their past experiences. Clinicians may use the timeline to help patients reflect on how they have navigated significant life events and encourage the identification of self-resilience. For example, an older patient who has lived longer than the practitioner may have faced adversity and dealt with life experiences (e.g. loss of spouse, changes to physical health and independence, role change) that the practitioner may not have faced (Laidlaw, 2015; Laidlaw and Kishita 2015). Despite often being viewed as a barrier, these experiences can actually inform treatment as older adults have the ability to benefit from their experiences and the sagacity to put that experience to good use in the here and now. In practical terms, life experiences foster resilience and provide emotional and psychological resources that may be especially helpful during support sessions (Chapter 6) for the LICBT practitioner to draw upon when the older patient is experiencing difficulties engaging with the LICBT intervention. Consequently, through recognising and respecting patients' lifeskills a strong rapport can be established. Recognising the clinical benefit of lifeskills may be especially beneficial for the LICBT practitioner within the IAPT programme given that this workforce tends to be younger (Chapter 20).

Supporting Home Practice Plans

LICBT practitioners who are inexperienced working with older adults should consider several factors when reviewing home practice plans during each support session (Chapter 6). This involves the need for the LICBT practitioner to consider completion within a context of what is possible with older adults and therefore an understanding of demographic change and ageing is important knowledge for the practitioner.

Rationale to Support Home Practice Plans

Older adults can profitably employ self-regulatory emotional strategies to optimise levels of functioning and enhanced satisfaction with life (Sims et al., 2015). According to Freund, 'Although we strive to maximize gains, losses are an inevitable part of life. Successfully managing this changing ratio of gains and losses can, therefore, be seen as the essence of successful development' (Freund, 2008: 102). In LICBT, supporting older adults engage with home practice plans may therefore be about optimising and maintaining functioning in the presence of significant losses and challenges. Home practice plans may therefore involve the LICBT practitioner supporting the older patient carry out a series of tasks to assess optimal levels of functioning. Moreover, home practice plans may serve to help older patients set appropriate goals and expectations for themselves in light of the reality of some changes and inform support for LICBT interventions.

Clinical Example

Using A Home Practice Plan to Inform Support for Behavioural Activation

Mr Caan was seeking treatment for low mood after developing memory problems and being treated for cancer. The LICBT practitioner and Mr Caan collaboratively decided that behavioural activation may represent the best intervention to address the low mood and started to schedule activities in the worksheet. During the first support session, however, the LICBT practitioner noted that Mr Caan was better able to complete tasks in the morning, but due to increasing fatigue he often struggled with activities scheduled later in the day. This helped the LICBT practitioner and Mr Caan recognise that activities were better scheduled earlier in the day and in particular *necessary* activities were always scheduled at the beginning of each day when they needed to be completed.

Summary

Access and outcomes following CBT for the treatment of common mental health difficulties in older adults are no worse, and possibly better, than those for working-age adults. However, several common misconceptions may serve as barriers for older people to seek or access treatment. This chapter has identified and challenged these misconceptions regarding CBT for older adults and highlighted several adaptations to LICBT that offer promise to enhance engagement and facilitate support for LICBT interventions.

Assessing Your Understanding

Declarative

Multiple Choice Questions

1. Which of the following are associated with the Five Cs [Select all that apply]
   (a) Complexity
   (b) Chronicity
   (c) Compassion
   (d) Compensation
   (e) Continuity
2. Which of the following are recognised benefits of CBT for older people [Select all that apply]
   (a) Simplistic explanations
   (b) Appreciation of available personal resources
   (c) Reduced need to recognise problematic cognitions
   (d) Empowers belief that change is possible
   (e) Promotes self-management

Procedural

Self-Practice/Self-Reflection

Role play a support session where an older person engaging with behavioural activation begins to face difficulties engaging with the intervention and attributes this solely to their age.

- Reflect upon any challenges you experienced.
- Consider ways in which a consideration of the patient's lifeskills may inform support.

Answers to Assessing Your Understanding questions can be found in the appendix on p. 338.

Further Reading and Resources

Baltes, P.B. and Baltes, M.M. (1990) Psychological perspectives on successful aging: the model of selective optimization with compensation. *Successful Aging: Perspectives from the Behavioral Sciences*, 1, 1–34.

Bryant, C. and Koder, D. (2015) Why psychologists do not want to work with older adults – and why they should… *International Psychogeriatrics*, 27, 351–4.

Chand, S.P. and Grossberg, G.T. (2013) How to adapt cognitive-behavioral therapy for older adults. *Current Psychiatry*, 12, 10–15.

Laidlaw, K. (2015) *CBT for Older People: An Introduction.* London: Sage.

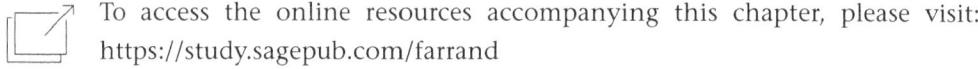 To access the online resources accompanying this chapter, please visit: https://study.sagepub.com/farrand

Part IV
Progress Takes Place Outside the Comfort Zone

20

Low-Intensity CBT

New Horizon or False Dawn?

Paul Farrand and Ursula James

Learning Objectives

By the end of this chapter you should be able to:

- Demonstrate an understanding regarding outcomes achieved by the Improving Access to Psychological Therapies Programme
- Critically appreciate challenges experienced following implementation of the low-intensity CBT practitioner role and consider solutions
- Demonstrate an awareness of areas of current research-informed developments in low-intensity CBT
- Appreciate guidance applied to inform the evaluation of low-intensity CBT interventions

---

Background

Following implementation within the Improving Access to Psychological Therapies (IAPT) programme, low-intensity CBT (LICBT) has truly come of age. Within the IAPT programme it has demonstrated value as an evidence-based psychological therapy for the treatment of many common mental health problems and established itself as the powerhouse driving improved access. Since initial implementation within the pilot Doncaster and Newham demonstration sites in 2006 (Clark et al., 2009), innovation in LICBT has encouraged ongoing developments with success leading to new avenues of research.

The Value of Data

From relatively humble beginnings, the IAPT programme has grown considerably across England. Since the beginning of the programme in 2008, the annual number of referrals has steadily grown to over 1.6 million (Figure 20.1).

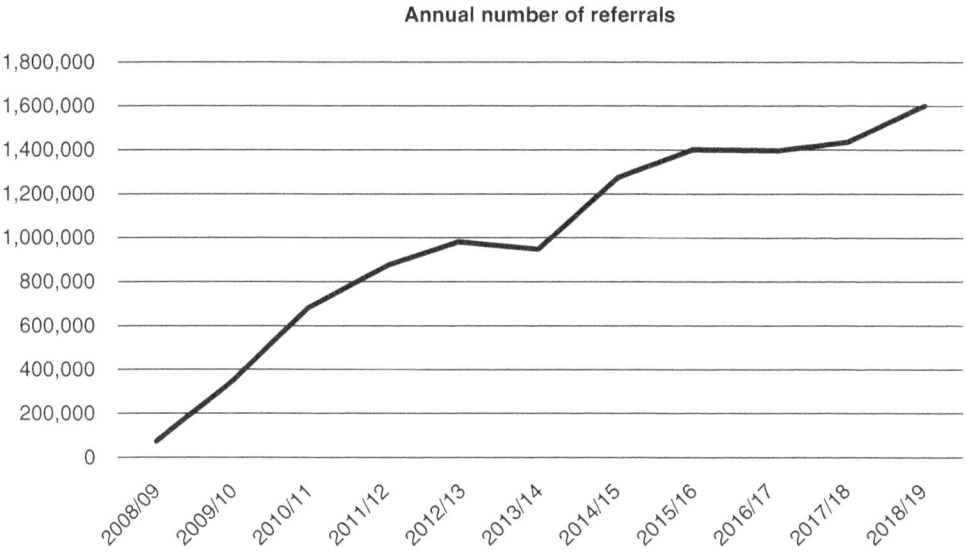

Figure 20.1 Annual number of referrals into the IAPT programme

In an unprecedented example of public transparency, pseudo-anonymised data from IAPT services is submitted every month to an NHS central body accountable to the government to publish monthly, quarterly and annual data. The reports published comprise access, recovery and waiting times for services across the country and provide a rich array of variables and metrics including data on equalities, therapy type and session numbers. The 2018–19 Annual Report (NHS Digital, 2019) highlights the following data regarding the operation of the IAPT programme.

Key Point

Operation of the IAPT Programme in 2018-19

Of those completing a course of treatment:

- 37.5 per cent received low intensity interventions only
- 23.1 per cent received high intensity interventions only
- 39.4 per cent received both low and high intensity interventions.

Average number of sessions:

- LICBT 4.8
- HICBT 7.7
- Both LICBT and HICBT 8.8.

Recovery

Patients are considered to have recovered if scores on both the PHQ9 and GAD7 taken at assessment (Chapter 2) and every support session (Chapter 6) fall below the clinical cut-off. This strict criterion emphasises the importance of treating the person rather than a single disorder. The recovery rate IAPT services have achieved since the start of the programme has been steadily improving and has exceeded the national standard since 2017 (Figure 20.2).

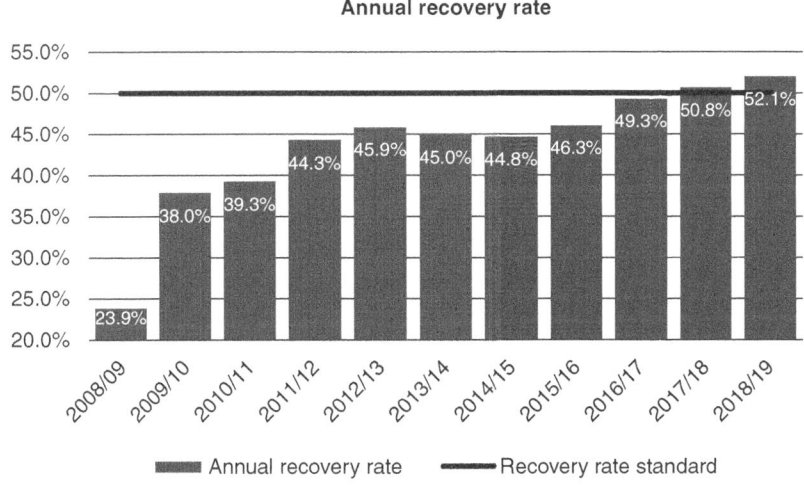

Figure 20.2 Annual recovery rate achieved by the IAPT programme (NHS Digital, 2018)

Whilst published data on clinical recovery now exceed national standards, variability at both the level of services and clinical commissioning groups varies between 33 per cent and 66 per cent (NHS Digital, 2018).

High Performing Services

Characteristics associated with high performing IAPT services that may serve to reduce variation between service performance have been identified (Clark, 2018; Clark et al., 2018; Gyani et al., 2011).

Key Point

High-Performing IAPT Services

- LICBT practitioner (Psychological Wellbeing Practitioner) supported to deliver a full course of treatment, as recommended in NICE guidance.
- Practitioner working within competencies developed during training and ensuring fidelity to the LICBT clinical method.
- Low referral attrition rates achieved by having low waiting times between different steps in the stepped care pathway (Chapter 1) and not just to assessment.
- No reluctance to step a patient up to a Step 3 HI intervention when appropriate.
  - On occasions, reluctance can depend on the LICBT practitioner being aware that the patient will experience a long waiting time before stepping up.
- Appropriate provision of clinical skills alongside outcome-focused case management supervision to monitor clinical decision-making (Chapters 4 and 9).
  - Enables LICBT practitioners to reflect and maintain fidelity with the LICBT intervention
  - Allows supervisors to identify where further training would be useful or encourage following up on areas of interest.
- Support for the LICBT practitioner to engage in continuing professional development.
- Good leadership and supportive supervision (Chapter 9).

Reflection Point

Reflect upon the role that LICBT practitioners have played in delivering clinical outcomes associated with the IAPT programme.

Challenges

Whilst outcomes associated with the IAPT programme highlight many successes, several challenges have been identified.

Practitioner Attrition

The LICBT practitioner role has developed considerably since 2008 and the benefits of this way of working have implications across many mental health areas of delivery. Attrition from the practitioner role, however, has the potential to destabilise services and threaten outcomes currently delivered by the IAPT programme.

Key Point

Challenges Arising from High Attrition

- Difficulties maintaining recovery rates with a workforce largely comprising novice practitioners who have failed to enhance and develop competency in LICBT (Roth and Pilling, 2017a).
- Threatens and fragments the quality of care (Imison et al., 2016).
- Challenges the economic case for the IAPT programme and threatens long-term sustainability.

The LICBT practitioner workforce mainly comprises young white female graduates (CORE, 2017). This cohort of staff are highly motivated, ambitious and thrive in services where they can develop areas of special interest, lead on projects, gain skills working with long-term conditions and get involved in service development initiatives. Equally however, many practitioners with this background often choose to move onto further training, often HICBT or clinical psychology. In 2019, services reported that 24 per cent of their high-intensity staff in post had previously been PWPs within their service (Health Education England, 2020).

Solutions

Potential solutions are being implemented or encouraged to address the challenge of attrition from the LICBT workforce.

Key Point

Solutions to Address Attrition

- Make use of apprenticeship routes or part-time training options to suit the needs of a more diverse range of people with different backgrounds, ages and having different academic and vocational qualifications.
- Recognise, raise the profile and promote awareness of the psychological practitioner role, now being achieved by the Psychological Professions Network (Psychological Professions Network, 2018).
- Increase the number of options for practitioners to progress within the LICBT role – for example, senior LICBT roles offering experienced LICBT practitioners the opportunity to manage a team of LICBT practitioners and develop and implement service strategies and policies. Services managed by LICBT practitioners are emerging.

Prioritising, maintaining and developing the LICBT workforce is crucial. If this fails to happen it is likely that, access, waiting time, recovery (Chapter 1) and ambitious expansion targets will not be realised.

Resiliency

Working within a high-volume mental health environment, LICBT practitioners have higher patient caseloads alongside shorter contact durations (Chapter 1; Richards, 2010a). This places increased demands on the psychological practitioner workforce compared with therapists delivering high-intensity psychological therapies at Step 3 of the stepped care model (Chapter 1). To ensure safe and effective working with a high patient caseload, clinical case management supervision was developed for the LICBT practitioner working within the IAPT programme with clinical skills supervision focused on skills development (Chapter 9; Richards, 2010b). However, whilst both forms of supervision meet four purposes of supervision (Chapter 9; Turpin and Wheeler, 2011), the fifth function, associated with staff support and the prevention of burn-out may not be fully realised. Consequently, there may be failure to support the practitioner to better maintain their own health and wellbeing or to address their own emotional difficulties that are unrelated to work. This function of supervision may therefore need to be enhanced. To target resiliency within the IAPT workforce, a strength-based CBT intervention (Padesky and Mooney, 2012) adapted into a low-intensity format has been developed (Farrand and Stonebank, 2019) with potential to complement the supportive function of supervision.

Research-Informed Developments

Given LICBT's significant impact revolutionising mental health service delivery for the treatment of common mental health difficulties (Chapter 1), it is unsurprising that there are significant research developments. Interestingly, whilst initially forming a seminal feature of the IAPT programme implemented across England, LICBT has now gained interest as a core component of service delivery models in other countries and across different settings.

Criteria to Inform Recommendations for LICBT Interventions

Variation has emerged with the techniques adopted within LICBT interventions alongside therapeutic drift in the way interventions may be employed within support sessions (Chapter 1). To address these challenges and ensure fidelity between the training received by the IAPT LICBT practitioners and interventions adopted, criteria have been developed to evaluate LICBT interventions. These serve as the basis of recommendations for IAPT services to ensure consistency between LICBT interventions, training to support their use and service adoption. Ensuring fidelity between training and delivery represents one of the change strategies informing implementation (Raghaven et al., 2008).

Key Point

Criteria to Evaluate LICBT Interventions

- Scope consistent with LICBT
- Current
- Engagement
- Usability
- Behavioural principles.

Criteria serve to emphasise features of LICBT specified in the IAPT manual, revised *National Curriculum for the Education of Psychological Wellbeing Practitioners* (UCL, 2015) and informed by characteristics of LICBT addressed in Chapter 1. Criteria have further been informed by various guidance documents used to inform written health information for patients and the public with adaptations to evaluate CBT self-help books for common mental health problems.

Key Point

Criteria Informing LICBT Intervention Recommendations

- *DISCERN* (Charnock et al., 1999): Criteria used to evaluate the quality of information of a publication or website about treatment choices
- *EQIP* (Moult et al., 2004): Audit tool to evaluate the quality of written information given to patients within a hospital setting, with criteria adapted to accommodate the specific focus of the evaluation
- NHS *Patient Information Toolkit* (Department of Health, 2003)
- The POPPI Guide: Practicalities of Producing Patient Information (Duman and Farrell, 2000).

Adapting LICBT To Accommodate Diversity

Despite considerably improved access resulting in reduced waiting times, challenges continue to exist regarding access targets for patients representing diversity with respect to spiritual values, cultural norms and personal, family or social circumstances. This challenges the commitment of the National Health Service to equality and fairness espoused in the NHS Constitution (Department of Health, 2015). Now that the IAPT programme has been fully implemented, several research and pilot projects are being undertaken to ensure that the demands of the NHS Constitution are achieved. These have informed Department of Health Positive Practice Guides to enhance service delivery and clinical practice with groups representing diversity including armed forces veterans (Department of Health, 2013), people from Black, Asian and Minority Ethnic populations (Chapter 18; Department of Health, 2009), older people (Chapter 19; Department of Health, 2009), people with learning difficulties (Department of Health, 2013) or long-term conditions (Department of Health, 2008).

Accommodating Armed Forces Veterans

To overcome barriers to access for armed forces veterans and family members (Zinzow et al., 2012), research has explored preferences for Step 2 service delivery and LICBT interventions themselves. Focus groups highlighted several necessary adaptations to enhance acceptability of the LICBT interventions (Farrand et al., 2018). In particular, adaptations to ensure imagery was easily recognisable by the armed forces population, straightforward language avoiding technical jargon was adopted and that case studies and metaphors reflected the armed forces community were highlighted as important to enhance acceptability (Farrand et al., 2019). Following adaptation, an interesting outcome arising from this research was that armed forces veterans expressed a preference for LICBT compared to high-intensity psychological therapies (Farrand et al., 2019). LICBT's emphasis on self-management was considered to be highly consistent with armed forces culture and therefore responded to favourably (Farrand et al., 2018).

Peer Support to Enhance Opportunity and Accommodate Challenges with Capability

The potential for peers to provide support for LICBT interventions has been recognised (Turpin et al., 2010). Such an approach may be particularly suitable to provide opportunities for people who might otherwise struggle to access services or engage in treatment over the phone (e.g. people with long-term conditions). The approach may also support people experiencing capability issues, such as individuals with learning difficulties who might otherwise struggle with the demands of engaging with LICBT between support sessions (Chapter 6). Research is addressing the potential for informal carers of people with mild dementia to support LICBT behavioural activation (Chapter 11; Farrand et al., 2016b). This research has now informed ongoing research on adapting the intervention for implementation in Sweden (Svedin et al., Submitted). Interestingly, across all these developments a specific supporters guide has been developed to enable the informal caregiver to guide the patient through their own LICBT intervention whilst the LICBT practitioner supports the caregiver.

LICBT for Informal Caregivers

Developing a specific guide for the peer to support the LICBT intervention is a similar approach to that developed for clinicians to support the *Mind Over Mood* self-help intervention for depression (Padesky and Greenberger, 1995). However, it is important to recognise that informal caregivers themselves are at increased risk of experiencing common mental health difficulties. Research is therefore addressing the need to adapt LICBT interventions to provide opportunities for informal caregivers who struggle to access services due to lack of time, competing demands and prioritising the person they care for. Examples include LICBT for informal caregivers of stroke survivors (Farrand et al., 2020; Woodford et al., 2014), parents of children treated for cancer (Wikman et al., 2018), informal caregivers of adults with cancer (Woodford, personal communication) and adult daughters providing informal care for older parents (Woodford, personal communication).

Important Caveat

Whilst innovation breeds innovation and should be encouraged, there is an important caveat with respect to the need to maintain an evidence-based practitioner approach (Carr and McNulty, 2016). Whilst consideration is given to patient choice and practitioner expertise within evidence-based practice (EBP), it should not be at the expense of the evidence base (Sackett et al., 2000). Maintaining fidelity to the evidence base within a new organisation of care represents a fundamental feature serving as the foundation of the IAPT programme, setting it aside from mental health developments across the world.

Conclusions

You have used this text to train others or develop a declarative understanding of the theoretical basis or procedural knowledge to develop competency in LICBT for yourself. We hope it has enabled you to see the horizon of opportunity that LICBT has delivered on and promises in the future. If so, helping you *see further by standing on the shoulders of giants* whether as a trainee, practitioner, trainer, supervisor, policy maker or researcher will enable you as pioneers to further develop and broaden the application of LICBT.

Assessing Your Understanding

Declarative

Multiple Choice Questions

1. Which of the following are associated with high-performing IAPT services? [Select all that apply]
   (a) Fidelity to the LICBT model
   (b) Higher number of HICBT therapists
   (c) Reluctance to step up a patient
   (d) Weekly clinical skills supervision
   (e) Support for the LICBT practitioner to engage in CPD
2. Which of the following are useful criteria by which to evaluate LICBT interventions? [Select all that apply]
   (a) Scope consistent with CBT
   (b) Adopts a formal writing style to reflect professional practice
   (c) Adopts behavioural principles
   (d) Efforts are made to ensure specific factors are current
   (e) Largest focus placed on psychoeducation

Essay Questions

- Critically evaluate challenges that arise with the LICBT practitioner workforce and propose potential solutions.
- Critically evaluate the 'value of data' within the IAPT programme and how it is used to inform delivery.

Procedural

Self-Practice/Self-Reflection

- Consider a challenge you are struggling with in your clinical practice and work through *Enhancing Resiliency: Finding Inner Strength to Manage the Demands of Clinical Practice* (Farrand and Stonebank, 2019) to enhance your resiliency.
- Reflect upon your experience of working through the intervention. Did you learn anything that could enhance your practice supporting LICBT interventions with patients? Reflect upon ways the intervention could be implemented within your service to enhance staff wellbeing.

  Answers to **Assessing Your Understanding** questions can be found in the appendix on p. 338.

Further Reading and Resources

Department of Health. *IAPT Positive Practice Guides*. Available at www.england.nhs. uk/ltphimenu/mental-health/iapt-positive-practice-guides-for-targeted-groups (last accessed 3 April 2020).

National Collaborating Centre for Mental Health (NCCMH) (2020) *The Improving Access to Psychological Therapies Manual*. Available at https://www.england.nhs.uk/ wp-content/uploads/2020/05/iapt-manual-v4.pdf (accessed 11 July 2020).

NHS Digital (2019) *Psychological Therapies, Annual Report on the Use of IAPT Services 2018–19*. London: NHS England. Available online at: https://digital.nhs.uk/data-and-information/publications/statistical/psychological-therapies-annual-reports-on-the-use-of-iapt-services/annual-report-2018-19 (accessed 23 January 2020).

To access the online resources accompanying this chapter, please visit: https://study.sagepub.com/farrand

Appendix

Answers to Assessing Your Understanding

Chapter 1

Declarative – correct answers

1. C, E, F, M, P
2. G, H, P, U, Z
3. C, E, M, O, V

Procedural – correctly completed table

1. Introduced herself as a 'therapist'	2. Used 'downward arrow' technique
3. States 'deliver' CBT self-help, not 'support'	4. Should not work with Ms Lashmay as social anxiety not treated with LICBT
5. No options provided about types of support available	6. The dose of 60-minute treatment sessions would generally be more than the dose offered at LICBT
7. States time engaging with treatment less with LICBT than HICBT	8. Recommended CBT self-help intervention was certainly multi-strand

Chapter 2

Declarative – correct answers

1. a
2. a, c, d
3. e

Chapter 3

Declarative – correct answers

1. N, V, C, D, Q
2. S, I, P, G, T
3. E, X, S, Y, M

Procedural – correctly completed table

Probable diagnosis	Social anxiety disorder
Recommended treatment	There is no LICBT treatment recommended at present for this condition – therefore, consider for HICBT
Justifications	
Abdul is feeling quite low and is struggling with sleep and fatigue. A probable diagnosis of depression could be considered but given the fear and anxiety mentioned we should continue down the flow-chart to consider other possible diagnoses too.	
Abdul has said his anxiety is largely related to one particular type of situation, when he has to pitch products at meetings with his chief executive and board.	
Abdul does not fear a particular object. His fears are based around particular activities related to contributing to committees and meetings. During these activities he fears embarrassment and humiliation, and he describes intense fear which might be suggestive of a situation-specific panic attack.	
We should therefore consider asking further questions to identify the specific triggers to his anxiety. Abdul tells us that he has never liked being the centre of attention, that he can sometimes be uneasy interacting with people he does not know and that if it were possible to avoid having to give the pitches in meetings each week he certainly would do so. He is embarrassed both about blushing when feeling anxious, and about feeling anxious in the first place. He is concerned that it is very noticeable.	
To determine the specific anxiety disorder and rule out others I would specifically ask about the nature of triggers, funnelling down to identify the specific trigger leading to the current probable diagnosis.	

Chapter 4

Declarative – correct answers

1. a and c
2. b and e

Procedural – correct answers

Information to bring to supervision:
Changes in ROM scores (insufficient response)
Patient's subjective reports
Number of treatment sessions to date
Engagement with therapy (e.g. completion of homework tasks)
Patient's wishes

Chapter 5

Declarative – correct answers

True: A, C, D, E, F, G, H, J, L
False: B, I, K

Chapter 6

Declarative – correct answers

1. E, F, O, J
2. A, B, N, O
3. H, J, K, M, O
4. A, B, L, O, J

Chapter 7

Declarative – correct answers

1. c, d
2. a, b
3. b

Chapter 8

Declarative – correct answers

1. Automatic motivation
2. Physical opportunity
3. Psychological capability
4. Social opportunity
5. Reflective motivation
6. Physical capability

Chapter 9

Declarative – correct answers

1. D, R, Z
2. A, T
3. F, J, N
4. M, S
5. G, X
6. I, O, P

Chapter 10

Declarative – correct answers

1. a, c, e
2. c, e
3. a, c

Chapter 11

Declarative – correct answers

1. c, d
2. a, d
3. b, e

Chapter 12

Declarative – correct answers

1. c
2. b, d
3. a, b

Chapter 13

Declarative – correct answers

1. a, c, d
2. c, d

Chapter 14

Declarative – correct answers

1. a, c, e
2. b, c, d
3. b, d, e

Chapter 15

Declarative – correct answers

1. d
2. b
3. a, c

Chapter 16

Declarative – correct answers

1. b, d, e
2. a, b, d, e
3. a, b, c, d

Chapter 17

Declarative – correct answers

1. b
2. d

Chapter 18

Declarative – correct answers

1. a, c, e
2. a, b, c

Chapter 19

Declarative – correct answers

1. a, b, e
2. b, d, e

Chapter 20

Declarative – correct answers

1. a, c, e
2. c, d

References

Abramowitz, J.S. (2006) The psychological treatment of obsessive-compulsive disorder. *Canadian Journal of Psychiatry*, 51, 407–16.

Ali, S., Rhodes, L., Moreea, O., McMillan, D., Gilbody, S., Leach, C., et al. (2017) How durable is the effect of low intensity CBT for depression and anxiety? Remission and relapse in a longitudinal cohort study. *Behaviour Research and Therapy*, 94, 1–8.

Allgulander, C. (2006) Generalized anxiety disorder: what are we missing? *European Neuropsychopharmacology*, 16, S101–8.

American Psychiatric Association (APA) (2013) *Diagnostic and Statistical Manual of Mental Disorders* (5th ed.) Arlington, VA: American Psychiatric Association.

Anderson, K. (2018a) *How to Beat Insomnia and Sleep Problems One Step at a Time Using Evidence-Based Low-Intensity CBT*. London: Robinson.

Anderson, K.N. (2018b) Insomnia and cognitive behavioural therapy: how to assess your patient and why it should be a standard part of care. *Journal of Thoracic Disease*, 10, S94–S102.

Anderson, R.J., Freedland, K.E., Clouse, R.E. and Lustman, P.J. (2001) The prevalence of comorbid depression in adults with diabetes. *Diabetes Care*, 24, 1069–78.

Andersson, G. and Cuijpers, P. (2009) Internet-based and other computerized psychological treatments for adult depression: a meta-analysis. *Cognitive Behaviour Therapy*, 38, 196–205.

Andrews, G., Basu, A., Cuijpers, P., Craske, M., McEvoy, P., English, C. and Newby, J. (2018) Computer therapy for the anxiety and depression disorders is effective, acceptable and practical health care: an updated meta-analysis. *Journal of Anxiety Disorders*, 55, 70–8.

Applebaum, R.A. and Austin, C.D. (1990) *Long-Term Care Case Management: Design and Evaluation*. New York: Springer Publishing.

Arnedt, J.T., Cuddihy, L., Swanson, L.M., Pickett, S., Aikens, J. and Chervin, R.D. (2013) Randomized controlled trial of telephone-delivered cognitive behavioural therapy for chronic insomnia. *Sleep*, 36, 353–62.

Aspland, H., Llewelyn, S., Hardy, G.E., Barkham, M. and Stiles, W. (2008) Alliance ruptures and rupture resolution in cognitive–behavior therapy: a preliminary task analysis. *Psychotherapy Research*, 18, 699–710.

Ayuso-Mateos, J.L., Nuevo, R., Verdes, E., Naidoo, N. and Chatterji, S. (2010) From depressive symptoms to depressive disorders: the relevance of thresholds. *British Journal of Psychiatry*, 196, 365–371.

BABCP (2019) Improving Access to Psychological Therapies: Black, Asian and Minority Ethnic Service User Positive Practice Guide. NHS. Available at: https://www.babcp.com/files/IAPT-BAME-PPG-2019.pdf

Baguley, C., Farrand, P., Hope, R., Leibowitz, J., Lovell, K., Lucock, M., et al. (2010) *Good Practice Guidance on the Use of Self-Help Materials within IAPT Services. Technical Report. IAPT*. London: NHS.

Baker, C. (2018) *Mental Health Statistics for England: Prevalence, Services and Funding.* Available at https://researchbriefings.parliament.uk/ResearchBriefing/Summary/SN06988 (last accessed 2 April 2020).

Baldwin, D.S., Anderson, I.M., Nutt, D.J., Allgulander, C., Bandelow, B., Boer, J.A. et al. (2014) Evidence-based pharmacological treatment of anxiety disorders, post-traumatic stress disorder and obsessive-compulsive disorder: a revision of the 2005 guidelines from the British Association for Psychopharmacology. *Journal of Psychopharmacology,* 28, 403–39.

Baltes, P.B. and Baltes, M.M. (1990) Psychological perspectives on successful aging: the model of selective optimization with compensation. *Successful Aging: Perspectives from the Behavioral Sciences*, 1, 1–34.

Bandura, A. (1973) *Aggression: A Social Learning Analysis*. Englewood Cliffs, NJ: Prentice-Hall.

Barlow, D.H. and Durrand, V.M. (1999) *Abnormal Psychology*. Pacific Grove, CA: Brooks/Cole Publishing.

Beadel, J.R., Mathews, A. and Teachman, B.A. (2016) Cognitive bias modification to enhance resilience to a panic challenge. *Cognitive Therapy and Research*, 40, 799–812.

Bearman, S.K., Schneiderman, R.L. and Zolth, E. (2017) Building an evidence base for effective supervision practice: an analogue experiment of supervision to increase EBT fidelity. *Administration and Policy in Mental Health*, 44, 293–307.

Beauchamp, N., Irvine, A.B., Seeley, J. and Johnson, B. (2005) Worksite-based internet multimedia program for family caregivers of persons with dementia. *The Gerontologist*, 45, 793–801.

Beck, A. (2016) *Transcultural Cognitive Behaviour Therapy for Anxiety and Depression.* London: Routledge.

Beck, A.T., Rush, A.J., Shaw, B.F. and Emery, G. (1987) *Cognitive Therapy of Depression.* New York: Guilford Press.

Beck, J.S. (1995) *Cognitive Therapy: Basics and Beyond.* New York: Guilford Press.

Beckwith, A. and Crichton, J. (2010) The negotiation of the problem statement in cognitive behavioural therapy. *Communication & Medicine*, 7, 23–32.

Bee, P.E., Bower, P., Lovell, K., Gilbody, S., Richards, D., Gask, L. and Roach, P. (2008) Psychotherapy mediated by remote communication technologies: a meta-analytic review. *BMC Psychiatry*, 8, 60.

Bee, P.E., Lovell, K., Lidbetter, N., Easton, K. and Gask, L. (2010) You can't get anything perfect: 'user perspectives on the delivery of cognitive behavioural therapy by telephone'. *Social Science and Medicine*, 71, 1308–15.

Behar, E., Alcaine, O., Zuellig, A.R. and Borkovec, T.D. (2003) Screening for generalized anxiety disorder using the Penn State Worry Questionnaire: a receiver operating characteristic analysis. *Journal of Behavior Therapy and Experimental Psychiatry*, 34, 25–43.

Bell, A.C. and D'Zurilla, T.J. (2009) Problem-solving therapy for depression: a meta-analysis. *Clinical Psychology Review*, 29, 348–53.

Bendelin, N., Hesser, H., Dahl, J., Carlbring, P., Zetterqvist, K. and Andersson, G. (2011) Experiences of guided internet-based cognitive-behavioural treatment for depression: a qualitative study. *BMC Psychiatry*, 11, 107.

Bennett-Levy, J. (2003) Reflection: a blind spot in psychology? *Clinical Psychology Science and Practice*, 23, 16–19.

Bennett-Levy, J. (2006) Therapist skills: a cognitive model of their acquisition and refinement. *Behavioural and Cognitive Psychotherapy*, 34, 57–78.

Bennett-Levy, J., Butler, G., Fennell, M., Hackman, A., Mueller, M. and Westbrook, D. (eds) (2004) *Oxford Guide to Behavioural Experiments in Cognitive Therapy*. Oxford: Oxford University Press.

Bennett-Levy, J., McManus, F., Westling, B.E. and Fennell, M. (2009) Acquiring and refining CBT skills and competencies: which training methods are perceived to be most effective? *Behavioural and Cognitive Psychotherapy*, 37, 571–83.

Bennett-Levy, J., Turner, F., Beaty, T., Smith, M., Paterson, B. and Farmer, S. (2001) The value of self-practice of cognitive therapy techniques and self-reflection in the training of cognitive therapists. *Behavioural and Cognitive Psychotherapy*, 29, 203–20.

Bennion, M., Hardy, G., Moore, R. and Millings, A. (2017) E-therapies in England for stress, anxiety or depression: what is being used in the NHS? A survey of mental health services. *British Medical Journal Open*, 7, e014844.

Bernal, G. and Domenech Rodríguez, M.M. (eds) (2012) *Cultural Adaptations: Tools for Evidence-Based Practice with Diverse Populations*. Washington DC: American Psychological Association.

Bernal, G., Bonilla, J. and Bellido, C. (1995) Ecological validity and cultural sensitivity for outcome research: issues for the cultural adaptation and development of psychosocial treatments with Hispanics. *Journal of Abnormal Child Psychology*, 23, 67–82.

Bernal, G., Jiménez-Chafey, M. and Domenech Rodríguez, M. (2009) Cultural adaptation of treatments: a resource for considering culture in evidence-based practice. *Professional Psychology: Research and Practice*, 40, 361–8.

Binnie, J. (2011) Structured reflection on the clinical supervision of supervisees with and without a core mental health professional background. *Issues in Mental Health Nursing*, 32, 584–8.

Blanchflower, D.G. and Oswald, A.J. (2008) Is well-being U-shaped over the life cycle? *Social Science and Medicine*, 66, 1733–49.

BNF (2020) *British National Formulary (79)*. London: Pharmaceutical Press.

Bootzin, R.R. and Perlis, M.L. (2011) Stimulus control therapy. In M. Perlis, M. Aloia and B. Kuhn (eds), *Behavioral Treatments for Sleep Treatments: Practical Resources for the Mental Health Professional*. London: Academic Press. (pp. 21–30).

Borbély, A.A. (1982) A two process model of sleep regulation. *Human Neurobiology*, 1, 205–10.

Borkovec, T.D. (2002) Life in the future versus life in the present. *Clinical Psychology: Science and Practice*, 9, 76–80.

Borkovec, T.D. and Inz, J. (1990) The nature of worry in generalized anxiety disorder: a predominance of thought activity. *Behaviour Research and Therapy*, 28, 153–8.

Borkovec, T.D. and Newman, M.G. (1998) Worry and generalized anxiety disorder. *Comprehensive Clinical Psychology*, 6, 439–59.

Borkovec, T.D. and Roemer, L. (1995) Perceived functions of worry among generalized anxiety disorder subjects: distraction from more emotional topics? *Journal of Behavior Therapy and Experimental Psychiatry*, 26, 25–30.

Borkovec, T.D. and Sharpless, B. (2004) Generalized anxiety disorder: bringing cognitive behavioral therapy into the valued present. In S. Hayes, V. Follette and M. Linehan (eds), *New Directions in Behavior Therapy*. New York: Guilford Press. (pp. 209–42).

Borkovec, T.D., Wilkinson, L., Folensbee, R. and Lerman, C. (1983) Stimulus control applications to the treatment of worry. *Behaviour Research and Therapy*, 21, 247–51.

Bourne, E.J. (1998) *Overcoming Specific Phobia: A Hierarchy and Exposure-Based Protocol for the Treatment of all Specific Phobias*. Oakland, CA: New Harbinger.

Bourne, E.J. (2015) *The Anxiety and Phobia Workbook*. Oakland, CA: New Harbinger.

Bower, P. and Gilbody, S. (2005) Stepped care in psychological therapies: access, effectiveness and efficiency: narrative literature review. *British Journal of Psychiatry*, 186, 11–17.

Bower, P., Gilbody, S., Richards, D., Fletcher, J. and Sutton, A. (2006) Collaborative care for depression in primary care. Making sense of a complex intervention: systematic review and meta-regression. *British Journal of Psychiatry*, 189, 484–93.

Bowman, D., Scogin, F. and Lyrene, B. (1995) The efficacy of self-examination therapy and cognitive bibliotherapy in the treatment of mild to moderate depression. *Psychotherapy Research*, 5, 131–40.

Boyden, E. and Dobel-Ober, D. (2016) An exploratory evaluation of phone interventions in a primary care service (IAPT). *Journal of Psychological Therapies in Primary Care*, 4, 120–38.

Bryant, C. and Koder, D. (2015) Why psychologists do not want to work with older adults – and why they should… *International Psychogeriatrics*, 27, 351–4.

Buckman, J., Naismith, I., Saunders, R., Morrison, T., Linke, S., Leibowitz, J. and Pilling, S. (2018) The impact of alcohol use on drop-out and psychological treatment outcomes in improving access to psychological therapies services: an audit. *Behavioural and Cognitive Psychotherapy*, 46, 513–27.

Burroughs, H., Lovell, K., Morley, M., Baldwin, R., Burns, A. and Chew-Graham, C. (2006) 'Justifiable depression': how primary care professionals and patients view late-life depression. A qualitative study. *Family Practice*, 23, 369–77.

Bush, K., Kivlahan, D.R., McDonell, M.B., Fihn, S.D. and Bradley, K.A. (1998) The AUDIT alcohol consumption questions (AUDIT-C): an effective brief screening test for problem drinking. *Archives of Internal Medicine*, 158, 1789–95.

Buysse, D.J., Germain, A., Moul, D.E., Franzen, P.L., Brar, L.K., Fletcher, M.E., et al. (2011) Efficacy of brief behavioural treatment for chronic Insomnia in older adults. *Archives of Internal Medicine*, 171, 887–95.

Cahill, J., Barkham, M., Hardy, G., Gilbody, S., Richards, D., Bower, P., Audin, K. and Connell, J. (2008) A review and critical appraisal of measures of therapist–patient interactions in mental health settings. *Health Technology Assessment*, 12, 1–47.

Carl, E., Stein, A.T., Levihn-Coon, A., Pogue, J., Rothbaum, B., Emmelkamp, P., Asmundson, G.J.G., Carlbring, P. and Powers, M.B. (2019) Virtual reality exposure therapy for anxiety and related disorders: a meta-analysis of randomized controlled trials. *Journal of Anxiety Disorders*, 61, 27–36.

Carlbring, P., Andersson, G., Cuijpers, P., Riper, H. and Hedman-Lagerlöf, E. (2018) Internet-based vs face-to-face cognitive behavior therapy for psychiatric and somatic disorders: an updated systematic review and meta-analysis. *Cognitive Behavioural Therapy*, 47, 1–18.

Carr, A. and McNulty, M. (eds) (2016) *The Handbook of Adult Clinical Psychology: An Evidence Based Practice Approach.* London: Routledge.

Carstensen, L.L., Turan, B., Ram, N., Ersner-Hershfield, H., Samanez-Larkin, G.R., Brooks, K.P. and Nesselroade, J.R. (2011) Emotional experience improves with age: evidence based on over 10 years of experience sampling. *Psychology and Aging*, 26, 21–33.

Centre for Economic Performance. (2006) *The Depression Report: A New Deal for Depression and Anxiety Disorders*. London: London School of Economics and Political Centre for Economic Performance.

Cernis, E., Pimm, J. and Clark, D.M. (2016) Using IAPT data for service improvement. In D.M. Clark (ed.), *IAPT National Enhanced Recovery Workshop*. Birmingham: IAPT.

Chambless, D.L., Caputo, G.C., Jasin, S.E., Gracely, E.J. and Williams, C. (1985) The Mobility Inventory for Agoraphobia. *Behaviour Research and Therapy*, 23, 35–44.

Chand, S.P. and Grossberg, G.T. (2013) How to adapt cognitive-behavioral therapy for older adults. *Current Psychiatry*, 12, 10–15.

Chaplin, R., Farquharson, L., Clapp, M. and Crawford, M. (2015) Comparison of access, outcomes and experiences of older adults and working age adults in psychological therapy. *International Journal of Geriatric Psychiatry*, 30, 178–84.

Chapman, G.B. and Sonnenberg, F.A. (2003) *Decision Making in Health Care: Theory, Psychology and Applications*. Cambridge: Cambridge University Press.

Charnock, D., Shepperd, S., Needham, G. and Gann, R. (1999) DISCERN: an instrument for judging the quality of written consumer health information on treatment choices. *Journal of Epidemiology and Community Health*, 2, 105–11.

Christensen, H., Griffiths, K.M. and Farrer, L. (2009) Adherence in internet interventions for anxiety and depression: systematic review. *Journal of Medical Internet Research*, 11: e13.

Cipriani, A., Furukawa, T.A., Salanti, G., Chaimani, A., Atkinson, L.Z. and Ogawa, Y. (2018) Comparative efficacy and acceptability of 21 antidepressant drugs for the acute treatment of adults with major depressive disorder: a systematic review and network meta-analysis. *The Lancet,* 391, 1357–66.

Clark, D.A. (1996) Panic disorder: from theory to therapy. In P.M. Salkovskis, (ed.), *Frontiers of Cognitive Therapy*. New York: Guilford Press.

Clark, D.A. (2013) Cognitive restructuring. In S.G. Hoffman (ed.), *The Wiley Handbook of Cognitive Behavioral Therapy*. London: Wiley & Sons. (pp. 23–44).

Clark, D.M. (2001) A cognitive perspective on social phobia. In W.R. Crozier and L.E. Alden (eds), *International Handbook of Social Anxiety: Concepts, Research and Interventions Relating to the Self and Shyness*. Chichester: John Wiley & Sons.

Clark, D.M. (2018) Realizing the mass public benefit of evidence-based psychological therapies: the IAPT program. *Annual Review of Clinical Psychology*, 14, 159–83.

Clark, D.M., Canvin, L., Green, J., Layard, R., Pilling, S. and Janecka, M. (2018) Transparency about the outcomes of mental health services (IAPT approach): an analysis of public data. *The Lancet*, 391, 679–86.

Clark, D.M., Layard, R., Smithies, R., Richards, D.A., Suckling, R. and Wright, B. (2009) Improving access to psychological therapy: initial evaluation of two UK demonstration sites. *Behaviour Research and Therapy*, 47, 910–20.

Clark, L.A., Cuthbert, B., Lewis-Fernández, R., Narrow, W.E. and Reed, G.M. (2017) Three approaches to understanding and classifying mental disorder: ICD-11, DSM-5, and the National Institute of Mental Health's Research Domain Criteria (RDoC). *Psychological Science in the Public Interest*, 18, 72–145.

Cleare, A., Pariante, C.M., Young, A.H., Anderson, I.M., Christmas, D., Cowen, P.J., et al. (2015) Evidence-based guidelines for treating depressive disorders with antidepressants: a revision of the 2008 British Association for Psychopharmacology guidelines. *Journal of Psychopharmacology*, 29, 5. 459–525.

Connor, K.M., Davidson, J.R.T., Churchill, L.E., Sherwood, A., Foa, E. and Weisler, R.H. (2000) Psychometric properties of the Social Phobia Inventory (SPIN): new self-rating scale. *British Journal of Psychiatry*, 176, 379–86.

Corcoran, K.A., Leaderbrand, K., Jovasevic, V., Guedea, A.L., Kassam, F. and Radulovic, J. (2015) Regulation of fear extinction versus other affective behaviors by discrete cortical scaffolding complexes associated with NR2B and PKA signaling. *Translational Psychiatry*, 5, e657.

CORE (2017) *Widening Participation to Psychological Wellbeing Practitioner Training*. London: University College London. Available at: www.ucl.ac.uk/pals/sites/pals/files/widening_participation_to_pwp_training_-_project_final_report_draft_for_core_website.pdf

Corrie, S. and Lane, D.D. (2015) *CBT Supervision*. London: Sage.

Craske, M.G., Kircanski, K., Zelikowsky, M., Mystkowski, J. and Baker, A. (2008) Optimising inhibitory learning during exposure therapy. *Behaviour Research and Therapy*, 46, 5–27.

Craske, M.G., Treanor, M., Conway, C., Zbozinek, T. and Vervliet, B. (2014) Maximizing exposure therapy: an inhibitory learning approach. *Behaviour Research Therapy*, 58, 10–23.

Creamer, M., Bell, R. and Failla, S. (2003) Psychometric properties of the Impact of Events Scale – Revised. *Behaviour Research and Therapy*, 41, 1489–96.

Cuijpers, P., Berking, M., Andersson, G., Quigley, L., Kleiboer, A. and Dobson, K.S. (2013) A meta-analysis of cognitive-behavioural therapy for adult depression, alone and in comparison with other treatments. *Canadian Journal of Psychiatry*, 58, 376–85.

Cuijpers, P., De Wit, L., Kleiboer, A., Karyotaki, E. and Ebert, D. (2018) Problem-solving therapy for adult depression: an updated meta-analysis. *European Psychiatry*, 48, 27–37.

Cuijpers, P., Donker, T., van Straten, A. and Andersson, G. (2010) Is guided self-help as effective as face-to-face psychotherapy for depression and anxiety disorders? A systematic review and meta-analysis of comparative outcome studies. *Psychological Medicine*, 40, 1943–57.

Cuijpers, P., Driessen, E., Hollon, S.D., van Oppen, P., Barth, J. and Andersson, G. (2012) The efficacy of non-directive supportive therapy for adult depression: a meta-analysis. *Clinical Psychology Review*, 32, 280–91.

Cuijpers, P., Muñoz, R.F., Clarke, G.N. and Lewinsohn, P.M. (2009a) Psychoeducational treatment and prevention of depression: the 'Coping with Depression' course thirty years later. *Clinical Psychology Review*, 29, 449–58.

Cuijpers, P., Noma, H., Karyotaki, E., Cipriani, A. and Furukawa, T.A. (2019a) Effectiveness and acceptability of cognitive behavior therapy delivery formats in adults with depression: a network meta-analysis. *JAMA Psychiatry*, 76, 700–7.

Cuijpers, P., Reijnders, M. and Huibers, M.J. (2019b) The role of common factors in psychotherapy outcomes. *Annual Review of Clinical Psychology*, 15, 207–31.

Cuijpers, P., Sijbrandij, M., Koole, S.L., Andersson, G., Beekman, A.T. and Reynolds, C. F. (2014) Adding psychotherapy to antidepressant medication in depression and anxiety disorders: a meta-analysis. *World Psychiatry*, 13, 56–67.

Cuijpers, P., van Straten, A., Smit, F. and Andersson, G. (2009a) Is psychotherapy for depression equally effective in younger and older adults? A meta-regression analysis. *International Psychogeriatrics*, 21, 16–24.

Cuijpers, P., van Straten, A., Warmerdam, L. and Andersson, G. (2009b) Psychotherapy versus the combination of psychotherapy and pharmacotherapy in the treatment of depression: a meta-analysis. *Depression and Anxiety*, 26, 3, 279–88.

D'Zurrilla, T.J. and Goldfried, M.R. (1971) Problem solving and behaviour modification. *Journal of Abnormal Psychology*, 78, 107–26.

D'Zurilla, T.J. and Nezu, A. (1982) Social problem solving in adults. In P.C. Kendall (ed.), *Advances in Cognitive-Behavioral Research and Therapy*. New York: Academic Press. pp. 202–74.

D'Zurilla, T.J. and Nezu, A.M. (2007) *Problem-Solving Therapy: A Positive Approach to Clinical Intervention*. New York: Springer Publishing.

Dazzi, T., Gribble, R., Wessely, S. and Fear, N.T. (2014) Does asking about suicide and related behaviours induce suicidal ideation? What is the evidence? *Psychological Medicine*, 44, 16, 3361–3.

Delgadillo, J. (2018) Guided self-help in a brave new world. *British Journal of Psychiatry*, 212, 65–6.

Delgadillo, J., Gellatly, J. and Stephenson-Bellwood, S. (2015) Decision making in stepped care: how do therapists decide whether to prolong treatment or not? *Behavioural and Cognitive Psychotherapy*, 43, 328–41.

Delgadillo, J., Huey, D., Bennett, H. and McMillan, D. (2017a) Case complexity as a guide for psychological treatment selection. *Journal of Consulting and Clinical Psychology*, 85, 835–53.

Delgadillo, J., McMillan, D., Lucock, M., Leach, C., Ali, S. and Gilbody, S. (2014) Early changes, attrition, and dose-response in low intensity psychological interventions. *British Journal of Clinical Psychology*, 53, 114–30.

Delgadillo, J., Moreea, O. and Lutz, W. (2016) Different people respond differently to therapy: a demonstration using patient profiling and risk stratification. *Behaviour Research and Therapy*, 79, 15–22.

Delgadillo, J., Overend, K., Lucock, M., Groom, M., Kirby, N., McMillan, D., et al. (2017b) Improving the efficiency of psychological treatment using outcome feedback technology. *Behaviour Research and Therapy*, 99, 89–97.

Denys, D., Tenney, N., van Megen, H.J., de Geus, F. and Westenberg, H.G. (2004) Axis I and II comorbidity in a large sample of patients with obsessive-compulsive disorder. *Journal of Affective Disorders*, 80, 155–62.

Department of Health (2003) Patient Information Toolkit. Available at: http://ppitoolkit.org.uk/PDF/toolkit/patient_info_toolkit.pdf (last accessed 3 April 2020).

Department of Health (2008) *Long Term Conditions: Positive Practice Guide*. London: Department of Health.

Department of Health (2009) *Black and Minority Ethnic: Positive Practice Guide*. London: Department of Health.

Department of Health (2009) *Older People: Positive Practice Guide*. London: Department of Health.

Department of Health (2010) *Equity and Excellence: Liberating the NHS (Cm 7881)*. London: The Stationery Office.

Department of Health (2011) *No Health without Mental Health: A Cross-Government Mental Health Outcomes Strategy for People of All Ages*. London: Department of Health.

Department of Health (2013) *Learning Difficulties: Positive Practice Guide*. London: Department of Health.

Department of Health (2014) *Closing the Gap: Priorities for Essential Change in Mental Health*. London: Department of Health.

Department of Health (2015) *The NHS Constitution: The NHS Belongs to Us All*. London: Department of Health.

Dijk, D.J. (2010) Slow-wave sleep deficiency and enhancement: implications for insomnia and its management. *World Journal of Biological Psychiatry*, 11, 22–8.

Dolan-Sewell, R. T., Riley, W. T. and Hunt, C. E. (2005) NIH State-of-the-science conference on chronic Insomnia. *Journal of Clinical Sleep Medicine*, 1, 412–21. Available at: https://jcsm.aasm.org/doi/pdf/10.5664/jcsm.26356.

Dowrick, C., Dunn, G., Ayuso-Mateos, J.L., Dalgard, O.S., Page, H., Lehtinen, V., Casey, P., Wilkinson, C., Vazquez-Barquero, J.L. and Wilkinson, G. (2000) Problem solving treatment and group psychoeducation for depression: multicentre randomised controlled trial. *British Medical Journal*, 321, 1–6.

Dugas, M.J. and Ladouceur, R. (2000) Treatment of GAD: targeting intolerance of uncertainty in two types of worry. *Behavior Modification*, 24, 635–57.

Dugas, M.J. and Robichaud, M. (2007) *Cognitive-Behavioural Treatment for Generalized Anxiety Disorder: From Science to Practice*. New York: Routledge.

Dugas, M.J., Freeston, M.H. and Ladouceur, R. (1997) Intolerance of uncertainty and problem orientation in worry. *Cognitive Therapy and Research*, 21, 593–606.

Duman, M. and Farrell, C. (2000) *The POPPI Guide: Practicalities of Producing Patient Information*. London: King's Fund Publishing.

Edinger, J.D. and Sampson, W.S. (2003) A primary care 'friendly' cognitive behaviour therapy insomnia therapy. *Sleep*, 2, 177–82.

Egan, G. (2002) *The Skilled Helper: A Problem-Management and Opportunity-Development Approach to Helping*. Pacific Grove, CA: Brooks/Cole.

Ehlers, A. and Clark, D. (2000) A cognitive model of posttraumatic stress disorder. *Behavior Research Therapy*, 38, 319–45.

Ekers, D., Richards, D.A. and Gilbody, S. (2008) A meta-analysis of randomised trials of behavioural treatment of depression. *Psychological Medicine*, 38, 611–23.

Ekers, D., Webster, L., Van Straten, A., Cuijpers, P., Richards, D.A. and Gilbody, S. (2014) Behavioural activation for depression; an update of meta-analysis of effectiveness and sub group analysis. *PLoS One*, 9: e100100.

Elliott, R., Bohart, A.C., Watson, J.C. and Greenberg, L.S. (2011) Empathy. In J.C. Norcross (ed.), *Psychotherapy Relationships that Work*. New York: Oxford University Press. pp. 132–52.

Elwyn, G., Laitner, S., Coulter, A., Walker, E., Watson, P. and Thomson, R. (2010) Implementing shared decision making in the NHS. *British Medical Journal*, 341, c5146.

Epstein, D.A., Sidani, S., Bootzin, R.R. and Belyea, M.J. (2012) Dismantling multicomponent behavioural treatment for insomnia in older adults: a randomised controlled trial. *Sleep*, 35, 797–805.

Espie, C.A. (2006) *Overcoming Insomnia and Sleep Problems: A Self-Help Guide Using Cognitive Behavioural Therapy*. London: Constable Robinson.

Espie, C.A. (2009) 'Stepped care': a health technology solution for delivering cognitive behavioural therapy as a first line insomnia treatment. *Sleep*, 32, 1549–58.

Espie, C.A. (2010) *Overcoming Insomnia and Sleep Problems*. London: Robinson.

Espie, C.A., MacMahon, K.M., Kelly, H.L., Broomfield, N.M., Douglas, N.J., Engelman, H.M., et al. (2007) Randomised clinical effectiveness trial of nurse-administered small-group cognitive behaviour therapy for persistent Insomnia in general practice. *Sleep*, 30, 574–84.

Farrand, P. (2005) Development of a supported self-help book prescription scheme in primary care. *Primary Care Mental Health*, 3, 61–6.

Farrand, P. and Sheppard, M. (2018) *Facing Your Fears*. Exeter: CEDAR. Available at cedar.exeter.ac.uk/media/universityofexeter/schoolofpsychology/cedar/documents/liiapt/Facing_your_Fears.pdf (accessed 15 August 2019).

Farrand, P. and Stonebank, H. (2019) *Enhancing Resiliency: Finding Inner Strength to Manage the Demands of Clinical Practice*. Exeter: Exeter University.

Farrand, P. and Woodford, J. (2012) Impact of support on the effectiveness of written cognitive behavioural self-help: a systematic review and meta-analysis of randomised controlled trials. *Clinical Psychology Review*, 33, 182–95.

Farrand, P., Confue, P., Byng, R. and Shaw, S. (2009) Guided self-help supported by paraprofessional mental health workers: an uncontrolled before–after cohort study. *Health and Social Care in the Community*, 17, 9–17.

Farrand, P., Jeffs, A., Bloomfield, T., Greenberg, N., Watkins, E. and Mullan, E. (2018) Mental health service acceptability for the armed forces veteran community. *Occupational Medicine*, 68, 6, 391–8.

Farrand, P., Mullan, E., Rayson, K., Engelbrecht, A., Mead, K. and Greenberg, N. (2019a) Adapting CBT to treat depression in armed forces veterans: qualitative study. *Behavioural and Cognitive Psychotherapy*, 47, 530–40.

Farrand, P., Pentecost, C., Greaves, C., Taylor, R.S., Warren, F., Green, C., Hillsdon, M., Evans, P., Welsman, J. and Taylor, A.H. (2014) A written self-help intervention for depressed adults comparing behavioural activation combined with physical activity promotion with a self-help intervention based upon behavioural activation alone: study protocol for a parallel group pilot randomised controlled trial (BAcPAc). *Trials*, 29, 15, 196.

Farrand, P., Perry, J. and Linsley, S. (2010) Enhancing self-practice/self-reflection (SP/SR) approach to cognitive behaviour training through the use of reflective blogs. *Behavioural and Cognitive Psychotherapy*, 38, 473–7.

Farrand, P., Rayson, K. and Lovis, L. (2016a) Reflection in low intensity CBT: challenges and practice-based innovations. In B. Haarhoff and R. Thwaites (eds), *Reflection in CBT*. London: SAGE. pp. 141–59.

Farrand, P., Woodford, J., Coumoundouros, C. and Svedin, F. (2020) Supported cognitive-behavioural therapy self-help versus treatment-as-usual for depressed informal caregivers of stroke survivors (CEDArS): feasibility randomised controlled trial. *The Cognitive Behavioural Therapist*, 13, e23.

Farrand, P., Woodford, J., Llewellyn, D., Anderson, M., Venkatasubramanian, S., Ukoumunne, O.C., Adlam A., et al. (2016b) Behavioural activation written self-help to improve mood, wellbeing and quality of life in people with dementia supported by informal carers (PROMOTE): a study protocol for a single-arm feasibility study. *Pilot and Feasibility Studies*, 2, 42.

Farrand, P., Woodford, J. and Jackson, K. (2019a) *Unhelpful Thoughts: Challenging and Testing Them Out*. Exeter: CEDAR.

Farrand, P., Woodford, J. and Small, F. (2019b) *Managing Your Worries*. Exeter: Exeter University.

Farrand, P., Woodford, J. and Small, F. (2019c) *From Problems to Solutions*. Exeter: Exeter University.

Fear, N.T., Jones, M., Murphy, D., Hull, L., Iversen, A.C., Coker, B., Machell, L. et al. (2010) What are the consequences of deployment to Iraq and Afghanistan on the mental health of the UK armed forces? A cohort study. *The Lancet*, 375, 1783–97.

Fennell, M.J.V. (1989) Depression. In K. Hawton, P. Salkovskis, J. Kirk and D. Clark (eds), *Cognitive Behaviour Therapy for Psychiatric Problems: A Practical Guide*. Oxford: Oxford University Press.

Fergusson, D., Doucette, S., Glass, K.C., Shapiro, S., Healy, D., Hebert, P. and Hutton, B. (2005) Association between suicide attempts and selective serotonin reuptake inhibitors: systematic review of randomised controlled trials. *BMJ*, 330, 7488, 396.

Finning, K., Richards, D.A., Moore, L., Ekers, D., McMillan, D., Farrand, P., O'Mahen, H.A. et al. (2017) Cost and outcome of behavioural activation versus cognitive behavioural therapy for depression (COBRA): a qualitative process evaluation. *BMJ Open*, 7, 4, e014161.

Firth, N., Barkham, M., Kellett, S. and Saxon, D. (2015) Therapist effects and moderators of effectiveness and efficiency in psychological wellbeing practitioners: a multilevel modelling analysis. *Behaviour Research and Therapy*, 69, 54–62.

Fiske, A., Wetherell, J.L. and Gatz, M. (2009) Depression in older adults. *Annual Review of Clinical Psychology*, 5, 363–89.

Foa, E.B. and Kozak, M.J. (1986) Emotional processing of fear: exposure to corrective information. *Psychological Bulletin*, 99, 20–35.

Foa, E.B., Kozak, M.J., Salkovskis, P.M., Coles, M.E. & Amir, N. (1998) The validation of a new obsessive-compulsive disorder scale: the Obsessive-Compulsive Inventory. *Psychological Assessment*, 10, 3, 206–14.

Freund, A.M. (2008) Successful aging as management of resources: the role of selection, optimization, and compensation. *Research in Human Development*, 5, 94–106.

Frost, R., Nair, P., Aw, S., Gould, R.L., Kharicha, K., Buszewicz, M. and Walters, K. (2019) Supporting frail older people with depression and anxiety: a qualitative study. *Aging & Mental Health*, 1–8, DOI: 10.1080/13607863.2019.1647132

Frude, N. (2004) A book prescription scheme in primary care. *Clinical Psychology, Science and Practice*, 39, 11–14.

Garcia-Palacios, A., Botella, C., Hoffman, H. and Bagregat, S. (2007) Comparing acceptance and refusal rates of virtual reality exposure vs in vivo exposure by patients with specific phobias. *Cyberpsychology and Behavior*, 10, 722–4.

Geiger-Brown, J.M., Rogers, V.E., Liu, W., Ludeman, E.M., Downton K.D. and Diaz-Abad, M. (2015) Cognitive Behavioural Therapy in persons with comorbid insomnia: a meta-analysis. *Sleep Medicine Review*, 23, 54–67.

Gellatly, J., Bower, P., Hennessy, S., Richards, D., Gilbody, S. and Lovell, K. (2007) What makes self-help interventions effective in the management of depressive symptoms? Meta-analysis and meta-regression. *Psychological Medicine*, 37, 1217–28.

Gellatly, J., Pedley, R., Molloy, C., Butler, J., Lovell, K. and Bee, P. (2017) Low intensity interventions for obsessive-compulsive disorder (OCD): a qualitative study of mental health practitioner experiences. *BMC Psychiatry*, 17, 77.

Gilbert, P. (2009) *Overcoming Depression: A Self-Help Guide Using Cognitive Behavioural Techniques.* London: Constable Robinson.

Glasgow, R.E. and Rosen, G.M. (1978) Behavioural bibliotherapy: a review of self-help behavior therapy manuals. *Psychological Bulletin*, 8, 1–23.

Gordon, P.K. (2012) Ten steps to cognitive behavioural supervision. *The Cognitive Behaviour Therapist*, 5, 71–82.

Gorman, J.M. (1997) Comorbid depression and anxiety spectrum disorders. *Depression and Anxiety*, 4, 160–8.

Gould, R.A. and Clum, G.A. (1993) A meta-analysis of self-help treatment approaches. *Clinical Psychology Review*, 13, 169–86.

Gould, R.L., Coulson, M.C. and Howard, R.J. (2012) Cognitive behavioral therapy for depression in older people: a meta-analysis and meta-regression of randomized controlled trials. *Journal of the American Geriatric Society*, 60, 1817–30.

Gowling, S., Persson, J., Holt, G., Ashbourne, S., Bloomfield, J., Shortland, H. and Bate, C. (2016) Richmond Wellbeing Service Access Strategy for Older Adults. *BMJ Open Quality*, 5, 1, u206099-w2510.

Graham, C.R. (2006) Blended learning systems: definition, current trends and future directions. In C.J. Bonk and C.R. Graham, *The Handbook of Blended Learning; Global Perspectives, Local Designs.* San Francisco: John Wiley & Sons.

Green, H., Barkham, M., Kellett, S., and Saxon, D. (2014) Therapist effects and IAPT psychological wellbeing practitioners (PWPs): a multilevel modelling and mixed methods analysis. *Behaviour Research and Therapy*, 63, 43–54.

Griner, D. and Smith, T.B. (2006) Culturally adapted mental health interventions: a meta-analytic review. *Psychotherapy: Theory, Research, Practice, Training*, 43, 531–48.

Gum, A.M., Areán, P.A., Hunkeler, E., Tang, L., Katon, W., Hitchcock, P., Steffens, D.C., Dickens, J. and Unützer, J. (2006) Depression treatment preferences in older primary care patients. *The Gerontologist*, 46, 14–22.

Gunn, J.E. and Pistole, M.C. (2012) Trainee supervisor attachment: explaining the alliance and disclosure in supervision. *Training and Education in Professional Psychology*, 6, 229–37.

Gunnell, D., Saperia, J. and Ashby, D. (2006) Selective serotonin reuptake inhibitors (SSRIs) and suicide in adults: meta-analysis of drug company data from placebo controlled, randomised controlled trials submitted to the MHRA's safety review. *Journal of Urology*, 175, 4, 1433–1434.

Gyani, A., Shafran, R., Layard, R. and Clark, D.M. (2011) Enhancing Recovery Rates in IAPT Services: Lessons from Analysis of the Year One Data. *Behaviour Research and Therapy*, 51, 597–606.

Hadjistavropoulos, H.D., Schneider, L.H., Klassen, K., Dear, B.F. and Titov, N. (2018) Development and evaluation of a scale assessing therapist fidelity to guidelines for delivering therapist-assisted internet-delivered cognitive behaviour therapy. *Cognitive Behaviour Therapy*, 47, 447–461.

Harmer, C., Bhagwagar, Z., Perrett, D., Vollm, B.A., Cowen, P.J. and Goodwin, G.M. (2003) Acute SSRI administration affects the processing of social cues in healthy volunteers. *Neuropsychopharmacology*, 28, 148–52.

Harmer, C. J., O'Sullivan, U., Favaron, E., Massey-Chase, R., Ayres, R., Reinecke, A., et al. (2009) Effect of acute antidepressant administration on negative affective bias in depressed patients. *American Journal of Psychiatry*, 166, 1178–84.

Harmer, C.J., Shelley, N.C., Cowen, P.J. and Goodwin, G.M. (2004) Increased positive versus negative affective perception and memory in healthy volunteers following selective serotonin and norepinephrine reuptake inhibition. *American Journal of Psychiatry*, 161, 1256–63.

Hayes, S.C. and Hofmann, S.G. (2017) The third wave of cognitive behavioural therapy and the rise of process-based care. *World Psychiatry*, 16, 245–6.

Hazlett-Stevens, H. and Craske, M.G. (2004) Brief cognitive-behavioural therapy: definition and scientific foundations. In F.W. Bond and W. Dryden (eds), *Handbook of Brief Cognitive Behaviour Therapy*. Chichester: Wiley and Sons.

Health Education England (2020) *IAPT Benchmarking Survey*. London.

Hepgul, N., King, S., Amarasinghe, M., Breen, G., Grant, N., Grey, N., et al. (2016) Clinical characteristics of patients assessed within an Improving Access to Psychological Therapies (IAPT) service: results from a naturalistic cohort study (Predicting Outcome Following Psychological Therapy; PROMPT). *BMC Psychiatry*, 16, 1–10.

Hides, L., Carroll, S., Lubman, D.I. and Baker, A. (2010) Brief motivational interviewing for depression and anxiety. In J. Bennett-Levy, D.A. Richards, P. Farrand, H. Christensen, K.M. Griffiths, D.J. Kavanagh, et al. (eds), *Oxford Guide to Low Intensity CBT Interventions*. Oxford: Oxford University Press. pp. 129–36.

Hirschfeld, R.M.A. (2001) The comorbidity of major depression and anxiety disorders: recognition and management in primary care. *Primary Care Companion to The Journal of Clinical Psychiatry*, 3, 244–54.

Hirshkowitz, M., Whiton, K., Albert, S.M., Alessi, C., Bruni, O., DonCarlos, L., et al. (2015) National Sleep Foundation's updated sleep duration recommendations: final report. *Sleep Health*, 1, 233–43.

Ho, F.Y.Y., Chung, K.F., Yeung, W.F., Ng, T.H., Kwan, K.S., Yung, K.P. and Cheng, S.K. (2015) Self-help cognitive-behavioural therapy for insomnia: a meta-analysis of randomised controlled trials. *Sleep Medicine Reviews*, 19, 17–28.

Hogarth, T., Hasluck, C., Gambin, L., Behle, H., Li, Y. and Lyonette, C. (2013) *Evaluation of Employment Advisers in the Improving Access to Psychological Therapies Programme* (Department for Work and Pensions Research Report no. RR826). Available at https://assets.publishing.service.gov.uk/government/uploads/system/uploads/attachment_data/file/221217/826summ.pdf (accessed 9 October 2019).

Hollander, E., Broatch, J., Himelein, C., Rowland, C., Stein, D. and Kwon, J. (1997) Psychosocial function and economic costs of obsessive-compulsive disorder. *CNS Spectrums*, 2, 16–25.

Hollon, S.D., DeRubeis, R.J., Fawcett, J., Amsterdam, J.D., Shelton, R.C., Zajecka, J., et al. (2014) Effect of cognitive therapy with antidepressant medications vs antidepressants alone on the rate of recovery in major depressive disorder: a randomized clinical trial. *JAMA Psychiatry*, 71, 10, 1157–64.

Hopko, D.R., Armento, M.E.A., Robertson, S.M.C., Ryba, M.M., Carvalho, J.P., Colman, L.K. et al. (2011) Brief behavioural activation and problem-solving therapy for depressed breast cancer patients: randomized trial. *Journal of Consulting and Clinical Psychology*, 79, 834–49.

Hopko, D.R., Lejuez, C.W., Ruggiero, K.J. and Eifert, G.H. (2003) Contemporary behavioural activation treatments for depression: procedures, principles, and progress. *Clinical Psychology Review*, 23, 699–717.

Hopko, D.R., Ryba, M.M., McIndoo, C. and File, A. (2015) Behavioral activation. In A.M. Nezu and C.M. Nezu (eds), *The Oxford Handbook of Cognitive and Behavioral Therapies*. New York: Oxford University Press.

Horvath, A.O., Del Re, A.C., Flückiger, C. and Symonds, D. (2011) Alliance in individual psychotherapy. *Psychotherapy*, 48, 9–16.

Huang, T.T., Liu, C.B., Tsai, Y.H., Chin, Y.F. and Wong, C.H. (2015) Physical fitness exercise versus cognitive behavior therapy on reducing the depressive symptoms among community-dwelling elderly adults: a randomized controlled trial. *International Journal of Nursing Studies*, 52, 1542–52.

Imison, C., Castle-Clarke, S. and Watson, R. (2016) *Reshaping the Workforce to Deliver the Care Patients Need. Research Report.* London: Nuffield Trust.

Improving Access to Psychological Therapies (IAPT) (2009) *Black and Minority Ethnic (BME) Positive Practice Guide.* Department of Health. Available at: https://www.uea.ac.uk/documents/246046/11919343/black-and-minority-ethnic-bme-positive-practice-guide.pdf

Insel, T., Cuthbert, B., Garvey, M., Heinssen, R., Pine, D., Quinn, K., Sanislow, C. and Wang, P. (2010) Research Domain Criteria (RDoC): Toward a new classification framework for research on mental disorders. *American Journal of Psychiatry*, 167, 748–51.

Inskipp, F. and Proctor, B. (1993) *The Art, Craft and Tasks of Counselling Supervision, Part 1. Making the Most of Supervisors.* Twickenham, UK: Cascade Publications.

Jacobson, N.S., Martell, C.R. and Dimidjian, S. (2001) Behavioral activation therapy for depression: returning to contextual roots. *Clinical Psychology: Science and Practice*, 8, 255–70.

Jacoby, R.J., Leonard, R.C., Riemann, B.C. and Abramowitz, J.S. (2014) Predictors of quality of life and functional impairment in obsessive-compulsive disorder. *Comprehensive Psychiatry*, 55, 1195–1202.

Johns, L., Jolley, S., Garety, P., Khondoker, M., Fornells-Ambrojo, M., Onwumere, J., et al. (2019) Improving access to psychological therapies for people with severe mental illness (IAPT-SMI): lessons from the South London and Maudsley psychosis demonstration site. *Behaviour Research and Therapy*, 116, 104–10.

Karel, M.J., Gatz, M. and Smyer, M.A. (2012) Aging and mental health in the decade ahead: what psychologists need to know. *American Psychologist*, 67, 184.

Karenga, M. (1980) *Kawaida Theory*. Los Angeles, CA: Kawaida Publications.

Karenga, M. (1998) *The African American Holiday of Kwanzaa: A Celebration of Family, Community and Culture*. Los Angeles, CA: University of Sankore Press.

Kasckow, J., Klaus, J., Morse, J., Oslin, D., Luther, J., Fox, L., Reynolds, C. and Haas, G.L. (2014) Using problem solving therapy to treat veterans with subsyndromal depression: a pilot study. *International Journal of Geriatric Psychiatry*, 29, 1255–61.

Katon, W.J., Von Koff, M., Lin, E.H.B., Simon, G., Ludman, E., Russo, J. et al. (2004) The pathways study. A randomized trial of collaborative care in patients with diabetes and depression. *Archives of General Psychiatry*, 61, 1042–9.

Kazantzis, N., Deane, F.P. and Ronan, K.R. (2000) Homework assignments in cognitive and behavioral therapy: a meta-analysis. *Clinical Psychology: Science and Practice*, 7, 189–202.

Kazantzis, N., Deane, F.P., Ronan, K.R. and L'Abate, L. (eds) (2005) *Using Homework Assignments in Cognitive Behaviour Therapy*. London: Routledge.

Keijsers, G.P.J., Schaap, C.P.D.R. and Hoogduin, C.A.L. (2000) The impact of interpersonal patient and therapist behavior on outcome in cognitive-behavior therapy: a review of empirical studies. *Behavior Modification*, 24, 264–97.

Kennerley, H., Kirk, J. and Westbrook, D. (2016) *An Introduction to Cognitive Behaviour Therapy: Skills and Applications*. London: SAGE.

Kenwright, M. (2010) Introducing and supporting written and internet-based guided CBT. In J. Bennett-Levy, D.A. Richards, P. Farrand, H. Christensen, K.M. Griffiths, D.J. Kavanagh, et al. (eds), *Oxford Guide to Low Intensity CBT Interventions*. Oxford: Oxford University Press. pp.129–36.

Kenwright, M., Burrowes, J., Wilson, K., Sharma, K., Barrass, B. and Ewart, E. (2008) *Outcomes from the Ealing IAPT Pathfinder Site 2007-08*. London: West London Mental Health NHS Trust.

Kessler, R.C., Chiu, W.T., Demler, O. and Walters, E.E. (2005) Prevalence, severity, and comorbidity of 12-Month DSM-IV Disorders in the National Comorbidity Survey Replication. *Archives of General Psychiatry*, 62, 617–27.

Khan, N., Bower, P. and Rogers, A. (2007) Guided self-help in primary care mental health: meta-synthesis of qualitative studies of patient experience. *British Journal of Psychiatry*, 191, 206–11.

Kirkham, J.G., Choi, N. and Seitz, D.P. (2016) Meta-analysis of problem-solving therapy for the treatment of major depressive disorder in older adults. *International Journal of Geriatric Psychiatry*, 31, 526–35.

Kirschner, S.R. (2013) Diagnosis and its discontents: Critical perspectives on psychiatric nosology and the DSM. *Feminism and Psychology*, 23, 1, 10–28.

Knopp-Hoffer, J., Knowles, S., Bower, P., Lovell, K. and Bee, P.E. (2016) 'One man's medicine is another man's poison': a qualitative study of user perspectives on low intensity interventions for obsessive-compulsive disorder (OCD). *BMC Health Services Research*, 18, 16, 188.

Knowles, S.E., Lovell, K., Bower, P., Gilbody, S., Littlewood, E. and Lester, H. (2015) Patient experience of computerised therapy for depression in primary care. *BMJ Open*, 5, e008581.

Knutson, B., Wolkowitz, O.M., Cole, S.W., Chan, T., Moore, E.A., Johnson, R.C. et al. (1998) Selective alteration of personality and social behavior by serotonergic intervention. *American Journal of Psychiatry*, 155, 373–9.

Koffel, E.A., Koffel, J.B. and Gehrman, P.R. (2015) A meta-analysis of group cognitive behavioural therapy for insomnia. *Sleep Medicine Reviews*, 19, 6–16.

Kroenke, K., Spitzer, R.L. and Williams, J.B.W. (2001) The PHQ-9: Validity of a brief depression severity measure. *Journal of General Medicine*, 16, 606–13.

Ladany, N., Ellis, M.V. and Friedlander, M.L. (1999) The supervisory working alliance, trainee self-efficacy and satisfaction. *Journal of Counseling & Development*, 77, 447–55.

Ladany, N., Hill, C.E., Corbett, M.M. and Nutt, A.A. (1996) Nature, extent, and importance of what psychotherapy trainees do not disclose to their supervisors. *Journal of Counseling Psychology*, 43, 10–24.

Laidlaw, K. (2010) Are attitudes to ageing and wisdom enhancement legitimate targets for CBT for late life depression and anxiety? *Nordic Psychology*, 62, 27–42.

Laidlaw, K. (2015) *CBT for Older People: An Introduction*. London: Sage.

Laidlaw, K. and Kishita, N. (2015) Age-appropriate augmented cognitive behavior therapy to enhance treatment outcome for late-life depression and anxiety disorders. *Geropsych*, 28, 57–66.

Laidlaw, K. and McAlpine, S. (2008) Cognitive behaviour therapy: how is it different with older people? *Journal of Rational-Emotive and Cognitive-Behavior Therapy*, 26, 250–62.

Laidlaw, K., Davidson, K., Toner, H., Jackson, G., Clark, S., Law, J. et al. (2008) A randomised controlled trial of cognitive behaviour therapy vs treatment as usual in the treatment of mild to moderate late life depression. *International Journal of Geriatric Psychiatry*, 23, 843–50.

Laidlaw, K., Thompson, L.W., Gallagher-Thompson, D. and Dick-Siskin, L. (2003) *Cognitive Behaviour Therapy with Older People*. London: Wiley and Sons.

Lambert, J., Greaves, C., Farrand, P., Price, L.R.S., Haase, A. and Taylor, A. (2018) Web-based intervention using behavioral activation and physical activity for adults with depression (the eMotion study): pilot randomised controlled trial. *Journal of Medical Internet Research*, 20, 120–36.

Lambert, M.J. (1992) Psychotherapy outcome research: implications for integrative and eclectic therapists. In J.C. Norcross and M.R. Goldfield (eds), *Handbook of Psychotherapy Integration*. New York: Basic Books. pp. 94–129.

Lancee, J., Effting, M., van der Zweerde, T., van Daal, L., van Straten, A. and Kamphuis, J.H. (2019) Cognitive processes mediate the effects of insomnia treatment: evidence from a randomized wait-list controlled trial. *Sleep Medicine*, 54, 86–93.

LaSalle, V.H., Cromer, K.R., Nelson, K.N., Kazuba, D., Justement, L. and Murphy, D.L. (2004) Diagnostic interview assessed neuropsychiatric disorder comorbidity in 334 individuals with obsessive-compulsive disorder. *Depression and Anxiety*, 19, 163–73.

Lastella, M., O'Mullan, C., Paterson, J.L. and Reynolds, A.C. (2019) Sex and sleep: perceptions of sex as a sleep promoting behaviour in the general adult population. *Front Public Health*, 7, 33.

Layard, R. and Clark, D. (2015) *Thrive: The Power of Psychological Therapy*. London: Penguin.

Layard, R., Clark, D., Knapp, M. and Mayraz, G. (2007) Cost-benefit analysis of psychological therapy. *National Institute Economic Review*, 202, 90–8.

Leahy, R.L. and Rego, S.A. (2012) Cognitive restructuring. In W.T. O'Donohue and J.E. Fisher (eds), *Cognitive Behavior Therapy: Core Principles for Practice*. New Jersey: John Wiley and Sons.

Leahy, R.L., Holland, J.F. and McGinn, L.K. (2012) *Treatment Plans and Interventions for Depression and Anxiety Disorders*. New York: Guilford Press.

Lee, H., Yoon, J.Y., Lim, Y., Jung, H.Y., Kim, S., Yoo, Y. et al. (2015) The effect of nurse-led problem solving therapy on coping, self-efficacy and depressive symptoms for patients with chronic obstructive pulmonary disease: a randomised controlled trial. *Age and Ageing*, 44, 397–403.

Leichsenring, F., Salzer, S., Jaeger, U., Kachele, H., Kreischle, R., Leweke, F. et al. (2009) Short-term psychodynamic psychotherapy and cognitive-behavioral therapy in generalized anxiety disorder: a randomized, controlled trial. *American Journal of Psychiatry*, 166, 875–81.

Leigh, S. and Flatt, S. (2015) App-based psychological interventions: friend or foe? *Evidence-Based Mental Health*, 18, 97–9.

Lenzenweger, M.F., Lane, M.C., Loranger, A.W. and Kessler, R.C. (2007) DSM-IV personality disorders in the National Comorbidity Survey Replication. *Biological Psychiatry*, 62, 6, 553–64.

Lewinsohn, P.M. (1975) The behavioural study and treatment of depression. In M. Hersen, R.M. Eisler and P.M. Miller (eds), *Progress in Behavior Modification*. New York: Academic Press. pp. 19–64.

Lewinsohn, P.M., Clarke, G.N. and Hoberman, H.M. (1989) The coping with depression course: review and future directions. *Canadian Journal of Behavioural Science*, 21, 470–93.

Lewis, C., Pearce, J. and Bisson, J.I. (2012) Efficacy, cost-effectiveness and acceptability of self-help interventions for anxiety disorders: systematic review. *British Journal of Psychiatry*, 200, 15–21.

Lexis, M.A.S., Jansen, N.W.H., Huibers, M.J.H., van Amelsvoort, L.G.P.M., Berkouwer, A., Ton, G.T.A. et al. (2011) Prevention of long-term sickness absence and major depression in high-risk employees: a randomised controlled trial. *Occupational and Environmental Medicine*, 68, 400–7.

Lieblich, S.M., Castle, D.J., Pantelis, C., Hopwood, M., Young, A. H. and Everall, I. P. (2015) High heterogeneity and low reliability in the diagnosis of major depression will impair the development of new drugs. *British Journal of Psychiatry Open*, 1, e5–e7.

Liese, B.S. and Beck, J.S. (1997) Cognitive therapy supervision. In C.E. Watkins (ed.), *Handbook of Psychotherapy Supervision*. Chichester: John Wiley & Sons. pp. 114–33.

Linden, M., Zubraegel, D., Baer, T., Franke, U. and Schlattmann, P. (2005) Efficacy of cognitive behaviour therapy in generalized anxiety disorders. *Psychotherapy and Psychosomatics*, 74, 36–42.

Liness, S. and Muston, J. (2011) *National Curriculum for High Intensity Cognitive Behavioural Therapy Training Course*. London: Department of Health. Available at www.uea.ac.uk/documents/246046/11919343/national-curriculum-for-high-intensity-cognitive-behavioural-therapy-courses.pdf/e893a788-8df2-4f2b-a1bd-a1c9c0ae37a1 (accessed 11 January 2019).

Livni, D., Crowe, T.P. and Gonsalvez, C. J. (2012) Effects of supervision modality and intensity in alliance and outcomes for the supervisee. *Rehabilitation Psychology*, 57, 178–86.

Longmore, R.J. and Worrell, M. (2007) Do we need to challenge thoughts in cognitive behavior therapy? *Clinical Psychology Review*, 27, 173–87.

Lorenzo-Luaces, L. and Dobson, K.S. (2019) Is behavioral activation (BA) more effective than cognitive therapy (CT) in severe depression? A reanalysis of a landmark trial. *International Journal of Cognitive Therapy*, 12, 73–82.

Lovell, K. (1999) *Overcoming Agoraphobia: A Self-Help Manual*. Available at www.anxietyuk.org.uk/wp-content/uploads/2010/05/overcoming-agoraphobia-lovell-1999.pdf (accessed 10 May 2019).

Lovell, K. and Bee, P. (2008) Implementing NICE OCD/BDD guidelines. *Psychology and Psychotherapy: Theory, Research and Practice*, 81, 365–76.

Lovell, K. and Gega, L. (2011) *Obsessive Compulsive Disorder: A Self-Help Book*. Manchester: University of Manchester.

Lovell, K. and Richards, D.A. (2012) *A Recovery Programme for Depression*. London: Rethink Mental Illness.

Lovell, K., Bower, P., Gellatly, J., Byford, S., Bee, P., McMillan, D., et al. (2017) Clinical effectiveness, cost-effectiveness and acceptability of low-intensity interventions in the management of obsessive compulsive disorder: the Obsessive-Compulsive Treatment Efficacy Randomised Controlled Trial (OCTET). *Health Technology Assessment*, 21, 37.

Lovell, K., Cox, D., Haddock, G., Jones, C., Raines, D., Garvey, R. et al. (2006) Telephone administered cognitive behaviour therapy for treatment of obsessive compulsive disorder: randomised controlled non-inferiority trial. *British Medical Journal*, 333, 7574, 883.

Lucock, M.P., Barber, R., Jones, A. and Lovell, J. (2007) Service users' views of self-help strategies and research in the UK. *Journal of Mental Health*, 16, 795–805.

Lucock, M., Kirby, R. and Wainwright, N. (2011) A pragmatic randomized controlled trial of a guided self-help intervention versus a waiting list control in a routine primary care mental health service. *British Journal of Clinical Psychology*, 50, 298–309.

Lucock, M., Padgett, K., Noble, R., Westley, A., Atha, C., Horsefield, C. and Leach, C. (2008) Controlled clinical trial of a self-help for anxiety intervention for patients waiting for psychological therapy. *Behavioural and Cognitive Psychotherapy*, 36, 541–51.

Ludman, E., Gregory, S., Tutty, S. and Von Korff, M. (2007) A randomized trial of telephone psychotherapy and pharmacotherapy for depression: continuation and durability of effects. *Journal of Consulting and Clinical Psychology*, 75, 257–66.

Macy, A.S., Theo, J.N., Kaufmann, S.C., Ghazzaoui, R.B., Pawlowski, P.A., Fakhry, H.I. et al. (2013) Quality of life in obsessive compulsive disorder. *CNS Spectrums*, 18, 21–33.

Malouff, J.M., Thorsteinsson, E.B. and Schutte, N.S. (2007) The efficacy of problem-solving therapy in reducing mental and physical health problems: a meta-analysis. *Clinical Psychology Review*, 27, 46–57.

Markarian, Y., Larson, M.J., Aldea, M.A., Baldwin, S.A., Good, D., Berkeljon, A. et al. (2010) Multiple pathways to functional impairment in obsessive-compulsive disorder. *Clinical Psychology Review*, 30, 78–88.

Marks, I.M. (1973) New approaches to the treatment of obsessive-compulsive disorders. *Journal of Nervous and Mental Disease*, 156, 420–6.

Marks, I.M. and Matthews, A.M. (1979) Brief standard self-rating for phobic patients. *Behaviour Research and Therapy*, 17, 3, 263–7.

Marques, L., LeBlanc, N.J., Weingarden, H.M., Timpano, K.R., Jenike, M. and Wilhelm, S. (2010) Barriers to treatment and service utilization in an internet sample of individuals with obsessive-compulsive symptoms. *Depression and Anxiety*, 27, 470–5.

Martell, C.R., Addis, M.E. and Jacobson, N.S. (2001) *Depression in Context: Strategies for Guided Action*. New York: Norton.

Martinez, C., Rietbrock, S., Wise, L., Ashby, D., Chick, J., Moseley, J. et al. (2005) Antidepressant treatment and the risk of fatal and non-fatal self harm in first episode depression: nested case-control study. *BMJ*, 330, 389.

Martinez, R. and Williams, C. (2010) Matching clients to CBT self-help resources. In J. Bennett-Levy, D. Richards, P. Farrand, H. Christensen, K. Griffiths, D. Kavanagh et al. (eds), *Oxford Guide to Low-intensity CBT Interventions*. Oxford: Oxford University Press.

Martinez, R., Whitfield, G., Dafters, R. and Williams, C. (2008) Can people read self-help manuals for depression? A challenge for the stepped care model and book prescription schemes. *Behavioural and Cognitive Psychotherapy*, 36, 89–97.

McFarlane, A.C. and Papay, P. (1992) Multiple diagnoses in posttraumatic stress disorder in the victims of a natural disaster. *Journal of Nervous and Mental Disease*, 180, 498–504.

McManus, S., Bebbington, P., Jenkins, R. and Brugha, T. (eds) (2016) *Mental Health and Wellbeing in England: Adult Psychiatric Morbidity Survey 2014*. Leeds: NHS Digital.

McMillan, D. and Lee, R. (2010) A systematic review of behavioral experiments vs exposure alone in the treatment of anxiety disorders: a case of exposure while wearing the emperor's new clothes? *Clinical Psychology Review*, 30, 467–78.

Medical Research Council (2019) *Developing and Evaluating Complex Interventions*. London: Medical Research Council.

Meisel, S., Drury, H. and Perera-Delcourt, R. (2018) Therapists' attitudes to offering eCBT in an inner-city IAPT service: a survey study. *The Cognitive Behaviour Therapist*, 11, e11.

Mental Health Foundation (2016) *Fundamental Facts About Mental Health 2016*. London: Mental Health Foundation.

Meyer, V. (1966) Modification of expectations in cases with obsessional rituals. *Behaviour Research and Therapy*, 4, 273–80.

Michie, S., Atkins, L. and West, R. (2014) *The Behaviour Change Wheel: A Guide to Designing Interventions*. Sutton, Surrey: Silverback Publishing.

Michie, S., Richardson, M., Johnston, M., Abraham, C., Francis, J., Hardeman, W. and Wood, C.E. (2013) The behavior change technique taxonomy (v1) of 93 hierarchically clustered techniques: building an international consensus for the reporting of behavior change interventions. *Annals of Behavioral Medicine*, 46, 81–95.

Michie, S., van Stralen, M.M. and West, R. (2011) The behaviour change wheel: a new method for characterising and designing behaviour change interventions. *Implementation Science*, 6, 42.

Michie, S., West, R., Campbell, R., Brown, J. and Gainforth, H. (2014) *ABC of Behaviour Change Theories*. Sutton, Surrey: Silverback Publishing.

Miller, R.W. and Rollnick, S. (2013) *Motivational Interviewing: Helping People Change*. New York: Guilford Press.

Milne, D. (2009) *Evidence-Based Clinical Supervision: Principles and Practice*. Oxford: BPS Blackwell.

Miskowiakn, K.W., Ott, C.V., Petersen, J.Z. and Kessing, L.V. (2016) Systematic review of randomized controlled trials of candidate treatments for cognitive impairment in depression and methodological challenges in the field. *European Neuropsychopharmacology*, 26, 1845–67.

Mitchell, M.D., Gehrman, P., Perlis, M. and Umscheid, C.A. (2012) Comparative effectiveness of cognitive behavioural therapy for insomnia: a systematic review. *BMC Family Practice*, 13, 40.

Modini, M., Joyce, S., Mykletun, A., Christensen, H., Bryant, R.A., Mitchell, P.B. and Harvey, S.B. (2016) The mental health benefits of employment: results of a systematic review. *Australasian Psychiatry,* 24, 331–6.

Mohr, D.C., Ho, J., Duffecy, J., Reifler, D., Sokol, L., Burns, N.N. et al. (2012) Effect of telephone-administered vs face-to-face cognitive behavioral therapy on adherence to therapy and depression outcomes among primary care patients: a randomized trial. *JAMA*, 307: 2278–85.

Morgan, K., Dixon, S., Mathers, N., Thompson, J. and Tomeny, M. (2004) Psychological treatment for insomnia in the management of long-term hypnotic drug use: a pragmatic randomised controlled trial. *British Journal of General Practice*, 53, 923–8.

Morgenthaler, T., Kramer, M., Alessi, C., Friedman, L., Boehlecke, B., Brown, T., et al. (2006) Practice parameters for the psychological and behavioural treatment of insomnia: an update. An American Academy of Sleep Medicine report. *Sleep*, 29, 1415–19.

Moult, B., Franck, L.S. and Brady, H. (2004) Ensuring quality information for patients: development and preliminary validation of a new instrument to improve the quality of written health care information. *Health Expectations*, 7, 165–75.

Mowrer, O.H. (1939) A stimulus-response analysis of anxiety and its role as a reinforcing agent. *Psychology Review*, 46: 553–65.

Mowrer, O.H. (1947) On the dual nature of learning – a reinterpretation of 'conditioning' and 'problem solving'. *Harvard Educational Review*, 17, 102–48.

Mulder, R., Murray, G. and Rucklidge, J. (2017) Common versus specific factors in psychotherapy: opening the black box. *The Lancet Psychiatry,* 4, 953–62.

Mundt, J.C., Marks, I.M., Shear, M.K. and Greist, J.H. (2002) The Work and Social Adjustment Scale: a simple measure of impairment in functioning. *British Journal of Psychiatry*, 180, 461–4.

Myles, P.J. and Shafran, R. (2015) *The CBT Handbook: A Comprehensive Guide to Using Cognitive Behavioural Therapy to Overcome Depression, Anxiety and Anger.* London: Robinson.

Mynors-Wallis, L. and Lau, M.A. (2010) Problem solving as a low-intensity intervention. In J. Bennett-Levy, D.A. Richards, P. Farrand, H. Christensen, K.M. Griffiths, D.J. Kavanagh, et al. (eds), *Oxford Guide to Low Intensity CBT Interventions.* Oxford: Oxford University Press. pp.151–8.

Mynors-Wallis, L.M., Gath, D.H., Day, A. and Baker, F. (2000) Randomised Control Trial of problem solving treatment, antidepressant medication, and combined treatment for major depression in primary care. *British Medical Journal*, 320, 26–30.

Mynors-Wallis, L.M., Gath, D.H., Lloyd-Thomas, A.R. and Tomlinson, D. (1995) Randomised controlled trial comparing problem solving treatment with amitriptyline and placebo for major depression in primary care. *British Medical Journal*, 310, 441–5.

Nancarrow, S.A. and Borthwick, A.M. (2005) Dynamic professional boundaries in the healthcare workforce. *Sociology of Health and Illness*, 27, 897–919.

National Collaborating Centre for Mental Health (NCCMH) (2018) *The Improving Access to Psychological Therapies Manual.* Available at www.england.nhs.uk/publication/the-improving-access-to-psychological-therapies-manual (accessed 6 October 2019).

National Collaborating Centre for Mental Health (NCCMH) (2020) *The Improving Access to Psychological Therapies Manual.* Available at https://www.england.nhs.uk/wp-content/uploads/2020/05/iapt-manual-v4.pdf (accessed 11 July 2020).

National Health Service (NHS) Digital (2019) *Psychological Therapies, Annual Report on the Use of IAPT Services 2018–19.* London: NHS England. Available online at: https://digital.nhs.uk/data-and-information/publications/statistical/psychological-therapies-annual-reports-on-the-use-of-iapt-services/annual-report-2018-19 (accessed 23 January 2020).

National Institute for Health and Care Excellence (NICE) (2005) *Obsessive-Compulsive Disorder and Body Dysmorphic Disorder: Treatment (CG31).* London: NICE.

National Institute for Health and Care Excellence (NICE) (2007) *Behaviour Change: The Principles for Effective Interventions (PH6).* London: NICE.

National Institute for Health and Care Excellence (NICE) (2009a) *Depression in Adults: Recognition and Management (CG90).* London: NICE.

National Institute for Health and Care Excellence (NICE) (2009b) *Depression in Adults with a Chronic Physical Health Problem: Recognition and Management (CG91).* London: NICE.

National Institute for Health and Care Excellence (NICE) (2011a) *Generalised Anxiety Disorder and Panic Disorder in Adults: Management (CG113)* London: NICE.

National Institute for Health and Care Excellence (NICE) (2011b) *Common Mental Health Disorders: Identification and Pathways to Care (CG123).* London: NICE.

National Institute for Health and Care Excellence (NICE) (2011c) *Alcohol-Use Disorders: Diagnosis, Assessment and Management of Harmful Drinking (High-Risk Drinking) and Alcohol Dependence (CG115).* London: NICE.

National Institute for Health and Care Excellence (NICE) (2013) *Social Anxiety Disorder: Recognition, Assessment and Treatment (CG159).* London: NICE.

National Institute for Health and Care Excellence (NICE) (2014a) *Psychosis and Schizophrenia in Adults: Prevention and Management (CG178)* London: NICE.

National Institute for Health and Care Excellence (NICE) (2014b) *Behaviour Change: Individual Approaches (PH49).* London: NICE.

National Institute for Health and Care Excellence (NICE) (2015a) *Obstructive Sleep Apnoea Syndrome. Scenario: Management of Sleep Apnoea.* London: NICE.

National Institute for Health and Care Excellence (2015b) *Managing Long Term Insomnia (>4 weeks).* Available at https://cks.nice.org.uk/insomnia#!scenario:1 (accessed 7 August 2019).

National Institute for Health and Care Excellence (NICE) (2016) *Restless Legs Syndrome. Scenario: Management of Restless Legs Syndrome.* London: NICE.

National Institute for Health and Care Excellence (NICE) (2017) *Depression in Adults: Treatment and Management. Methods, Evidence and Recommendations. Draft for Consultation.* London: NICE.

National Institute for Health and Care Excellence (NICE) (2018a) *Depression in Adults: Recognition and Management (CG90).* London: NICE.

National Institute for Health and Care Excellence (NICE) (2018b) *Post-Traumatic Stress Disorder (NG116).* London: NICE.

National Institute for Health and Care Excellence (NICE) (2019) *Depression in Adults: Recognition and Management (CG90).* London: NICE.

National Institute for Mental Health in England (2003) *Inside Outside: Improving Mental Health Services for Black and Minority Ethnic Communities in England.* London: Department of Health.

National Treatment Agency for Substance Misuse (2012) *IAPT Positive Practice Guide for Working with People Who Use Drugs and Alcohol.* Available at www.drugwise.org.uk/wp-content/uploads/iapt-drug-and-alcohol-positive-practice-guide.pdf (last accessed 3 April 2020).

Newman, M.G. and Borkovec, T.D. (2002) Cognitive behavioural therapy for worry and generalised anxiety disorder. In G. Simos (ed.), *Cognitive Behaviour Therapy: A Guide for the Practising Clinician*. New York: Taylor and Francis. pp. 150–72.

Nezu, A.M., Nezu, C.M., Saraydarian, L., Kalmar, K. and Ronan, M. F. (1986) Social problem solving as a moderating variable between negative life stress and depressive symptoms. *Cognitive Therapy and Research*, 10, 489–98.

Ngui, E.M., Khasakhala, L., Ndetei, D. and Weiss Roberts, L. (2010) Mental disorders, health inequalities and ethics: a global perspective. *International Review of Psychiatry*, 22, 235–44.

NHS (2018) *Treatment: Phobias*. Available at www.nhs.uk/conditions/phobias/treatment (accessed 15 May 2019).

NHS Digital (2019) *Psychological Therapies, Annual Report on the Use of IAPT Services 2018–19*. London: NHS England. Available online at: https://digital.nhs.uk/data-and-information/publications/statistical/psychological-therapies-annual-reports-on-the-use-of-iapt-services/annual-report-2018-19 (accessed 23 January 2020).

Nicolas, G., Arntz, D.L., Hirsch, B. and Schmiedigen, A. (2009) Cultural adaptation of a group treatment for Haitian American adolescents. *Professional Psychology: Research and Practice*, 40, 378–84.

Norcross, J.C. and Lambert, M.J. (2019) What works in the psychotherapy relationship: results, conclusions, and practices. In J.C. Norcross and M.J. Lambert (eds), *Psychotherapy Relationships that Work: Volume 1: Evidence-Based Therapist Contributions*. Oxford: Oxford University Press. pp. 631–46.

Office for National Statistics (ONS) (2011) *Ethnicity and National Identity in England and Wales*. Available online at: www.ons.gov.uk/peoplepopulationandcommunity/culturalidentity/ethnicity/articles/ethnicityandnationalidentityinenglandandwales/2012-12-11

Office of National Statistics (ONS) (2019) *Measuring National Well-being: At what age is Personal Well-being the highest? Statistical Bulletin*. London: ONS. Available online at: https://www.ons.gov.uk/peoplepopulationandcommunity/wellbeing/articles/measuringnationalwellbeing/internationalcomparisons2019

Ohayon, M., Wickwire, E.M., Hirshkowitz, M., Albert, S.M., Avidan, A., Daly, F.J. et al. (2017) National Sleep Foundation's sleep quality recommendations: first report. *Sleep Health*, 3, 6–19.

Olatunji, B.O., Davis, M.L., Powers, M.B. and Smits, J.A. (2013) Cognitive-behavioral therapy for obsessive-compulsive disorder: a meta-analysis of treatment outcome and moderators. *Journal of Psychiatric Research*, 47, 33–41.

Ost, L-G. (1989) One session treatment for specific phobias. *Behaviour Research and Therapy*, 27, 1–7.

Ost, L-G. and Sterner, U. (1989) Applied tension: a specific behavioral method for treatment of blood phobia. *Behaviour Research and Therapy*, 25, 25–9.

Ost, L-G., Havnen, A., Hansen, B. and Kvale, G. (2015) Cognitive behavioural treatments of obsessive-compulsive disorder. A systematic review and meta-analysis of studies published 1993–2014. *Clinical Psychology Review*, 40, 156–69.

Padesky, C.A. (1994) Schema change processes in cognitive therapy. *Clinical Psychology and Psychotherapy*, 1, 267–78.

Padesky, C.A. and Greenberger, D. (1995) *Clinician's Guide to Mind Over Mood*. New York: The Guilford Press.

Padesky, C.A. and Mooney, K.A. (1990) Presenting the cognitive model to clients. *International Cognitive Therapy Newsletter*, 6, 13–14.

Padesky, C.A. and Mooney, K.A. (2012) Strengths-based cognitive-behavioural therapy: a four-step model to build resilience. *Clinical Psychology and Psychotherapy*, 19, 283–90.

Painter, A. (2018) *Processing People! The Purpose and Pitfalls of Case Management Supervision Provided for Psychological Wellbeing Practitioners, Working Within Improving Access to Psychological Therapies (IAPT) Services: A Thematic Analysis*. PhD thesis, University of the West of England, Bristol.

Pampallona, S., Bollini, P., Tibaldi, G., Kupelnick, B. and Munizza, C. (2004) Combined pharmacotherapy and psychological treatment for depression: a systematic review. *Archives of General Psychiatry*, 61, 7, 714–9.

Papworth, M.A. (2019) Behaviour change and client engagement. In M. Papworth and T. Marrinan (eds), *Low Intensity Cognitive Behaviour Therapy: A Practitioner's Guide*. London: Sage.

Papworth, M.A. (2020) *How to Beat Fears and Phobias One Step at a Time*. London: Little Brown Books.

Papworth, M. and Marrinan, T. (2019) *Low Intensity Cognitive Behaviour Therapy: A Practitioner's Guide*. London: SAGE.

Papworth, M., Ward, A. and Leeson, K. (2015) Negative effects of self-help materials: three explorative studies. *The Cognitive Behaviour Therapist*, 8, e30.

Pavlov, I. (1903) *The Experimental Psychology and Psychopathology of Animals*. The 14th International Medical Congress, Madrid, Spain.

Pawluk, E.J., Koerner, N., Tallon, K. and Antony, M.M. (2017) Unique correlates of problem-solving effectiveness in individuals with generalized anxiety disorder. *Cognitive Therapy Research*, 41, 881–9.

Pearcy, C.P., Anderson, R.A., Egan, S.J. and Rees, C.S. (2016) A systematic review and meta-analysis of self-help therapeutic interventions for obsessive-compulsive disorder: is therapeutic contact key to overall improvement? *Journal of Behavior Therapy and Experimental Psychiatry*, 51, 74–83.

Pedley, R., Bee, P., Wearden, A. and Berry, K. (2019) Illness perceptions in people with obsessive-compulsive disorder: a qualitative study. *PLoS One*, 14 3, e0213495.

Pimm, J. (2016) Plan, do, study, act: a methodology for enhancing recovery in your service. Presented at IAPT National Enhancing Recovery Workshop, Birmingham, UK, March 16.

Pocklington, C. (2017) Depression in older adults. *British Journal of Medical Practitioners*, 10, a1007.

Proctor, B. and Inskipp, F. (2001) Group supervision. In J. Scaife (ed.), *Supervision in Clinical Practice. A Practitioner's Guide* (2nd edition). London: Routledge.

Psychological Professions Network. (2018) Delivering the Expansion in the Psychological Professions. Available online at: https://www.nwppn.nhs.uk/attachments/article/2578/PPN_Brochure_June18_Online_SinglePages.pd

Pullen, I. and Loudon, J. (2006) Improving standards in clinical record-keeping. *Advances in Psychiatric Treatment*, 12, 280–6.

Rachman, S. (1977) The conditioning theory of fear acquisition: a critical examination. *Behaviour Research and Therapy*, 15, 375–87.

Raghaven, R., Lyn Bright, C. and Shadoin, A.L. (2008) Toward a policy ecology of implementation of evidence-based practices in public mental health settings. *Implementation Science*, 3, 26.

Ramos-Sanchez, L., Esnil, E., Goodwin, A., Riggs, S., Osachy Touster, L., Wright, L.K. et al. (2002) Negative supervisory events: effects on supervision satisfaction and supervisory alliance. *Professional Psychology: Research and Practice*, 33, 197–202.

Richards, D.A. (2004) Self-help: empowering service users or aiding cash strapped mental health services? *Journal of Mental Health*, 13, 117–23.

Richards, D.A. (2010a) Access and organization: putting low intensity interventions to work in clinical services. In J. Bennett-Levy, D.A. Richards, P. Farrand, H. Christensen, K.M. Griffiths, D.J. Kavanagh, et al. (eds), *Oxford Guide to Low Intensity CBT Interventions*. Oxford: Oxford University Press. pp. 19–33.

Richards, D.A. (2010b) Supervising low-intensity workers in high volume clinical environments. In J. Bennett-Levy, D.A. Richards, P. Farrand, H. Christensen, K.M. Griffiths, D.J. Kavanagh, et al. (eds), *Oxford Guide to Low-intensity CBT Interventions*. Oxford: Oxford University Press. pp. 129–36.

Richards, D.A. (2010c) Behavioural activation. In J. Bennett-Levy, D.A. Richards, P. Farrand, H. Christensen, K.M. Griffiths, D.J. Kavanagh, et al. (eds), *Oxford Guide to Low Intensity CBT Interventions*. Oxford: Oxford University Press. pp. 141–51.

Richards, D.A. and Farrand, P. (2010) Choosing self-help books wisely: sorting the wheat from the chaff. In J. Bennett-Levy, D.A. Richards, P. Farrand, H. Christensen,

K.M. Griffiths, D.J. Kavanagh, et al. (eds), *Oxford Guide to Low Intensity CBT Interventions*. Oxford: Oxford University Press. pp. 202–7.

Richards, D.A. and Suckling, R. (2008) Improving access to psychological therapy: the Doncaster demonstration site organisational model. *Clinical Psychology Forum*, 181, 9–16.

Richards, D.A. and Whyte, M. (2008) *Reach Out: Educator Materials to Support the Delivery of Training for Psychological Wellbeing Practitioners Delivering Low Intensity Interventions*. London: Rethink.

Richards, D.A. and Whyte, M. (2011) *Reach Out: National Programme Student Materials to Support the Delivery of Training for Psychological Wellbeing Practitioners Delivering Low Intensity Interventions*. London: Rethink.

Richards, D.A., Ekers, D., McMillan, D., Taylor, R.S., Byford, S., Warren, F.C. et al. (2016) Cost and outcome of behavioural activation versus cognitive behavioural therapy for depression (COBRA): a randomised, controlled, non-inferiority trial. *The Lancet*, 388, 871–80.

Richards, D., Duffy, D., Blackburn, B., Early, C., Enrique, A., Palacios, J. et al. (2018) Digital IAPT: the effectiveness & cost-effectiveness of internet-delivered interventions for depression and anxiety disorders in the Improving Access to Psychological Therapies programme: study protocol for a randomised control trial. *BMC Psychiatry*, 18: 59. Available online at: https://doi.org/10.1186/s12888-018-1639-5

Richards, D., Farrand, P. and Chellingsworth, M. (2011) *National Curriculum for the Education of Psychological Wellbeing Practitioners*. London: Department of Health. Available at www.babcp.com/files/Accreditation/PWP/IAPT-PWP-National-Curriculum.pdf (accessed 17 January 2019).

Richardson, R., and Richards, D. A. (2006) Self-help: towards the next generation. *Behavioural and Cognitive Psychotherapy*, 34, 13–23.

Ritterband, L., Thorndike, F., Vasquez, D. and Saylor, D. (2010) Treatment credibility and satisfaction with internet interventions. In In J. Bennett-Levy, D.A. Richards, P. Farrand, H. Christensen, K.M. Griffiths, D.J. Kavanagh, et al. (eds), *Oxford Guide to Low Intensity CBT Interventions*. Oxford: Oxford University.

Rizq, R., Hewey, M., Salvo, L., Spencer, M., Varnaseri, H. and Whitfield, J. (2010) Reflective voices: primary care mental health workers' experiences in training and practice. *Primary Health Care Research and Development*, 11, 72–86.

Roberts, L. and Kwan, S. (2017) Putting the C into CBT: cognitive challenging with adults with mild to moderate intellectual disabilities and anxiety disorders. *Clinical Psychology and Psychotherapy*, 25, 662–71.

Robinson, A. (2018) Reading Well Books on Prescription programme. *Practice Nursing*, 29, 188.

Robinson, K.L., Rose, D. and Salkolvskis, P.M. (2017) Seeking help for obsessive compulsive disorder (OCD): a qualitative study of the enablers and barriers conducted by a researcher with personal experience of OCD. *Psychology and Psychotherapy: Theory, Research and Practice*, 90, 193–211.

Rogers, A., Oliver, D., Bower, P., Lovell, K. and Richards, D. (2004) Peoples' understanding of a primary care-based mental health self-help clinic. *Patient Education and Counseling*, 53, 1, 41–6.

Rogers, C.R. (1957) The necessary and sufficient conditions of therapeutic personality change. *Journal of Consulting Psychology*, 21, 95–103.

Roiser, J.P., Elliott, R. and Sahakian, B.J. (2012) Cognitive mechanisms of treatment in depression. *Neuropsychopharmacology*, 37, 117–36.

Rolfe, G., Freshwater, D. and Jasper, M. (2001) *Critical Reflection in Nursing and the Helping Professions: A User's Guide*. Basingstoke: Palgrave Macmillan.

Rosenzweig, S. (1936) Some implicit common factors in diverse methods of psychotherapy. *American Journal of Orthopsychiatry*, 6, 412–15.

Rosqvist, J. (2005) *Exposure Treatments for Anxiety Disorders: A Practitioner's Guide to Concepts, Methods and Evidence-Based Practice*. New York: Taylor and Francis.

Rost, T., Stein, J., Löbner, M., Kersting, A., Luck-Sikorski, C. and Riedel-Heller, S. (2017) User acceptance of computerized cognitive behavioral therapy for depression: systematic review. *Journal of Medical Internet Research*, 19, e309.

Roth, A.D. and Pilling, S. (2007a) *The Competences Required to Deliver Effective Cognitive and Behavioural Therapy for People with Depression and with Anxiety Disorders*. London: Department of Health.

Roth, A.D., and Pilling, S. (2007b) *CBT Competences Framework for Depression and Anxiety Disorders*. Available at www.ucl.ac.uk/clinical-psychology/competency-maps/cbt/Problem%20specific%20competences/GAD%20-%20Borkovec%20model.pdf (accessed 1 October 2019).

Roth, A.D. and Pilling, S. (2008) *A Competence Framework for the Supervision of Psychological Therapies*. University College London.

Rouf, K., Fennell, M., Westbrook, D., Cooper, M. and Bennett-Levy, J. (2015) Devising effective behavioural experiments. In J. Bennett-Levy, D.A. Richards, P. Farrand, H. Christensen, K.M. Griffiths, D.J. Kavanagh, et al. (eds), *Oxford Guide to Low Intensity CBT Interventions*. Oxford: Oxford University Press.

Royal College of Psychiatrists (2013) *Whole-Person Care: From Rhetoric to Reality: Achieving Parity Between Mental and Physical Health*. London: Royal College of Psychiatrists.

Ruscio, A.M., Stein, D.J., Chiu, W.T. and Kessler, R.C. (2010) The epidemiology of obsessive-compulsive disorder in the National Comorbidity Survey Replication. *Molecular Psychiatry*, 15, 53–63.

Sackett, D.L., Straus, S.E., Richardson, W.S., Rosenberg, W. and Haynes, R.B. (2000) *Evidence-Based Medicine: How to Practice and Teach EBM.* New York: Churchill-Livingstone.

Sadavoy, J. (2009) An integrated model for defining the scope of psychogeriatrics: the five Cs. *International Psychogeriatrics,* 21, 805–12.

Safran, J.D. and Safran, J.C. (2000) Resolving therapeutic alliance ruptures: diversity and integration. *Clinical Psychology,* 56, 233–43.

Safran, J.D., Muran, J.C. and Eubanks-Carter, C. (2011) Repairing alliance ruptures. *Psychotherapy,* 48, 80–7.

Salkovskis, P.M., Rimes, K.A., Warwick, H.M.C. and Clark, D.M. (2002) The Health Anxiety Inventory: development and validation of scales for the measurement of health anxiety and hypochondriasis. *Psychological Medicine,* 32, 843–53.

Scaife, J. (2001) *Supervision in Clinical Practice. A Practitioner's Guide.* London: Routledge.

Schön, D. (1983) *The Reflective Practitioner: How Professionals Think in Action.* Aldershot: Ashgate Arena.

Seligman, M.E.P. (1971) Phobias and preparedness. *Behavior Therapy,* 2, 307–20.

Serfaty, M.A., Haworth, D., Blanchard, M., Buszewicz, M., Murad, S. and King, M. (2009) Clinical effectiveness of individual cognitive behavioral therapy for depressed older people in primary care: a randomized controlled trial. *Archives of General Psychiatry,* 66, 1332–40.

Seward, J. and Clark, M. (2010) Establishing the Improved Access to Psychological Therapies programme: lessons from large-scale change in England. In J. Bennett-Levy, D.A. Richards, P. Farrand, H. Christensen, K.M. Griffiths, D.J. Kavanagh, et al. (eds), *Oxford Guide to Low Intensity CBT Interventions.* Oxford: Oxford University Press. pp. 479–86.

Seyffert, M., Lagisetty, P., Landgraf, J., Chopra, V., Pfeiffer, P.N., Conte, M.L. and Rogers, M.A.M. (2016) Internet-delivery cognitive behavioral therapy to treat insomnia: a systematic review and meta-analysis. *PLoS One,* 11, 2, e0149139.

Shear, M.K., Rucci, P., Williams, J., Frank, E., Grochonski, V., Vanderbilt, J. et al. (2001) Reliability and validity of the Panic Disorder Severity Scale. *Journal of Psychiatric Research,* 35, 293–6.

Shepherd, M. and Rosairo, M. (2008) Low-intensity workers: lessons learned from supervising primary care mental health workers and dilemmas associated with such roles. *Mental Health in Family Medicine,* 5, 237–45.

Shimokawa, K., Lambert, M.J. and Smart, D.W. (2010) Enhancing treatment outcome of patients at risk of treatment failure: meta-analytic and mega-analytic review of a psychotherapy quality assurance system. *Journal of Consulting and Clinical Psychology,* 78, 298–311.

Shiroma, P.R., Thuras, P., Johns, B. and Lim, K.O. (2014) Emotion recognition processing as early predictor of response to 8-week citalopram treatment in late-life depression. *International Journal of Geriatric Psychiatry,* 29, 11, 1132–9.

Sim, K., Lau, W.K., Sim, J., Sum, M.Y. and Baldessarini, R.J. (2016) Prevention of relapse and recurrence in adults with major depressive disorder: systematic review and meta-analyses of controlled trials. *International Journal of Neuropsychopharmacology*, 19, 10, pyw031.

Sims, T., Hogan, C. L. and Carstensen, L.L. (2015) Selectivity as an emotion regulation strategy: lessons from older adults. *Current Opinion in Psychology*, 3, 80–4.

Skapinakis, P., Caldwell, D., Hollingworth, W., Bryden, P., Fineberg, N., Salkovskis, P. et al. (2016) A systematic review of the clinical effectiveness and cost-effectiveness of pharmacological and psychological interventions for the management of obsessive-compulsive disorder in children/adolescents and adults. *Health Technology Assessment*, 20, 43, 1–392.

Skinner, B.F. (1938) *The Behavior of Organisms: An Experimental Analysis*. New York: Appleton-Century.

Skinner, B.F. (1969) *Contingencies of Reinforcement: A Theoretical Analysis*. New York: Appleton-Century-Crofts.

Skovholt, T.M. and Rønnestad, M.H. (2001) The long, textured path from novice to senior practitioner. In T.M. Skovholt (ed.), *The Resilient Practitioner: Burnout Prevention and Self-Care Strategies for Counselors, Therapists, Teachers, and Health Professionals*. Boston: Allyn and Bacon. pp. 25–54.

Sleep Council (2017) *The Great British Bedtime Report*. Skipton: The Sleep Council. Available at https://sleepcouncil.org.uk/wp-content/uploads/The-Great-British-Bedtime-Report-2017-1.pdf (accessed 29 April 2020).

Smiles, S. (1859) *Self-Help*. London: Seven Treasures Publications. Available at www.gutenberg.org/files/935/935-h/935-h.htm (accessed 25 January 2019).

Spitzer, R.L., Kroenke, K., Williams, J.B., and Lowe, B. (2006) A brief measure for assessing generalized anxiety disorder: The GAD-7. *Archives of Internal Medicine*, 166, 1092–7.

Stampfl, T.G. and Levis, D.J. (1967) Essentials of implosive therapy: a learning theory based psychodynamic behavioral therapy. *Journal of Abnormal Psychology*, 72, 496–503.

Steel, C., Macdonald, J., Schröder, T. and Mellor-Clark, J. (2015) Exhausted but not cynical: burnout in therapists working within Improving Access to Psychological Therapy Services. *Journal of Mental Health*, 24, 33–7.

Stevens, A. and Gabbay, J. (1991) Needs assessment. *Health Trends*, 23, 20–3.

Stutz, J., Eiholzer, R. and Spengler, C.M. (2019) Effect of evening exercise on sleep in healthy participants: a systematic review and meta-analysis. *Sports Medicine*, 49, 269–87.

Subramaniam, M., Soh, P., Vaingankar, J.A., Picco, L. and Chong, S.A. (2013) Quality of life in obsessive-compulsive disorder: impact of the disorder and of treatment. *CNS Drugs*, 27, 67–83.

Svedin, F., Brantnell, A., Farrand, P., Aberg, A.G., Blomberg, O., Coumoundouros, C., Von Essen, L. and Woodford, J. (Submitted) Adaptation of a guided low-intensity behavioural activation intervention for people with dementia and depression for the Swedish healthcare context (INVOLVERA): Study protocol utilising co-design and participatory action research. *BMJ Open*.

Teasdale, J.D. and Fennell, M.J.V. (1982) Immediate effects on depression of cognitive therapy interventions. *Cognitive Therapy and Research*, 6, 343–52.

Tee, J. and Kazantzis, N. (2011) Collaborative empiricism in cognitive therapy: a definition and theory for the relationship construct. *Clinical Psychology Science and Practice*, 18, 47–61.

Telford, J. and Wilson, R. (2010) From classroom to 'shop floor': challenges faced as a low-intensity practitioner. In J. Bennett-Levy, D.A. Richards, P. Farrand, H. Christensen, K.M. Griffiths, D.J. Kavanagh, et al. (eds), *Oxford Guide to Low Intensity CBT Interventions*. Oxford: Oxford University Press. pp. 129–36.

Thwaites, R. and Bennett-Levy, J. (2007) Conceptualizing empathy in cognitive behaviour therapy: making the implicit explicit. *Behavioural and Cognitive Psychotherapy*, 35, 591–612.

Thwaites, R., Bennett-Levy, J., Cairns, L., Lowrie, R., Robinson, A., Haarhoff, B. et al. (2017) Self-practice/self-reflection (SP/SR) as a training strategy to enhance therapeutic empathy in low intensity CBT practitioners. *New Zealand Journal of Psychology*, 46, 63–70.

Torres, A.R., Prince, M.J., Bebbington, P.E., Bhugra, D., Brugha, T.S., Farrell, M. et al. (2006) Obsessive-compulsive disorder: prevalence, comorbidity, impact, and help-seeking in the British National Psychiatric Morbidity Survey of 2000. *American Journal of Psychiatry*, 163: 1978–85.

Troxel, W.M., Germain, A. and Buysse, D.J. (2012) Clinical management of insomnia with Brief Behavioural Treatment (BBTI). *Behavioural Sleep Medicine*, 10, 266–79.

Tse, W.S. and Bond, A.J. (2002) Serotonergic intervention affects both social dominance and affiliative behaviour. *Psychopharmacology*, 161, 324–30.

Turner, J., Brown, J. and Carpenter, D. (2018) Telephone-based CBT and the therapeutic relationship: the views and experiences of IAPT practitioners in a low-intensity service. *Journal of Psychiatric and Mental Health Nursing*, 25, 285–96.

Turpin, G. and Wheeler, S. (2011) *IAPT Supervision Guidance*. London: Department of Health IAPT Programme. Available at https://webarchive.nationalarchives.gov.uk/20160302160224/http://www.iapt.nhs.uk/silo/files/iapt-supervision-guidance-revised-march-2011.pdf (accessed 25 May 2019).

Turpin, G., Baguley, C., Farrand, P., Hope, R., Leibowitz, J., Lovell, K. et al. (2010) *Good Practice Guidance on the Use of Self-Help Materials Within IAPT Services*. London: NHS Improving Access to Psychological Therapies.

Tutty, S., Spangler, D.L., Poppleton, L.E., Ludman, E.J. and Simon, G.E. (2010) Evaluating the effectiveness of cognitive-behavioral teletherapy in depressed adults. *Behavior Therapy*, 41, 229–36.

U.S. Department of Health and Human Services (2001) *Mental Health: Culture, Race and Ethnicity – A Supplement to Mental Health: A Report of the Surgeon General.* Rockville, MD: U.S. Department of Health and Human Services, Public Health Service, Office of the Surgeon General.

University College London (2015) *National Curriculum for the Education of Psychological Wellbeing Practitioners*, 3rd edn. Available at www.uea.ac.uk/documents/246046/ 11991919/PWP+Curriculum+3rd+Edition+2015.pdf/a300b754-7f0e-4241-8130- 7d729b2d8b13 (accessed 21 March 2020).

Unlu Ince, B., Cuijpers, P., van't Hof, E., van Ballegooijen, W., Christensen, H. and Riper, H. (2013) Internet-based, culturally sensitive, problem-solving therapy for Turkish migrants with depression: randomized controlled trial. *Journal of Medical Internet Research*, 15, e227.

Vallury, K.D., Jones, M. and Oosterbroek, C. (2015) Computerized cognitive behavior therapy for anxiety and depression in rural areas: a systematic review. *Journal of Medical Internet Research*, 17, e139.

Van Boeijen, C.A., van Oppen, P., van Balkom, A., Visser, S., Kempe, P.T., Blankenstein, N. and van Dyck, R. (2005) Treatment of anxiety disorders in primary care practice: a randomised controlled trial. *British Journal of General Practice*, 55, 763–69.

van Straten, A. and Cuijpers, P. (2009) Self-help therapy for insomnia: a meta-analysis. *Sleep Medicine Reviews*, 13, 61–71.

van Straten, A., Hill, J., Richards, D.A. and Cuijpers, P. (2015) Stepped care treatment delivery for depression: a systematic review and meta-analysis. *Psychological Medicine*, 45, 231–46.

van Straten, A., Tiemens, B., Hakkaart, L., Nolen, W.A. and Donker, M.C. (2006) Stepped care v. matched care for mood and anxiety disorders: a randomized trial in routine practice. *Acta Psychiatrica Scandinavica*, 113, 468–76.

van Straten, A., van der Zweerde, T., Kleiber, A., Cuijpers, P., Morin, C. M. and Lancee, J. (2018) Cognitive and behavioural therapies in the treatment of insomnia: a meta-analysis. *Sleep Medicine Reviews*, 38, 3–16.

van't Hof, E., Stein, D.J., Marks, I., Tomlinson, M. and Cuijpers, P. (2011) The effectiveness of problem solving therapy in deprived South African communities: results from a pilot study. *BMC Psychiatry*, 11, 156.

Vec, T., Vec, T.R. and Zorga, S. (2014) Understanding how supervision works and what it can achieve. In C.E. Watkins and D.L. Milne (eds) *The Wiley International Handbook of Clinical Supervision*. Chichester: John Wiley & Sons.

Visser, H.A., van Oppen, P., van Megen, H.J., Eikelenboom, M. and van Balkom, A.K. (2014) Obsessive-compulsive disorder: chronic versus non-chronic symptoms. *Journal of Affective Disorders*, 152–4, 169–74.

Vuong, T.M., Gellatly, J., Lovell, K. and Bee, P. (2016) The experiences of help-seeking in people with obsessive compulsive disorder: an internet survey. *The Cognitive Behaviour Therapist*, 9, 1–15.

Wakefield, A., Spilsbury, K., Atkin, K. and McKenna, H. (2010) What kind of work do assistant practitioners do and does this reflect the policy aspirations? *Nursing Times*, 106, 14–17.

Waller, G. (2009) Evidence-based treatment and therapist drift. *Behaviour Research and Therapy*, 47, 119–27.

Ward, E.C. and Brown, R. (2015) A culturally adapted depression intervention designed for African American adults experiencing depression: Oh happy day. *American Journal of Orthopsychiatry*, 85, 1, 11–22.

Ward, E.C., Clark, L. and Heidrich, S. (2009) African American Women's Beliefs, Coping Behaviors, and Barriers to Seeking Mental Health Services. *Qualitative Health Research*, 19, 1589–1601.

Warmerdam, L., van Straten, A., Jongsma, J., Twisk, J. and Cuijpers, P. (2010) Online cognitive behavioral therapy and problem-solving therapy for depressive symptoms: exploring mechanisms of change. *Journal of Behavior Therapy and Experimental Psychiatry*, 41, 41–70.

Weiland, M., Dammermann, C. and Stoppe, G. (2011) Selective optimization with compensation (SOC) competencies in depression. *Journal of Affective Disorders*, 133, 114–19.

Westbrook, D., Kennerley, H. and Kirk, J. (2007) *An Introduction to Cognitive Behaviour Therapy: Skills and Applications*. London: SAGE.

Westen, D. and Morrison, K. (2001) A multi-dimensional meta-analysis for treatments for depression, panic and generalised anxiety disorder: an empirical examination of the status of empirically supported therapies. *Journal of Consulting and Clinical Psychology*, 69, 875–99.

Wetherell, J.L., Gatz, M. and Craske, M.G. (2003) Treatment of generalized anxiety disorder in older adults. *Journal of Consulting and Clinical Psychology*, 71, 1, 31–40.

Whaley, A. and Davis, K. (2007) Cultural competence and evidence-based practice in mental health services: a complimentary perspective. *American Psychologist*, 6, 563–74.

Wikman, A., Kukkola, L., Börjesson, H., Woodford, J., Grönqvist, H. and von Essen, L. (2018) Development of an internet-administered cognitive behavior therapy program (ENGAGE) for parents of children previously treated for cancer: participatory action research approach. *Journal of Medical Internet Research*, 18, 4, e133.

Wilkinson, P., Alder, N., Juszczak, E., Matthews, H., Merritt, C., Montgomery, H. et al. (2009) A pilot randomised controlled trial of a brief cognitive behavioural group intervention to reduce recurrence rates in late life depression. *International Journal of Geriatric Psychiatry*, 24, 68–75.

Williams, C. (2012) *Overcoming Anxiety, Stress and Panic: A Five Areas Approach.* London: Hodder Arnold.

Williams, C.J. and Garland, A. (2002) A cognitive behavioural therapy assessment model for use in everyday clinical practice. *Advances in Psychiatric Treatment*, 8, 172–9.

Williams, C. and Morrison, J. (2010) A new language for CBT: new ways of working require new thinking, as well as new words. In J. Bennett-Levy, D.A. Richards, P. Farrand, H. Christensen, K.M. Griffiths, D.J. Kavanagh, et al. (eds), *Oxford Guide to Low Intensity CBT Interventions*. Oxford: Oxford University Press. pp. 129–36.

Williams, D.R., Gonzalez, H.M., Neighbors, H., Nesse, R., Abelson, J.M., Sweetman, J. and Jackson, J.S. (2007) Prevalence and distribution of major depressive disorder in African Americans, Caribbean Blacks, and Non-Hispanic Whites: Results from the National Survey of American Life. *Archives of General Psychiatry*, 64, 305–15.

Wilson, G.D. (1968) Reversal of differential GSR conditioning by instructions. *Journal of Experimental Psychology*, 76, 491–3.

Wilson, K., Mottram, P.G. and Vassilas, C. (2008) Psychotherapeutic treatments for older depressed people. *Cochrane Database of Systematic Reviews*, 1, CD004853.

Wohlgemuth, W.K. and Edinger, J.D. (2000) Sleep restriction therapy. In K.L. Lichstein and C.M. Morin (eds), *Treatment of Late-Life Insomnia*. Thousand Oaks, CA: Sage. pp. 147–66.

Wolitzky-Taylor, K.B., Horowitz, J.D., Powers, M.B. and Telch, M.J. (2008) Psychological approaches in the treatment of specific phobias: a meta-analysis. *Clinical Psychology Review*, 28, 1021–37.

Woodford, J., Farrand, P., Watkins, E.R., Richards, D.A. and Llewellyn, D.J. (2014) Supported cognitive-behavioural self-help versus treatment-as-usual for depressed informal carers of stroke survivors (CEDArS): study protocol for a feasibility randomized controlled trial. *Trials*, 15, 157.

Wootton, B. (2016) Remote cognitive–behavior therapy for obsessive-compulsive symptoms: A meta-analysis. *Clinical Psychology Review*, 43, 103–13.

World Health Organization (WHO) (1992) *International Statistical Classification of Diseases and Related Health Problems* 10th revision. Geneva: WHO. Available at www.who.int/classifications/icd/ICD-10_2nd_ed_volume2.pdf (last accessed 24 March 2020).

World Health Organization (WHO) (2017) *Depression and Other Common Mental Disorders: Global Health Estimates*. Geneva: WHO.

World Health Organization (2018) *International Statistical Classification of Diseases and Related Health Problems* 11th revision. Accessed at https://icd.who.int (accessed 9 October 2019).

Yaryura-Tobias, J.A. and Neziroglu, F.A. (1997) *Obsessive-Compulsive Disorder Spectrum: Pathogenesis, Diagnosis, and Treatment.* Arlington: American Psychiatric Association.

Yeragani, V., Ramachandraih, C., Subramanyam, N., Bar, K. and Baker, G. (2011) Antidepressants: from MAOIs to SSRIs and more. *Indian Journal of Psychiatry*, 53, 2, 180–2.

Yourman, D.B. (2003) Trainee disclosure in psychotherapy supervision: the impact of shame. *Journal of Clinical Psychology*, 59, 601–9.

Zayfert, C. and Becker, C.B. (2007) *Cognitive-Behavioral Therapy for PTSD: A Case Formulation Approach.* New York: Guilford Press.

Zinzow, H.M., Britt, T.W., McFadden, A.C., Burnette, C.M. and Gillispie, S. (2012) Connecting active duty and returning veterans to mental health treatment: interventions and treatment adaptations that may reduce barriers to care. *Clinical Psychology Review*, 32, 741–53.

Index

NOTE: Page numbers in *italic* type refer to figures, tables and worksheets.